Rob:
Hope you enjoy the book!
Great working w/ you!

Deadly Dermatologic Diseases

Deadly Dermatologic Diseases

Clinicopathologic Atlas and Text

Michael B. Morgan, MD
Bay Area Dermatopathology, Dermpath Diagnostics, Tampa, Florida
Professor, Department of Pathology, University of South Florida College of Medicine, Tampa, Florida

Bruce R. Smoller, MD
Department of Pathology, College of Medicine, Little Rock, Arkansas

Stephen C. Somach, MD
Departments of Dermatology and Pathology, MetroHealth Medical Center, Case Western Reserve University School of Medicine, Cleveland, Ohio

Foreword by Mark Allen Everett, MD

CD-ROM INCLUDED

Springer

Michael B. Morgan, MD
Bay Area Dermatopathology
Dermpath Diagnostics
Tampa, FL 33612
and
Professor
Department of Pathology
University of South Florida
College of Medicine
Tampa, FL 33612
USA

Bruce R. Smoller, MD
Department of Pathology
College of Medicine
Little Rock, AR 72205
USA

Stephen C. Somach, MD
Departments of Dermatology and Pathology
MetroHealth Medical Center
Case Western Reserve University
School of Medicine
Cleveland, OH 44109
USA

Library of Congress Control Number: 2005932087

ISBN-10: 0-387-25442-0
ISBN-13: 978-0387-25442-5

Printed on acid-free paper.

9 8 7 6 5 4 3 2 1

springer.com

To my parents, James and Glenda, who were first to inculcate an enduring fascination with books and their contents.

MBM

I would like to dedicate this work to my always loving and supportive family, Gabey, Jason, and Laura, without whom none of this would be worth doing.

BRS

This effort to highlight life-threatening skin diseases is made in the spirit of the dermatology training I received at MetroHealth Medical Center (formerly Cleveland Metropolitan General Hospital). This was a department of faculty members never seeking national recognition, but dedicated to outstanding training in medical dermatology. The department was headed by Dr. Jerome Pomeranz and given much of its energy by the tireless teaching of the residency director, Dr. Bryan Davis, who instilled his enthusiasm and passion for dermatology into scores of dermatologists who have received their training in the department. Another prominent member of this department to whom I owe thanks is the late Dr. Richard Belcher, whose personal photographs are included in this book. I would also like to thank my colleagues, Drs. Christine Jaworsky and Arlene Rosenberg, for reviewing the manuscript and providing valuable suggestions and my colleague and good friend, Dr. Michael Morgan, for giving me the opportunity to participate in this project.

I would like to dedicate this work to my parents, Roberta Fox Somach and Dr. Fredric Somach, for countless gifts, especially a love of teaching, music, and medicine.

SCS

Foreword

Almost exactly ten years ago, two young physicians joined me at the University of Oklahoma for the study of dermatopathology: Stephen C. Somach, a brilliant dermatologist-scholar from Cleveland, who was also a highly accomplished cellist, and Michael B. Morgan, an effervescent, newly minted pathologist from Florida, who was brimming with energy, curiosity, and zeal and was also sporting water skiis and a red Porsche! Bruce R. Smoller, whose impressive erudition is universally acknowledged, I met during a Residency Review committee visit to Stanford some fifteen years ago. Each of these men has made original contributions to the dermatopathology literature as well as to patient care in the clinical setting. Their publications have broadened our understanding of the biologic behavior of pigmented lesions, cutaneous lymphomas, vascular lesions, and soft tissue tumors. It is indeed a pleasure to welcome their volume, *Deadly Dermatologic Diseases*, a unique and stimulating outcome of their enthusiastic collaboration.

Deadly Dermatologic Diseases discusses a wide variety of entities–neoplastic, vascular, infectious, metabolic–each of which may eventuate in death of the patient. In addition, numerous tumors and dermatoses frequently associated with internal malignancies are reviewed. High-quality histologic photomicrographs and clinical pictures accompany many of the discussions. A unique initial summary page facilitates the reading of each presentation. Recent relevant genetic and biochemical findings in every chapter were particularly helpful to this reader. Finally, the detailed reviews of immunochemistry presented with each entity are highly practical. This volume is a welcome addition to the library of practicing dermatologists and pathologists.

Mark Allen Everett, MD
Regents' Professor Emeritus
Dermatology and Pathology

Preface

The last thing one settles in writing a book is what one should put in first.

—Blaise Pascal, 1654

Dermatology textbooks exist in abundance. They include classics, such as Lever's *Histopathology of the Skin*, which have gone through several editions, as well as a burgeoning number of newer titles. They have served practitioners of pathology and dermatology well. However, the diagnosis and treatment of deadly dermatologic disorders remains a relatively unexamined topic. In *Deadly Dermatologic Diseases*, we have attempted to address this void in the literature. A wide variety of dermatologic entities are capable of directly leading to or are associated with serious medical consequences, including death. Because entities present in a variety of clinical and pathologic guises or represent emerging pathogens (such as anthrax or smallpox), it is important that clinicians and pathologists are apprised of and able to quickly recognize and treat these important public health concerns. This book is comprised of disorders capable of causing the death of the patient.

The book is organized in four sections dealing with dermatologic diseases: serious cutaneous malignancies, including merkel cell carcinoma and paraneoplastic syndromes such as paraneoplastic pemphigus; life-threatening and/or emerging infectious pathogens, including anthrax and smallpox; endocrinologic disorders such as calciphylaxis; and, lastly, inborn errors of metabolism or life-threatening genodermatoses, such as ataxia telangiectasia. Each section of the book is organized alphabetically for easy reference. Approximately 50 disease states are discussed with accompanying full-color clinical and microscopic photographs. Each entity contains clinical photographs accompanied by photomicrographs detailing the diagnostic features of each case. Subsections detailing the demographic attributes, etiology, pathogenesis, clinical presentation, pathologic features, diagnostic adjuncts, treatment, and prognosis with a current bibliography of each disease state presented in a succinct bullet-style manner. Although comprehensive by design, this textbook is by no means exhaustive in scope. Several entities rarely capable of causing death or that are extremely uncommon have not been included due to space constraints.

This book should become a shelf reference work for primary care clinicians, including general practitioners and internists, dermatologists, and pathologists, who are responsible for the diagnosis of skin biopsy specimens. The book might also serve as a potential study source for dermatology and pathology residents preparing for board examinations and dermatopathologists in training.

Michael B. Morgan, MD
Bruce R. Smoller, MD
Stephen C. Somach, MD

Contents

Part I
Malignant Cutaneous Neoplasms

1 Angiosarcoma

■ Synonyms:	Hemangiosarcoma, lymphangiosarcoma, malignant hemangioendothelioma
■ Etiology:	Ultraviolet light, radiotherapy, lymphedema (Treves-Stewart syndrome), preexisting vascular malformations (Mafucci's syndrome)
■ Associations:	Mafucci's syndrome
■ Clinical:	Rapidly expanding bruise-like patch, erythematous papules, violaceous nodules
■ Histology:	Ill-defined anastomosing dermal network of atypical endothelial-lined spaces (most common) or defined diffusely arranged aggregates of epithelioid or spindled cells
■ IHC repertoire:	CD-31 (most sensitive and specific), CD-34, Ulex europaeus, Factor VIII
■ Staging:	None for cutaneous disease
■ Prognosis:	Overall 5-year ~10%
■ Adverse variables:	Size > 5 cm, depth of invasion > 3.0 mm, mitotic rate > 3 HPF, positive surgical margins, recurrence, and metastases
■ Treatment:	WLE/XRT for localized disease, XRT for systemic disease, limited role for CTX

Angiosarcoma (AS), otherwise known as hemangiosarcoma, lymphangiosarcoma, or malignant hemangioendothelioma, is a malignant tumor derived from endothelium that occurs in a variety of anatomic sites including the skin (1–3). Sixty percent of cases arise within the skin or superficial soft tissues. Although these tumors derive from the vascular endothelium, the exact vascular origin is unknown and likely derives from both the blood vessels and lymphatics.

AS is an extremely uncommon tumor, accounting for less than 1% of all sarcomas (4). With the exception of tumors that may arise in preexisting vascular lesions, AS predominantly afflicts the elderly and is seen more commonly in men. Males outnumber females by a ratio of approximately 2:1. Most patients described have been Caucasian. The etiology of AS is multifactorial and is influenced by the clinical setting. Fifty percent of cases occur on the head and neck and in particular the scalp of elderly men where ultraviolet light is thought to constitute an important risk factor. While tenable, investigators have argued that CA remains an extremely uncommon tumor among individuals with excessive ultraviolet light exposure and that other sun-prone anatomic sites are rarely afflicted by AS (5). In reconciling these contradictions, it has been recently hypothesized that factors unique to these anatomic locations might exist that predispose to its development. These factors might include the vascular density of the scalp or the anastomotic arrangement of the vessels in these areas. Unusual vascular arrangements or density might also combine with ultraviolet light or thermal (heat) effect potentiating oncogenesis. Ionizing radiation in the form of radiotherapy is a recognized risk factor for these tumors particularly involving the anterior chest wall of women who have undergone treatment for breast cancer (6). Lymphedematous extremities, particularly resulting from radical mastectomy for breast cancer, predispose to AS. Known as the Treves-Stewart syndrome, named after the surgeons who described this association among six patients in 1948, this condition has been reported in over 300 patients to date. Other causes of chronic lymphedema, including congenital lymphedema, and complications resulting from long-standing filariasis infection may eventuate in this tumor as well. Preexisting vascular lesions, including arteriovenous malformations, and hemangiomas including the Mafucci syndrome have been described in conjunction with this neoplasm. Interestingly, most of these cases have been described in children. AS has also been rarely described following foreign body implantation and in sites of recurring herpes zoster infection. Unlike identical tumors occurring in the viscera, there is no known association of cutaneous lesions with toxin exposure including Thoratrast, arsenic, polyvinyl chloride, or anabolic steroids.

The clinical presentation is varied and dependent upon the various risk factor(s). The classic presentation associated with ultraviolet exposure is of a rapidly centripetally expanding brown-to-erythematous patch situated on the forehead or scalp (Figure 1.1) (7). In time, the lesion is capable of producing an ulcerated erythematous-to-violaceous plaque or nodule. Later, there is a tendency to develop a centrifugal pattern of tumor satellites (8,9). Among the most common entities cited in the differential diagnosis are lymphoma and metastatic carcinoma. Although the scalp and face are most commonly afflicted, the ears, neck, and upper trunk may be involved as well. Lesions attributed to antecedent radiotherapy consist of rapidly growing papules and nodules classically located on the chest wall of women with a history of irradiated breast carcinoma. Radiotherapy-associated tumors may, however, arise in either sex and within the radiation field of a variety of anatomic sites. Most tumors arise following a 10-year or greater latent period. AS arising within a lymphedematous extremity is generally heralded by the development of a rapidly enlarging papule/nodule superimposed upon the brawny induration typical of longstanding lymphedema. Most lesions develop an average of 10 years following surgery. Lesions associated with congenital lymphedema generally occur in younger patients who have experienced lymphedema for greater than 20 years. AS associated with preexisting vascular lesion(s) is characterized by rapid eccentric growth and epidermal ulceration.

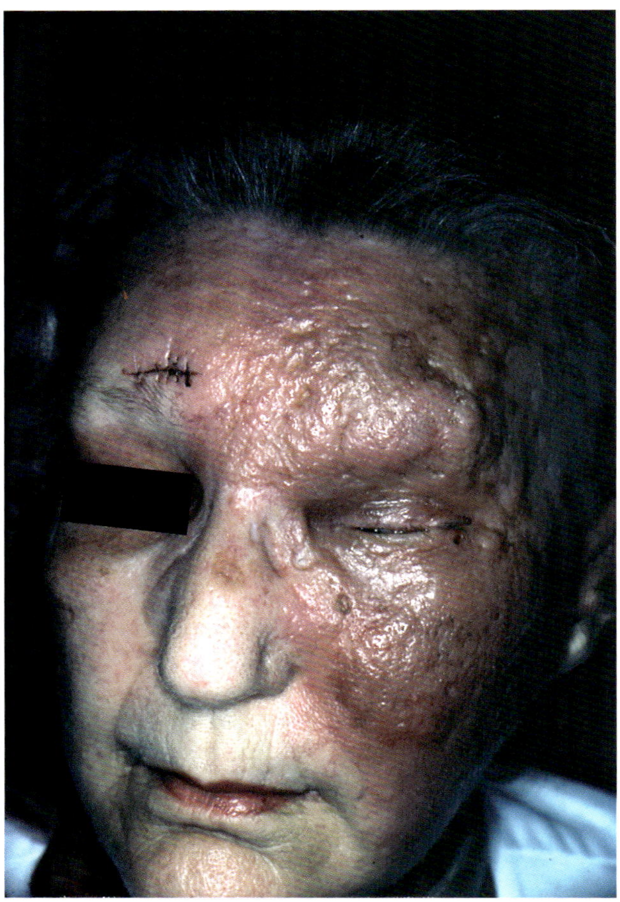

FIGURE 1.1. Violaceous plaque of angiosarcoma.

The histologic attributes of this lesion are varied. The most common pathologic alteration consists of a subtle increase in vascularity detected in the superficial and mid-dermis (5). The vascular channels diffusely ramify throughout the dermis, forming an anastomosing network of endothelial lined vascular spaces (Figures 1.2 and 1.3). The vascular channels may consist of sinusoids with parallel sides or gaping cavernous spaces. The vascular spaces are lined by a population of cuboidal to hobnailed cells possessing enlarged and hyperchromatic nuclei (Figures 1.4 and 1.5). The endothelial may stratify forming papillations. The intervening stroma often contains plasma cells and neutrophils as well as hemosiderin pigment. The tumor periphery is often bounded by a fringe of dilated and otherwise normal-appearing vascular spaces. Less common histologic presentations include a nested or diffusely arranged population of either spindled or enlarged epithelioid cells. In the latter setting, striking cellular pleomorphism may rarely be encountered. Although early lesions are confined to the dermis, well-developed lesions may extend laterally over a large expanse of dermis as well as deep into the subcutaneous fat and soft tissues. Microscopic extension of tumor is commonly seen well beyond what is deemed to be the clinical boundary of tumor.

Special techniques that may be employed in confirmation of the diagnosis include electron microscopy, and increasingly, immunohistochemistry (6). Ultrastructural features of endothelial derivation include the presence of prominent external laminae, pinocytotic vesicles, and specialized endothelial organelles termed Weibel-Palade bodies. These attributes are more commonly observed in well-differentiated and epithelioid tumors. Immunohistochemistry has become an indispensable diagnostic adjunct, particularly in the evaluation of poorly differentiated tumors and in the epithelioid variant. Among the

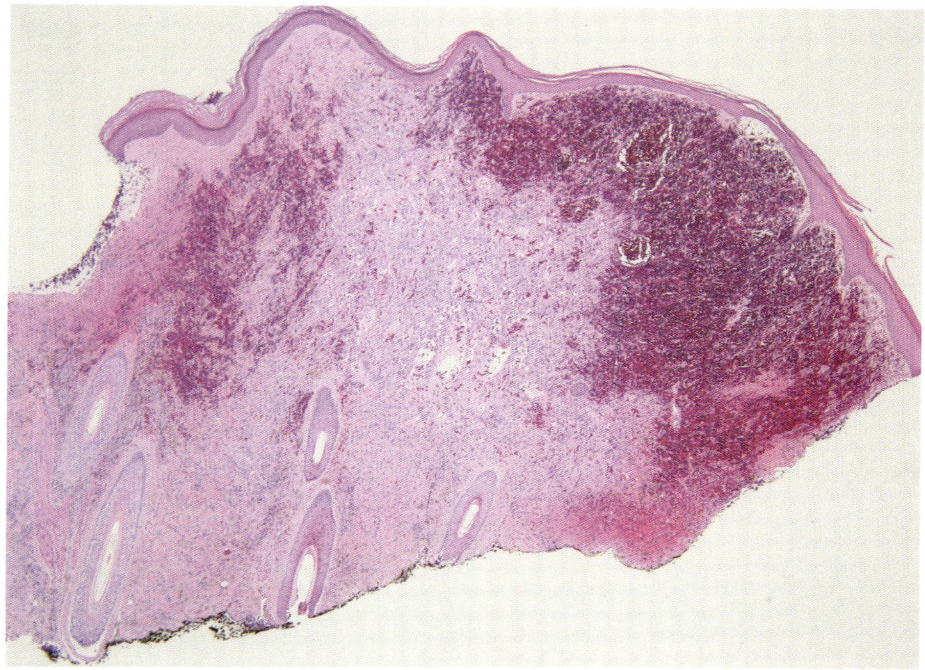

FIGURE 1.2. Low power photomicrograph depicting diffuse dermal hemorrhage.

various markers that include CD-31, CD-34, Ulex europaeus, Factor VIII, CD-31 is regarded as the most specific marker for endothelial derivation with Ulex europaeus as the most sensitive (4). An important pitfall to consider is that approximately one-third of cases stain with keratin antibodies, prompting consideration for carcinoma.

Important entities to consider in the histologic differential diagnosis include benign entities such as the tufted angioma (TA) and targetoid hemosiderotic hemangioma (THH), low-grade vascular tumors of intermediate prognosis such as epithelioid hemangioendothelioma (EHA) and Kaposi's sarcoma (KS), as well as malignant entities

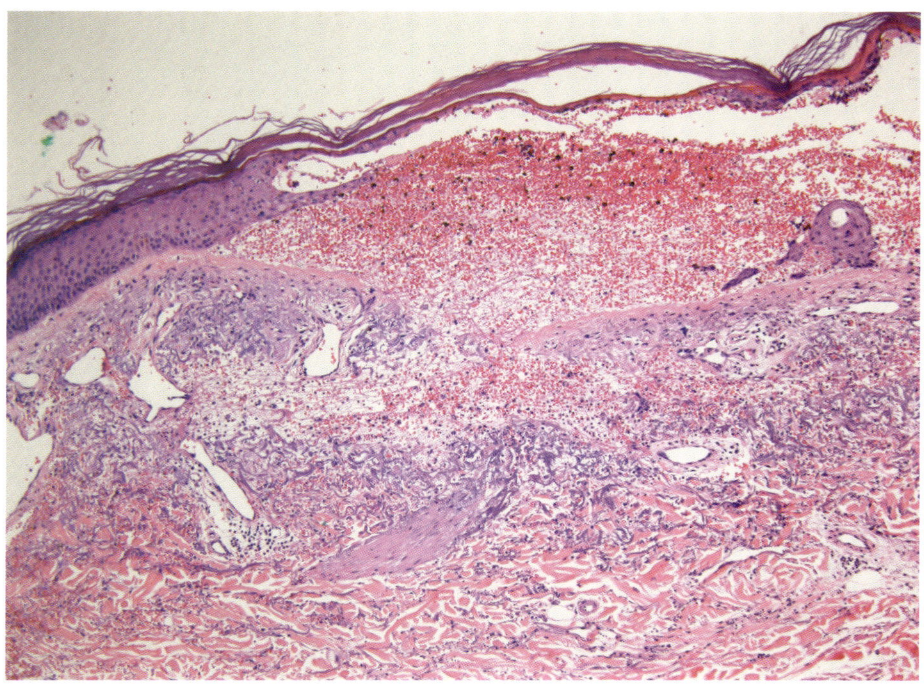

FIGURE 1.3. Medium power photomicrograph depicting subtle proliferation of endothelial-lined dermal vascular channels.

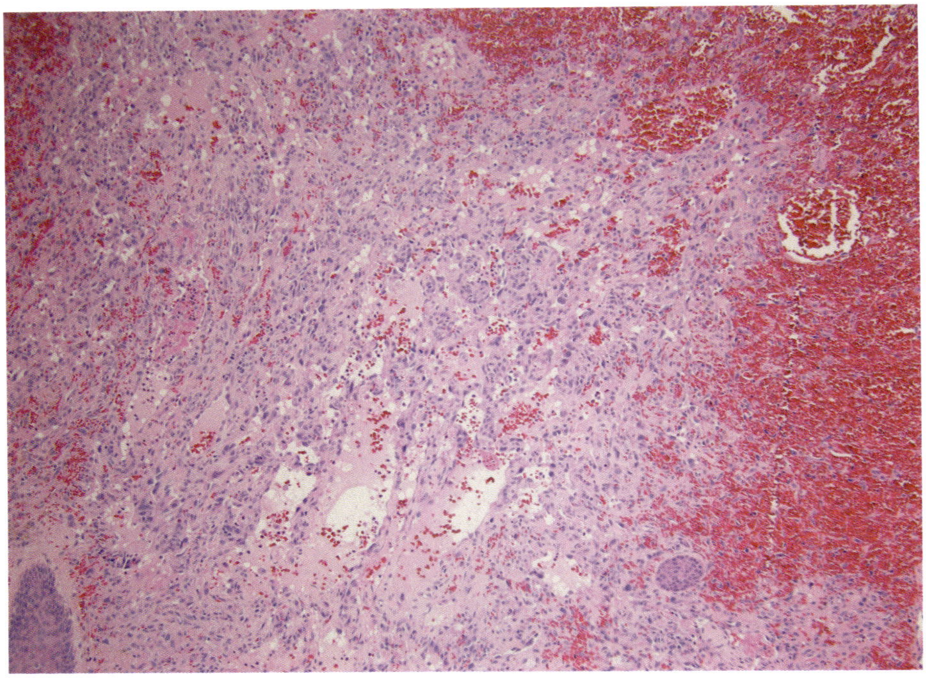

FIGURE 1.4. Medium power photomicrograph depicting deeper dermis with gaping vascular channels lined by atypical hyperchromatic endothelial cells.

such as poorly differentiated carcinoma. THH consists of a superficial papillary dermal central focus of hobnail-lined vascular spaces and surrounding progressively inconspicuous and attenuated vascular channels. TA consists of discrete nests or tufts of epithelioid endothelia situated throughout the dermis. Endothelial atypia and/or extensive dermal or subcutaneous fat extension are not seen in these lesions. EHA is an uncommon tumor comprised of dermal and subcutaneous nests, strands, and diffusely arranged epithelioid cells often possessing intracytoplasmic lumina that contain erythrocytes. KS consists of a diffusely spindled cell population that char-

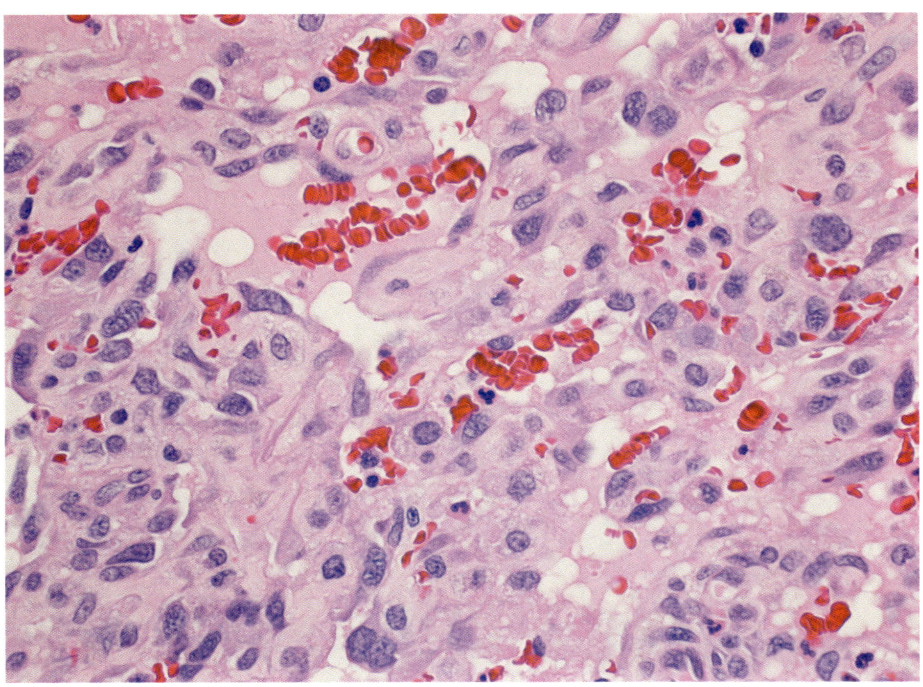

FIGURE 1.5. High power photomicrograph depicting cytologic detail of vascular channels lined by atypical endothelial cells.

acteristically forms slit-like vascular spaces and is punctuated by plasma cells and extracellular hyaline globules. Metastatic and poorly differentiated carcinoma may closely simulate AS. Epithelial connection, intercellular bridges, and glandular formation favor carcinoma. Difficult cases may require immunohistochemical characterization. Carcinomas should not stain with antibodies to CD-31.

AS is an aggressive tumor. It tends to recur locally, later metastasizing despite aggressive multimodal therapy. Because of its predilection for multifocality and inapparent spread, complete surgical resection is often unattainable. Overall prognosis is poor, with reported 5-year survival rates of 10%–35%. Usual metastatic sites are the skin, lung, lymph nodes, spleen, liver, and bone. The development of metastases is ominous, as most patients eventually succumb to their disease. Metastases and recurrences usually develop within 2 years of diagnosis. Histologic appearance, tumor grade, demographic factors such as age and gender, anatomic location, and clinical setting, do not influence prognosis (10). The diameter of the lesion at the time of initial diagnosis is the most important factor in influencing survival. Lesions of less than 5 centimeters have a better prognosis (5). Generally, smaller tumors are more accessible to treatment with surgery. Other potential factors responsible for this observation include shorter clinical duration and limited vascular access with the attendant risk of metastases. Other favorable attributes recently shown to influence survival include average tumor mitotic rate of less than 3 per microscopic high power field, a tumor depth of less than 3 millimeters, and absence of recurrence and metastases.

Patients need clinical examination every 3 months for the first year following diagnosis to detect early recurrence. Lymph node survey and imaging studies including CT or MRI of the head and neck should be considered at these time intervals as well (11). Due to the rarity of this tumor, there are no widely adopted standard protocols for therapy (11). Localized disease is generally treated with wide local excision or in combination with radiotherapy if the anatomic site and health status of the patient permits. Those who cannot tolerate surgery can be palliated with radiotherapy. Most radiation protocols employ fractionalized megavoltage dosing of between 180 and 300 centigray per day for a total of between 3000 and 7000 centigray. Systemic disease can also be palliated with radiotherapy. The use of various chemotherapeutic agents, including methotrexate, doxorubixin, cyclophosphamide, and vincristine, has been reported with varying success. The role of chemotherapy is not well defined and requires further investigation. Future developments include the use of anti-angiogenic drugs, anti-endothelial antibodies conjugated with cytotoxins, and XRT radiosensitizers.

References

1. Cooper P. Angiosarcomas of the skin. *Semin Diagn Pathol* 1987; 4: 2.
2. Haustein U. Angiosarcoma of the face and scalp. *Int J Dermatol* 1991; 30: 851.
3. Meis-Kindblom J, Kindblom L. Angiosarcoma of soft tissue: A study of 80 cases. *Am J Surg Pathol* 1998; 22: 683.
4. Antman K, Eilber F, Shiu M. Soft tissue sarcomas: Current trends in diagnosis and management. *Curr Probl Cancer* 1989; 14: 340.
5. Weiss S, Goldblum J. *Soft Tissue Tumors*. St. Louis: C.V. Mosby Company, 2002.
6. Mark P, Poen J, Tran L, et al. Angiosarcoma: A report of 67 patients and a review of the literature. *Cancer* 1996; 77: 2400.
7. Maddox J, Evans H. Angiosarcoma of the skin and soft tissue: A study of 44 cases. *Cancer* 1981; 48: 1907.
8. Lydiatt W, Shaha A, Shah J. Angiosarcoma of the head and neck. *Am J Surg* 1994; 168: 451.
9. Cerroni L, Peris K, Legge A, et al. Angiosarcoma of the face and scalp, prognosis, and treatment. *J Dermatol Surg Oncol* 1991; 17: 539–542.
10. Morgan MB, Swann M, Somach S, et al. Cutaneous angiosarcoma of the skin: A case series with prognostic correlation. *J Am Acad Dermatol* 2004; 50: 867.
11. Holden C, Spittle M, Wilson Jones E. Angiosarcoma of the face and scalp, prognosis, and treatment. *Cancer* 1987; 59: 1046.
12. Budd G. Management of angiosarcoma. *Curr Oncol Rep* 2002; 4: 515.

2
Cutaneous B-Cell Lymphoma

■ Synonyms:	Lymphoma cutis, marginal zone lymphoma, follicular lymphoma, large cell lymphoma, malignant angioendotheliomatosis
■ Etiology:	Unknown
■ Associations:	Systemic lymphoma
■ Clinical:	Violaceous nodules, most common on head and neck
■ Histology:	Malignant lymphocytes in dermis, diffusely or in patchy distribution
■ IHC repertoire:	Lymphocyte surface markers and light chains
■ Staging:	Systemic work-up required
■ Prognosis:	Excellent if limited to skin
■ Adverse variables:	Systemic involvement
■ Treatment:	Radiation, intralesional chemotherapy; systemic chemotherapy if systemic involvement

Cutaneous B-cell lymphoma is not a single disease, but rather a family of neoplastic processes characterized by a proliferation of malignant B lymphocytes. These lymphomas may arise *de novo* on the skin (primary cutaneous B cell lymphoma) or spread to the skin as part of a systemic disease (secondary cutaneous B-cell lymphoma). It is not possible to make this distinction based purely on histologic findings, and a systemic work-up is required in all of these patients in order to determine the extent of disease. The prognosis is greatly altered depending upon this extent. As subtypes of lymphoma correlate with clinical correlation, histologic findings, and prognosis, several of the most prevalent subtypes will be described individually.

Marginal Zone Lymphoma (Immunocytoma)

Marginal zone lymphoma (MZL) is reported to be the most common B-cell lymphoma that occurs in the skin. This type of lymphoma may be closely related to mucosa-associated lymphoid tissue (MALT) lymphomas. There is a slight male predominance and the mean age of onset is approximately 50 years (1). The usual presentation is that of one or several red-brown papules or nodules, most commonly on the upper extremities or head and neck (Figure 2.1).

Histologic findings include diffuse infiltrates of lymphocytes within the dermis and subcutaneous fat. A Grenz zone is present in most cases (Figure 2.2).

The lymphocytes are often admixed with scattered plasma cells and plasmacytoid cells, which provide a clue to the diagnosis (Figure 2.3).

In more than 75% of cases, reactive germinal centers may be present, often masking the diagnosis (1). Areas containing a relatively monomorphous infiltrate of plasmacytoid lymphocytes constitute the neoplastic population. These marginal zones may demonstrate pallor at lowest magnification. This is often quite subtle, especially in early lesions. Rare eosinophils are occasionally present, further complicating the diagnosis.

Lymphocyte immunophenotyping is helpful in making the diagnosis, but the findings may be subtle. The neoplastic lymphocytes express both CD79a and CD20 and fail to express T cell markers. Light chain restriction can be detected in areas with neoplastic cells in some cases, though in others, the tumor cells fail to produce any light chains (2). In most cases of MZL, there is a brisk reactive

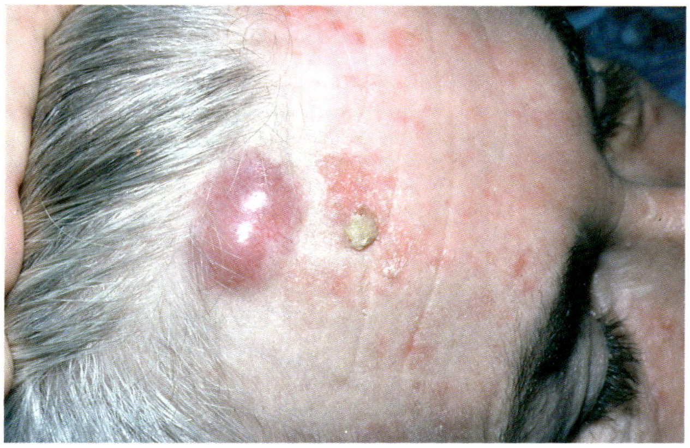

FIGURE 2.1. Erythematous nodule located at hairline biopsy showed marginal zone lymphoma.

T cell infiltrate that may obscure the diagnostic population.

The differential diagnosis mainly includes a reactive lymphoid hyperplasia. The presence of reactive germinal centers and plasma cells makes this distinction especially difficult. The presence of abundant plasmacytoid cells within greatly expanded interfollicular regions favors MZL, but this is not always apparent. In many cases, immunostains are helpful in detecting subtle light chain restrictions that reveal a clonal population not apparent with routine sections. Gene rearrangement studies are best reserved for cases in which there is a high degree of suspicion for lymphoma and when routine sections and immunostains are not helpful in arriving at a firm diagnosis (see Table 2.1).

The prognosis for patients with MZL is excellent. Aggressive chemotherapy is not necessary. Local excision and/or radiotherapy have been used with a great deal of success. The five-year survival rate is >95%.

Follicular Cell Lymphoma

Follicular cell lymphoma (FCL) occurs with approximately the same frequency as does MZL, but has a tendency to involve the head and neck, rather than the upper extremities. There is a slight female predominance for patients with FCL and these tumors occur most commonly in middle-aged adults (3). The most common presentation is that of one or several papules or nodules. There may be some clustering of lesions.

The histologic changes in FCL can be separated into several histologic patterns. Similar to the subtypes seen in node-based FCL, the neoplastic infiltrate can involve the dermis diffusely or with a tendency to form neoplastic follicles (Figure 2.4).

The neoplastic follicles can be distinguished from reactive germinal centers based upon the lack of surrounding mantle zone, absence of tingible-body macrophages, and uniformity of the follicular cells. The cells may be small or

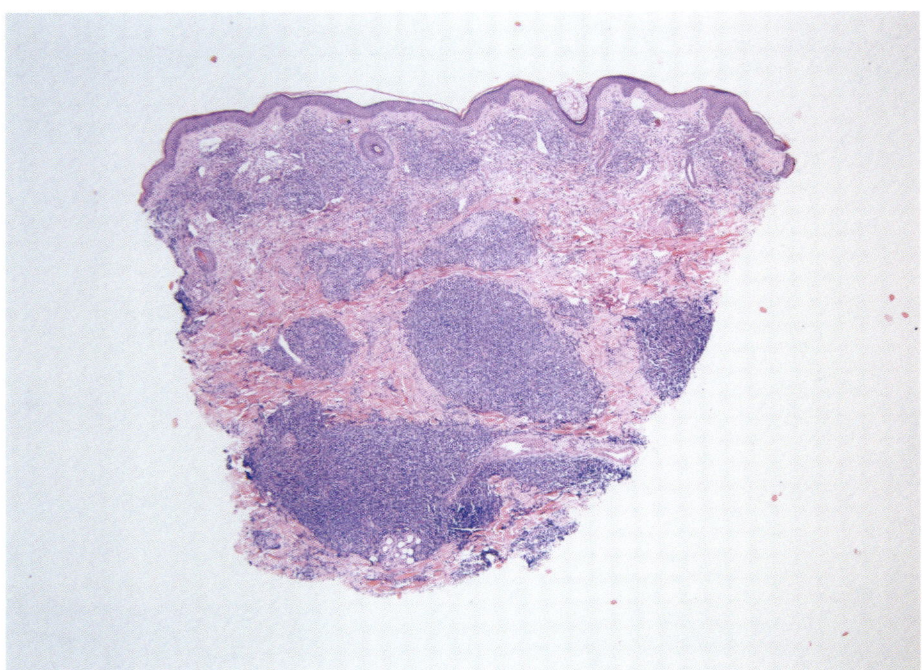

FIGURE 2.2. MZL demonstrating a dense dermal lymphocytic infiltrate separated from the epidermis by a Grenz zone.

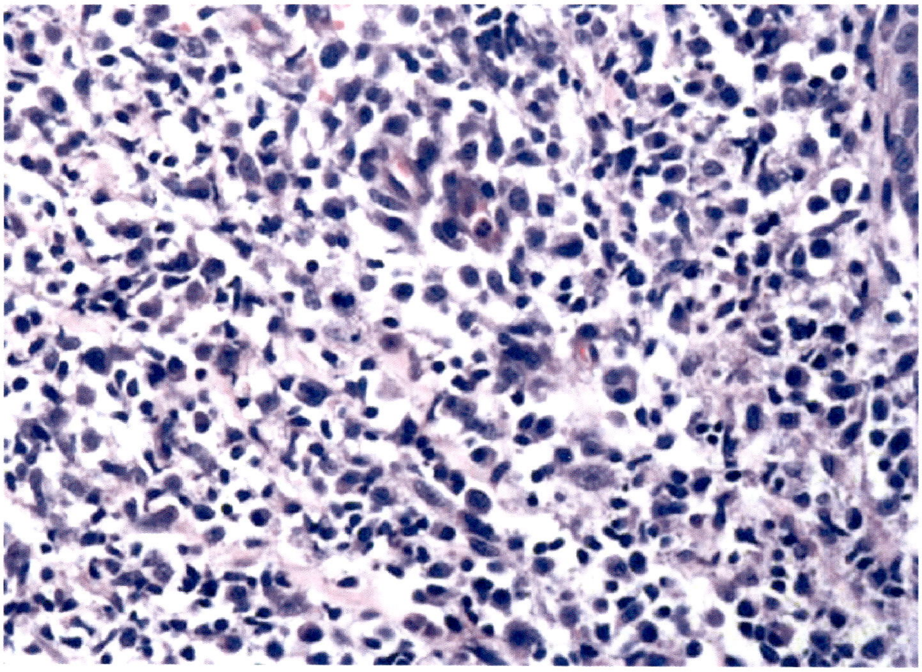

FIGURE 2.3. Abundant plasma cells and plasmacytoid lymphocytes are present in MZL in the interfollicular regions.

large, round or cleaved, similar to the appearances described in the nodal counterparts to this family of lymphomas. More commonly, however, FCL does not demonstrate a follicular growth pattern. Rather, the most common appearance is that of a diffuse, dense infiltrate of a uniform population of lymphocytes coursing though the dermis and the subcutaneous fat. There is no tendency for involvement of the epidermis or appendageal epithelium, and a Grenz zone may be present. Plasma cells and eosinophils are usually not present in FCL (Figures 2.5 and 2.6).

TABLE 2.1.

	Marginal Zone Lymphoma	Follicular Center Lymphoma	Large Cell Lymphoma	Intravascular Lymphoma
Histologic features	Expansion of interfollicular regions with abundant plasmacytoid lymphocytes	Neoplastic follicles devoid of histiocytes or diffuse uniform population of lymphocytes throughout dermis	Markedly atypical lymphocytes with abundant mitoses and necrosis	Large, atypical cells largely confined to within lymphatic vessels
Immunostains	Many CD79a+ cells in interfollicular regions; often light chain restriction	Large areas of CD79a+ cells; frequent light chain restriction	Sheets of CD79a+ cells; occasionally fail to express lymphocyte surface antigens	Intravascular CD79+ lymphocytes
Gene rearrangements	Positive in some cases; early cases often negative	Positive for clonal population in most cases	Positive for clonal population in most cases	Positive for clonal population in most cases.

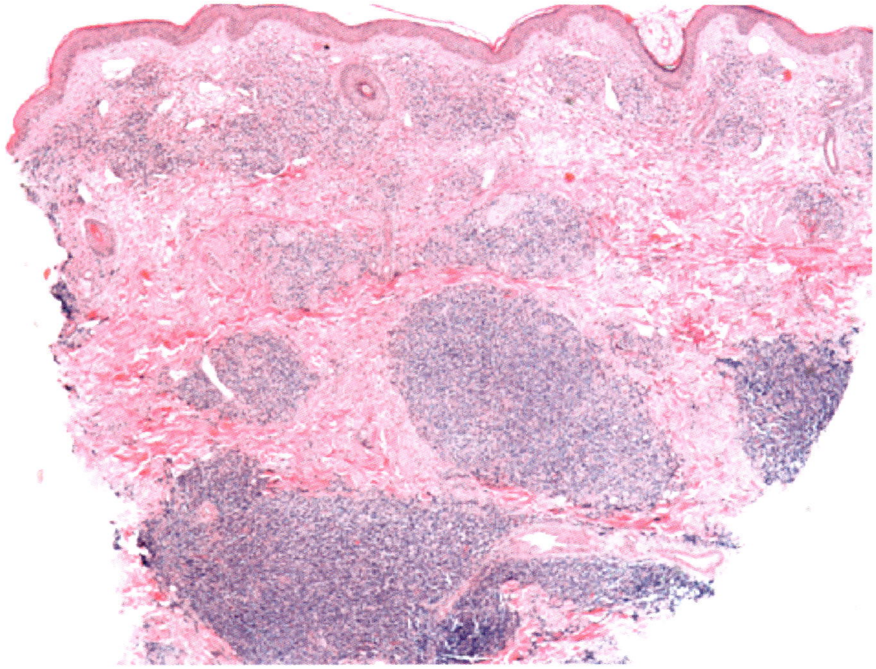

FIGURE 2.4. Low power photomicrograph depicting nodular lymphoid infiltrate of FCL.

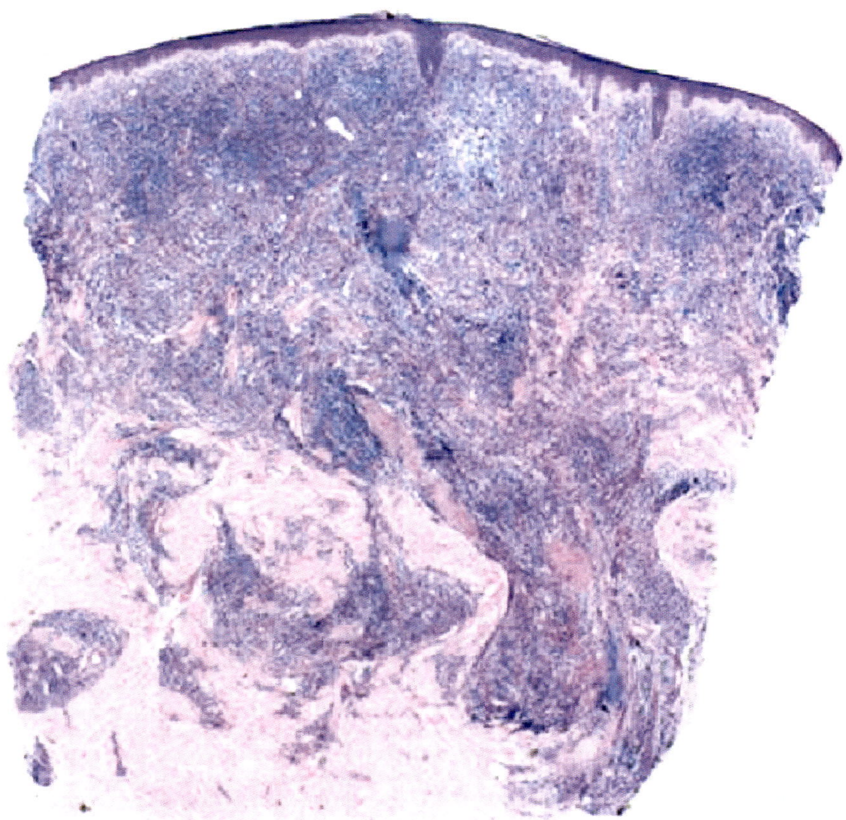

FIGURE 2.5. FCL with a diffuse dermal disposition. Note sparing or Grenz zone.

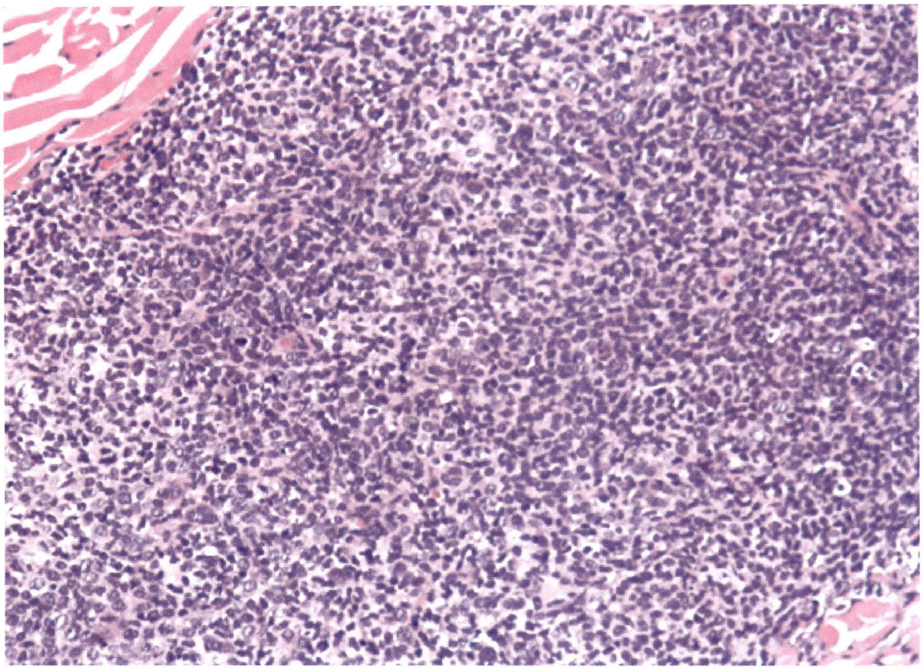

FIGURE 2.6. FCL with a monomorphous infiltrate of relatively small lymphocytes and lack of eosinophils or plasma cells.

Immunostains reveal the infiltrating lymphocytes to express CD79a and CD20. Most T cell markers are negative, but coexpression with CD43 has been described in FCC. Light chain restriction is found in some cases, but lack of any light chain production is also common in primary cutaneous FCL. Bcl-2, a good marker for node-based FCL, is seen only in a minority of cases of primary cutaneous FCL; further, as this marker is constitutively expressed by T lymphocytes, interpretation may be difficult in dermal infiltrates (4).

The major differential diagnosis includes cutaneous lymphoid hyperplasia. The presence of histiocytes, plasma cells, and eosinophils favors a reactive process, as does heterogeneity in the size and shape of the lymphocytes. In many cases, immunostains are helpful in demonstrating large sheets of B lymphocytes. The presence of significant numbers of B lymphocytes in the skin in any pattern other than confined to a reactive germinal center is concerning for lymphoma.

As is the case with MZL, patients with primary cutaneous FCL have an excellent prognosis and aggressive systemic chemotherapy is not required. The five-year survival rate exceeds 95% (5).

Large Cell Lymphoma of the Leg

This is a controversial form of B-cell lymphoma that involves the legs of elderly patients. Some investigators believe this subtype of lymphoma to be a variant of FCL. Others cite differences in histologic pattern and overall survival in supporting the contention that this should be considered a separate subtype of lymphoma (6).

The clinical presentation is that of one or several large erythematous to violaceous nodules with occasional ulceration in a linear distribution on a lower extremity. Bilateral involvement occurs in some cases, but rarely do tumor nodules extend beyond the lower extremities at the time of initial presentation. This subtype of lymphoma may be more common in women (6).

The histologic appearance is that of a diffuse infiltrate of large, atypical cells filling the entire papillary and reticular dermis. There is no tendency for involvement of the epidermis and a Grenz zone may be present. The tumor cells are large, with vesicular nuclei, occasional nucleoli, and abundant cytoplasm (Figure 2.7). Mitotic activity may be brisk, and individual cell necrosis is common (Figure 2.8).

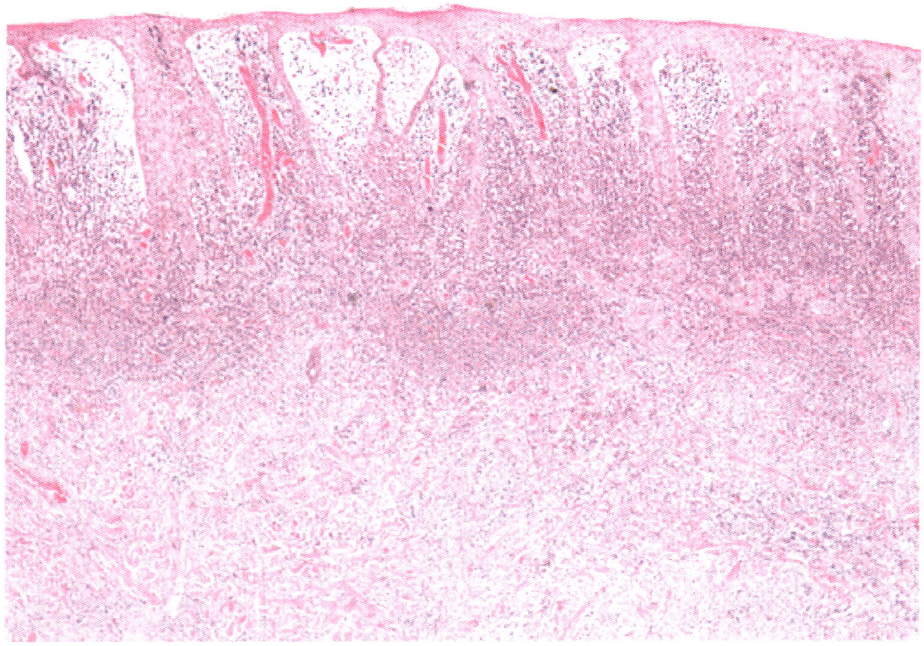

FIGURE 2.7. Large cell lymphoma is characterized by a dense dermal infiltrate for epidermotropism.

Immunostains demonstrate CD20 and CD79a expression by the neoplastic lymphocytes. Light chain restriction is seen in many cases, though in some cases there may be no light chain production. The neoplastic cells in large cell lymphomas all variably express bcl-2, CD10, and bcl-6 (7).

The main differential diagnosis includes large cell anaplastic lymphoma. This type of lymphoma is a T cell lymphoma in which the great majority of neoplastic lymphocytes express CD30. Immunostains make this distinction straightforward in virtually all cases.

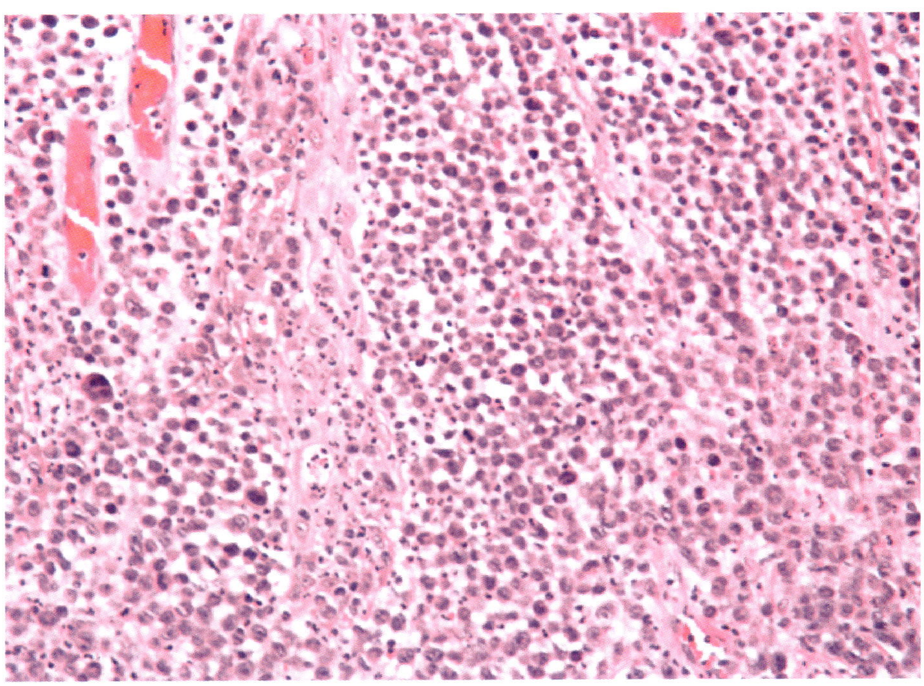

FIGURE 2.8. Large cell lymphoma shows large lymphocytes with vesicular nuclei, abundant mitoses and individual cell apoptosis.

The prognosis tends to be much worse for patients with this type of lymphoma than for the very favorable FCL (7). If considered a distinct subtype, it is classified as an intermediate grade lymphoma (6).

Intravascular Lymphoma

This extremely rare subtype of CBCL was previously known as malignant endotheliomatosis based upon its histologic appearance. (Immunostains have subsequently proven that the tumor cells are not endothelial in nature, but rather, are B lymphocytes (8,9). Exceedingly rare cases are T cell lymphomas (10)). Intravascular lymphoma (IVL) affects primarily elderly adults who present with a diffuse hemorrhagic cutaneous eruption and signs of central nervous system thromboi. They are generally acutely ill at the time of presentation and require immediate clinical intervention.

The histologic features include a proliferation of large, markedly atypical lymphocytes that are confined almost exclusively to within vascular spaces. The tumor cells display little tendency to extend beyond vessels, and in most cases, the dermis is completely devoid of lymphomatous infiltrate beyond the vessels. Affected vessels are significantly distended and occluded by the neoplastic cells, and signs of infarction may be present.

Immunostains reveal that the large tumor cells are CD20+, CD79a+ B lymphocytes. In most cases, there is not sufficient cellularity to attempt demonstration of light chain restriction.

The major differential diagnosis is metastatic carcinoma within lymphatics. Immunostains are helpful in making this distinction in virtually all cases.

The prognosis for patients with IVL is very poor. Mortality rates exceed 80% and the mean survival has been reported to be about 13 months (11). Many of these patients succumb to consequences of ischemic episodes within the central nervous system caused by occlusion of these vessels by tumor cells. Rapid cytoreductive therapy is required, but rarely does this result in long-term survival.

References

1. Cerroni L, Signoretti S, Hofler G, Annessi G, Putz B, Lackinger E, Metze D, Giannetti A, Kerl H. Primary cutaneous marginal zone B-cell lymphoma: A recently described entity of low-grade malignant cutaneous B-cell lymphoma. *Am J Surg Pathol* 1997; 21: 1307–1315.
2. Tomaszewski M-M, Abbondanzo SL, Lupton GL. Extranodal marginal zone B-cell lymphoma of the skin: A morphologic and immunophenotypic study of 11 cases. *Am J Dermatopathol* 2000; 22: 205–211.
3. Cerroni L, Kerl H. Cutaneous follicle center cell lymphoma, follicular type. *Am J Dermatopathol* 2001; 23: 370–373.
4. Cerroni L, Volkenandy M, Rieger E, Soyer HP, Kerl H. bcl-2 proteinexpressionandcorrelationwiththeinterchromosomal 14:18 translocation in cutaneous lymphomas and pseudolymphomas. *J Invest Dermatol* 1994; 102: 231–235.
5. Rijlaarsdam JU, Toonstra J, Meijer OWM, Noordijk EM, Willemze R. Treatment of primary cutaneous B-cell lymphomas of follicular center cell origin. *J Clin Oncol* 1996; 14: 549–555.
6. Vermeer MH, Geelen FAMJ, van Haselen CW, van Voorst Vader PC, Geerts M-L, van Vloten WA, Willemze R (for the Dutch Lymphoma Working Group). Primary cutaneous large B-cell lymphomas of the legs. *Arch Dermatol* 1996; 132: 1304–1308.
7. Goodlad JR, Krajewski AS, Batstone PJ, McKy P, White JM, Benton EC, Kavanagh GM, Lucraft HH (on behalf of the Scotland and Newcastle Lymphoma Group). Primary cutaneous diffuse large B-cell lymphoma: Prognostic significance of clinicopathological subtypes. *Am J Surg Pathol* 2003; 27: 1538–1545.
8. Bhawan J, Wolff SM, Ucci AA, Bhan AK. Malignant lymphoma and malignant angioendotheliomatosis: One disease. *Cancer* 1985; 55: 570–576.
9. Wick MR, Mills SE, Sheithauer BW, Cooper PH, Davitz MA, Parkinson K. Reassessment of malignant "angioendotheliomatosis": Evidence in favor of its reclassification as "intravascular lymphomatosis." *Am J Surg Pathol* 1986; 10: 112–123.
10. Sangueza O, Hyder DM, Sangueza P. Intravascular lymphomatosis: Report of an unusual case with T cell phenotype occurring in an adolescent male. *J Cutan Pathol* 1992; 19: 226–231.
11. Sepp N, Schuler G, Romani N, Geissler D, Gattringer C, Burg G, Bartram CR, Fritsch P. "Intravascular lymphomatosis" (angioendotheliomatosis): Evidence for a T-cell origin in two cases. *Hum Pathol* 1990: 20: 1051–1058.

3
Granulomatous Slack Skin

■ Synonyms:	Cutaneous T-cell lymphoma, granulomatous mycosis fungoides
■ Etiology:	Unknown
■ Associations:	Hodgkin's disease, mycosis fungoides, non-Hodgkin's lymphoma, leukemia, Langerhans cell histiocytosis
■ Clinical:	Pendulous folds in axilla and inguinal regions
■ Histology:	Epidermotropic, hyperchromatic lymphocytes in epidermis with admixed granulomatous areas and elastolysis in dermis
■ IHC repertoire:	CD4, CD8, C7 in some cases
■ Staging:	Systemic work-up required
■ Prognosis:	Controversial; possibly better than conventional mycosis fungoides
■ Adverse variables:	Anaplasia of T cells, nodal involvement
■ Treatment:	Electron beam irradiation, topical and systemic chemotherapy

Granulomatous slack skin (GSS) is a subtle variant of mycosis fungoides that is easily overlooked on initial biopsy due to its well-formed granulomatous appearance (1). The initial clinical presentation is similar to that of conventional mycosis fungoides in that patients present with erythematous-to-violaceous patches and plaques. As the lesions progress, however, pendulous folds develop on flexural surfaces of extremities, especially the axillae and inguinal regions (Figure 3.1). Less commonly, the skin on the trunk is affected. At this point in the course of the disease, the clinical appearance is similar to that of cutis laxa. This extremely rare variant of mycosis fungoides affects middle-aged adults with a slight predilection for women in some, but not all, series (2–5). It is most common in Caucasians.

The histologic findings consist of a dense dermal infiltrate of lymphocytes that are morphologically similar to those seen in mycosis fungoides (Figure 3.2). The lymphocytes are slightly enlarged, hyperchromatic and hyperconvoluted or cerebriform. These atypical lymphocytes intercolate through the dermal interstitium. Pautrier's microabscesses may be present in some cases.

Admixed is a population of multinucleated giant cells that demonstrate lymphophagocytosis (5) (Figure 3.3).

These multinucleated giant cells have been reported to have up to forty nuclei (3) (Figures 3.4 and 3.5).

The confusing histologic pattern is the accompanying presence of well-formed granulomas comprised of mature lymphocytes and histiocytes. In the granulomatous areas, there is degeneration of elastic tissue fibers and some of these may be seen within reactive histiocytes.

Caseation is not present. Plasma cells and eosinophils are present in most cases. These granulomas are believed to be reactive in nature, perhaps as a response to the infiltrating neoplastic T lymphocytes (3). Identical histologic changes have been reported in the spleen and lymph nodes in patients with GSS (6).

Immunophenotyping reveals that the neoplastic lymphocytes are all CD3- and CD4-positive T helper cells that may demonstrate loss of CD7. Most commonly, T-cell gene rearrangement studies demonstrate a clonal population (7). Trisomy 8 has been reported within the neoplastic cells in several cases (3).

The histologic differential diagnosis includes sarcoidosis, though GSS demonstrates far more of a lymphocytic infiltrate than is usual for sarcoidosis. Histiocytic proliferations such as Rosai-Dorfman disease and reticulohistiocytoma may also present diagnostic difficulties, but the atypical lymphocytes are not present in these conditions. There is extensive histologic overlap between granulomatous mycosis fungoides and GSS, and many authors consider them to be identical or closely related entities (8).

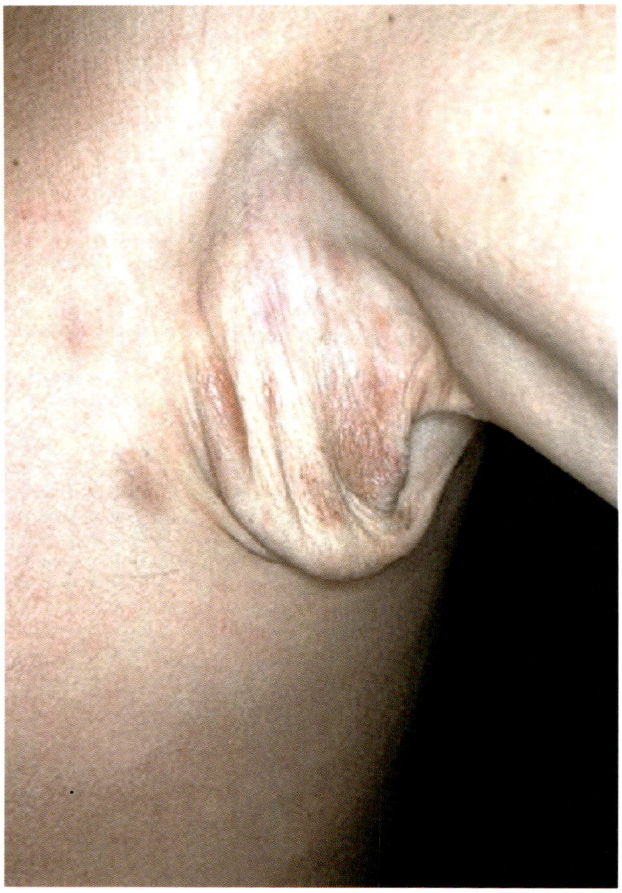

FIGURE 3.1. Pendulous skin folds typical of granulomatous slack skin. Note surface erythematous patches in the involved areas.

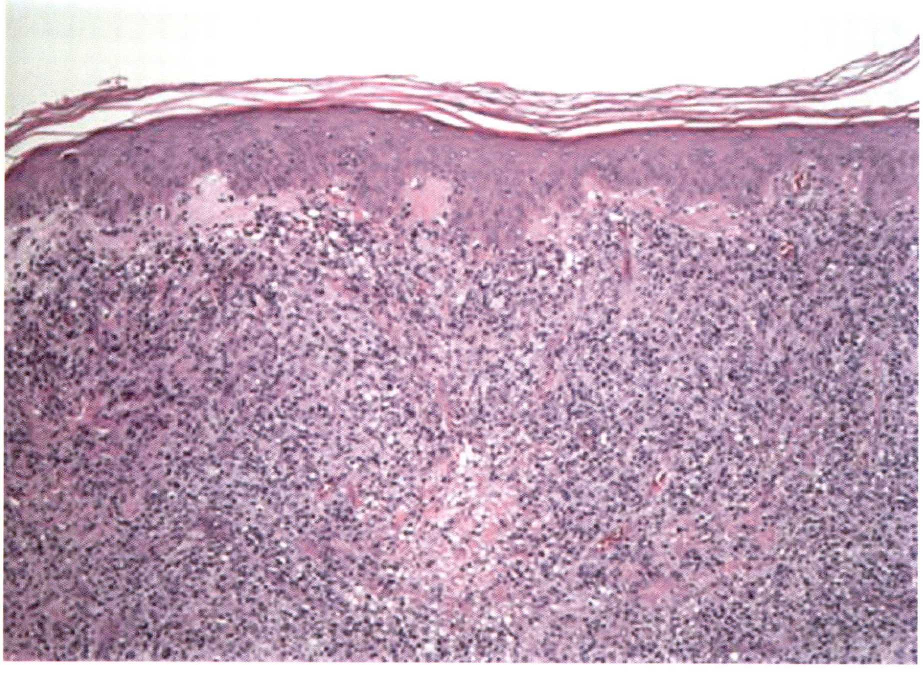

FIGURE 3.2. Low power photomicrograph depicting dense dermal infiltrate. Note the sparing of the superficial dermis (Grenz zone).

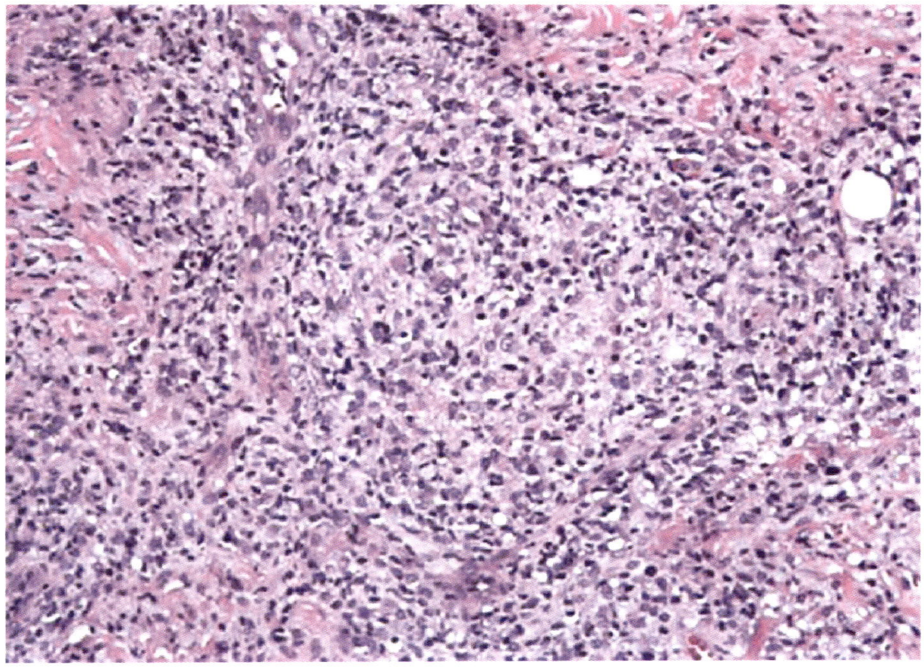

FIGURE 3.3. High power photomicrograph depicting nodular disposition of infiltrate in the deep dermis. Note the aggregates of larger, clearer histiocytes and smaller, darker lymphocytes.

The granulomatous response is more prominent in GSS than in granulomatous mycosis fungoides for those who view the entities as differing (9). Further, elastolysis involving the entire dermis is not a feature of granulomatous mycosis fungoides. The sharpest distinction between these entities is clinical in that granulomatous mycosis fungoides does not demonstrate the pendulous skin folds characteristic of GSS (5).

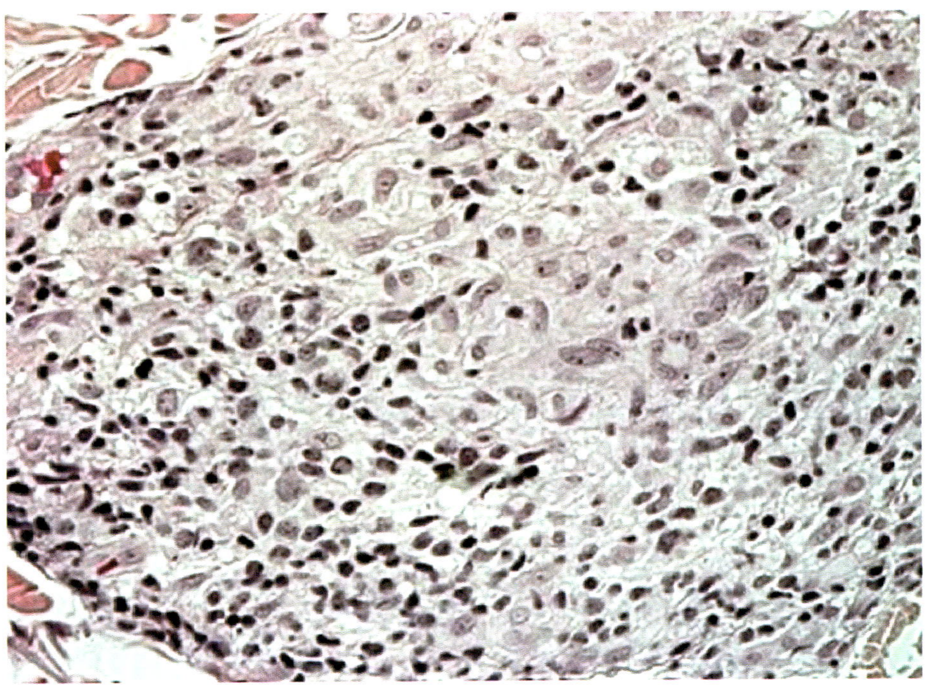

FIGURE 3.4. High power detail of granuloma with interspersed hyperchromatic convoluted T-cells.

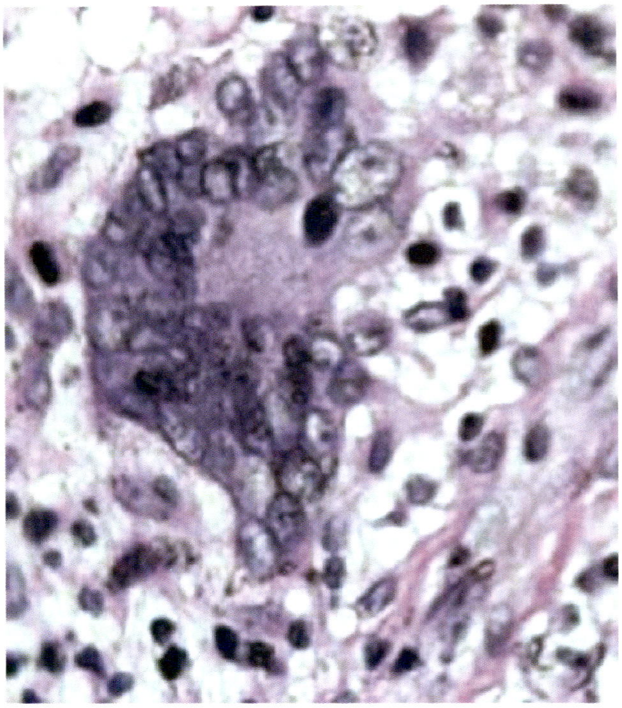

FIGURE 3.5. High power photomicrograph depicting bizarre giant cells with engulfed atypical lymphocytes.

Patients with GSS may have concomitant, preceding, or subsequent development of other hematopoietic malignancies including Hodgkin's lymphoma, non-Hodgkin's lymphoma, mycosis fungoides, leukemia, and Langerhans cell histiocytosis. Hodgkin's lymphoma is the most frequent association (10).

There is no effective therapy for GSS, though treatment regimens for mycosis fungoides and other lymphomas are frequently attempted.

References

1. Scarabello A, Leinweber B, Ardigo M, Rutten A, Feller AC, Kerl H, Cerroni L. Cutaneous lymphomas with prominent granulomatous reaction: A potential pitfall in the histopathologic diagnosis of cutaneous T- and B-cell lymphomas. *Am J Surg Pathol* 2002; 26: 1259–1268.
2. Topar G, Zelger B, Schmuth M, Romani N, Thaler J, Sepp N. Granulomatous slack skin: A distinct disorder or a variant of mycosis fungoides? *Acta Derm Veneereol* 2001; 81: 42–44.
3. Balus L, Manente L, Remotti D, Grammatico P, Bellocci M. Granulomatous slack skin: Report of a case and review of the literature. *Am J Dermatopathol* 1996; 18: 199–206.
4. van Haselen CW, Toonstra J, van der Putte SJC, van Dongen JJ, van Hees CL, van Vloten WA. Granulomatous slack skin: Report of three patients with an updated review of the literature. *Dermatology* 1998; 196: 382–391.
5. LeBoit PE, Zackheim HS, White CR, Jr. Granulomatous variants of CTCL: The histopathology of granulomatous mycosis fungoides and granulomatous slack skin. *Am J Surg Pathol* 1988; 12: 83–95.
6. Schot JDL. Granulomatous slack skin. *Br J Dermatol* 1989; 121: 807.
7. LeBoit PE, Beckstead JH, Bond B, Epstein WL, Frieden IJ, Parslow TG. Granulomatous slack skin: Clonal rearrangement of the T-cell receptor beta gene is evidence for the lymphoproliferative nature of a cutaneous elastolytic disorder. *J Invest Dermatol* 1987; 89: 183–186.
8. Chen M, Qui B, Kong J. Granulomatous slack skin: A case of unusual variant of mycosis fungoides. *Chin Med J (Engl)* 2000; 113: 189–192.
9. Metzler G, Schlagenhauff B, Krober SM, Kaiserling E, Schaumburg-Lever G, Lischka G. Granulomatous mycosis fungoides: Report of a case with some histopathologic features of granulomatous slack skin. *Am J Dermatopathol* 1999; 21: 156–160.
10. Noto G, Pravata G, Micceli S, Arico M. Granulomatous slack skin: Report of a case associated with Hodgkin's disease and review of the literature. *Br J Dermatol* 1994; 131: 275–279.

4
Langerhans Cell Histiocytosis

■ Synonyms:	Histiocytosis X, Langerhans cell granulomatosis, eosinophilic granuloma, Hand-Schüller-Christian disease, Letterer-Siwe disease, self-healing reticulohistiocytosis, Hashimoto-Pritzker syndrome
■ Etiology:	Unknown, a clonal or reactive expansion of Langerhans cells infiltrating various organs
■ Associations:	May coexist, precede, or follow the development of various solid tumors and hematopoietic malignancies
■ Clinical:	Polymorphous: red-brown purpuric scaly papules, lichenoid papules, purpura, vesicles, pustules, erosions, ulcers of head, neck, trunk, mucosa, sometimes prominently involving intertriginous areas; may be solitary or extensive
■ Histology:	Superficial dermal mononuclear cells with abundant eosinophilic cytoplasm, lobulated and clefted nucleus often with "coffee-bean" or reniform appearance; epidermotropism common
■ IHC:	CD 1a+, S100+, CD68+
■ Ultrastructure:	Deep nuclear cleaving, Birbeck granules (cytoplasmic linear tubular structures with inner serrations and terminal bulbous dilations, "tennis racquet-like")
■ Evaluation:	Radionuclide studies, chest radiograph, radiographs of areas of bone pain, urine specific gravity
■ Treatment:	Excision of solitary lesions, curettage of solitary bone lesions, with or without low-dose irradiation; for multifocal disease, observation or prednisone, vinblastine, or methotrexate
■ Prognosis:	Excellent for unifocal disease if no progression to multifocal disease within two years; multifocal disease is associated with limited mortality, primarily due to respiratory failure or cor pulmonale

Langerhans cell histiocytosis (LCH) refers to a collection of syndromes, characterized by infiltration of various tissues by Langerhans cells. In 1941, Farber suggested that eosinophilic granuloma, Letterer-Siwe disease, and Hand-Schüller-Christian disease all represent different manifestations of a single pathologic process, and in 1953, Lichtenstein used the term "histiocytosis X" to encompass these entities (1,2). Subsequent to the description of Birbeck granules as a specific ultrastructural marker for Langerhans cells (3), the infiltrating cells of histiocytosis X were identified as Langerhans cells. In 1987, the Writing Group of the Histiocyte Society proposed that *Langerhans cell histiocytosis* replace the term *histiocytosis X* as more appropriate (4).

Paul Langerhans first observed the cell that bears his name in the epidermis in 1868. The function of the Langerhans cell remained a mystery until recently. Langerhans cells are dendritic antigen-presenting cells that normally reside within squamous epithelium, periepithelial connective tissue, lymphatics, and in areas of lymph node.

They are important in antigen processing that occurs in the development of contact dermatitis.

Studies to date suggest that LCH is a heterogeneous disease with an unclear etiology. A clonal expansion of Langerhans cells has been demonstrated in many cases (5,6). However, an analysis of pulmonary LCH found that the majority of nodules were not clonal, suggesting that some forms of the disorder may be reactive (7). Cigarette smoking was suggested as a possible stimulus in reactive cases. Also supporting a reactive nature in some cases of LCH is the observation of a close pathological association of lesions of LCH with associated malignancies, particularly lymphomas and lung carcinomas (8). Nodular collections of LC have also been observed in close association with lymph node metastatic melanoma (9).

A possible infectious etiology of LCH has been explored. One investigation identified human herpesvirus-6 in lesional tissue (10), but another did not find any evidence of genomes for adenovirus, cytomegalovirus, Epstein-Barr virus, herpes simplex virus, human herpesvirus-6, human immunodeficiency virus, human T-cell leukemia viruses, or parvovirus (11). A familial clustering has been reported, supporting a genetic factor in the development of the disease (12). Chromosomal translocations and an increase in chromosome breaks have been reported in LCH lesions, possibly due to genetic chromosomal instability, viral infection, or chromosomal injury from toxic environmental exposures (13). There is some epidemiologic evidence linking LCH to cigarette smoking, solvent exposure, family history of benign tumors, blood transfusions, and urinary tract infections during pregnancy. Cigarette smoking, in particular, has been linked to pulmonary LCH (14). LCH has also been reported in association with malignant neoplasms (8,15,16). Approximately two-thirds occur in association with lymphomas or leukemia, and one-third, with solid tumors, most commonly lung carcinoma (8). Most cases of malignancy-associated LCH occur after the malignant diagnosis, suggesting a possible therapy-related etiology.

Cutaneous lesions of LCH have a wide range of morphologies. These include papules or plaques that may be scaly or eroded, bullae, vesicles, ulcers, petechiae or purpura (Figures 4.1 and 4.2). The lesions may be solitary, but in widespread disease tends to favor scalp and intertriginous areas, following an anatomic distribution similar to that of seborrheic dermatitis, which it may resemble. Solitary or multiple lesions of the external genitalia may also occur. Because patterns of cutaneous LCH do not appear to be predictive of underlying disease, diagnostic studies should be undertaken in all cases, even if there is limited cutaneous involvement (see evaluation listing below).

Biopsy specimens of LCH contain an infiltrate of Langerhans cells (LC), usually within the papillary and superficial reticular dermis, sometimes in greater density around adnexal structures (17), often demonstrating varying degrees of epitheliotropism (Figure 4.3A and 4.3B). The individual cells are 10–12 μm, with eosinophilic cytoplasm and convoluted, sometimes reniform nuclei. Small nucleoli may be apparent. Mitotic figures are uncommon. By contrast, foci of necrosis are common, and

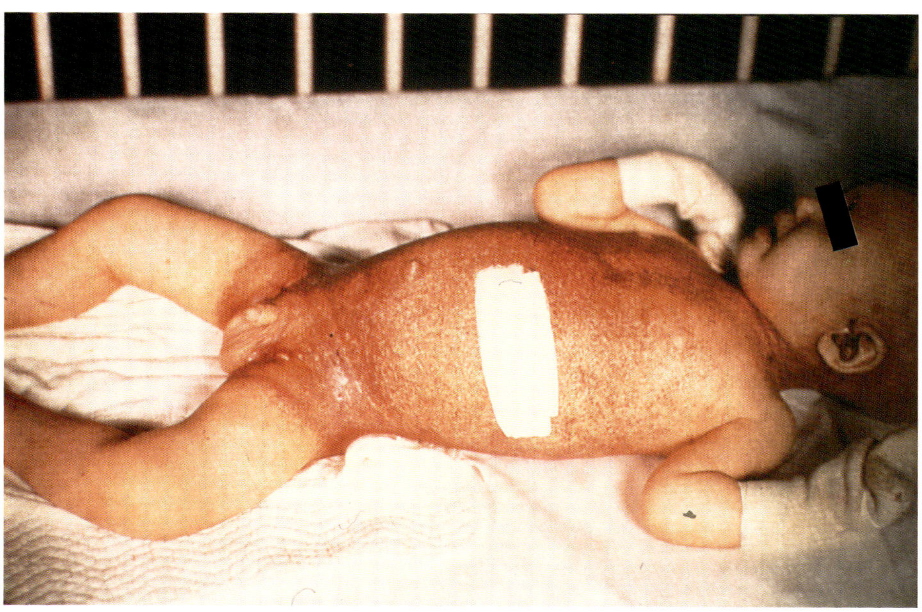

FIGURE 4.1. Coalescing red-brown papules with flexural accentuation.

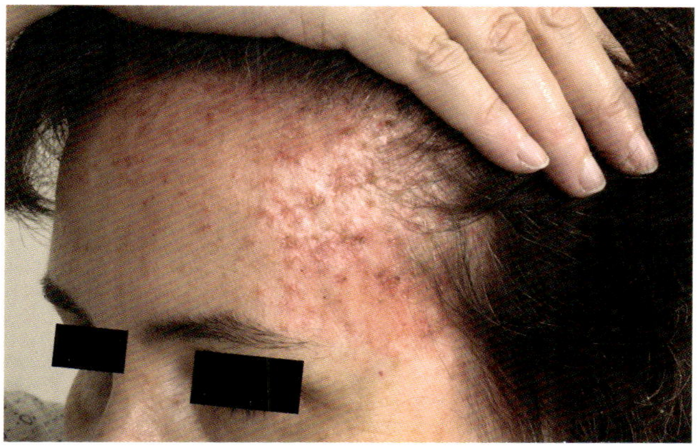

FIGURE 4.2. Red-violaceous scaly papules with hemorrhagic crust.

correlate with the frequent clinical scenario of erosion and sometimes ulceration. LC are frequently admixed with eosinophils. Multinucleated cells and lipidized macrophages are seen in some lesions, but there is no evidence that these are LC (15,18). Given overlapping morphology with other cells, additional confirmatory studies should be undertaken. These include immunohistochemical staining with antibodies to CD1a, displaying a membranous pattern (18). LC are also labeled by antibodies to S100 and peanut agglutinin, but not by histiocytic markers such as muramidase or HAM56 (15). Prior to the development of antibodies to CD1a, a specific diagnosis of LC required ultrastructural identification of Birbeck granules. Birbeck granules are linear cytoplasmic granules with interior serrations and occasional bulbous "tennis racquet-like" terminal dilations that are thought to arise from cell membrane and may show membrane connections. Their formation is known to be induced by a C-type lectin cell surface receptor, langerin. Langerin (CD207) is a more specific marker of LC than is CD1a and may eventually supplant its use as a diagnostic tool (19). The role of langerin and Birbeck granules is unknown, but they do not appear to be necessary for principal LC functions (20).

Mucocutaneous involvement in LCH should be taken in the context of involvement of other organ systems. Combining the two largest single center series, 67% of LCH cases involve a single organ system, bone being by far the most frequent (15,16). When looking at both single-system and multisystem disease, bone involvement occurs in 70%, followed by pulmonary in 18%, and mucocutaneous involvement in 16%. Of those with mucocutaneous involvement, approximately one fifth have disease limited to the skin (15). Evaluation of data from the French Langerhans' Cell Histiocytosis Study Group, a pediatric population, and the adult cases from the International Registry of the Histiocyte Society, suggests a greater incidence of pulmonary disease in adults (58%, versus 9% in the pediatric population) (21,22).

Having made a diagnosis of cutaneous Langerhans cell histiocytosis, it is important to perform an additional diagnostic evaluation for multisystem disease, since most cutaneous presentations are accompanied by other organ system involvement. Appropriate evaluation is directed by clinical symptoms and signs. General guidelines are suggested:

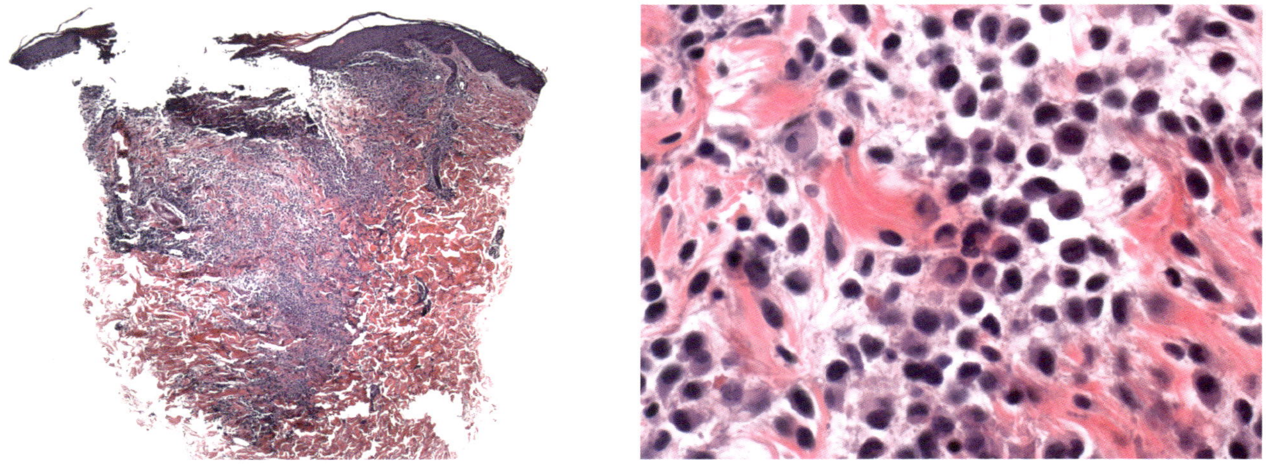

A B

FIGURE 4.3. (A and B) Ulcerated papule with wedge-shaped and epitheliotropic infiltrate of Langerhans cells with amphophilic cytoplasm and eccentric reniform nuclei.

Evaluation of the Patient Presenting with Cutaneous Langerhans Cell Histiocytosis

1. Thorough physical examination with attention to lymph nodes, liver, spleen
2. Bone scan with radiographs of symptomatic areas
3. Chest radiograph
4. Random urine specific gravity and serum uric acid as screen for diabetes insipidus; vasopressin challenge test to confirm if screen suggests
5. Complete blood count with differential, platelets
6. Liver enzyme tests if hepatomegaly is present

Should no evidence of multifocal disease be present, close clinical follow-up in the first two years is advised since additional foci of disease are most likely to become apparent in that time period (15).

Prognosis in LCH is generally favorable. Large series have shown low mortality directly due to disease, the most frequent cause being respiratory failure associated with pulmonary disease (15,16). There may be considerable morbidity and mortality associated with treatment (15). Deaths due to overwhelming LCH are exceptional. Long-term complications from the disease include pituitary dysfunction or diabetes insipidus, each occurring in approximately 25% of patients, and a neurodegenerative syndrome occurring in approximately 10% of patients with long-term follow-up (23).

Treatment for LCH is determined by extent and type of organ system involvement. Isolated bone lesions are best treated with curettage. If the lesions are in critical weight-bearing bones, low-dose irradiation may be added. Systemic treatment most commonly consists of prednisone, followed by vinblastine, or methotrexate. It has been emphasized that doses associated with bone marrow depression or other toxicities are not generally required for a good therapeutic response (15). 2-deoxychloro-adenosine administration has also produced favorable outcomes (24). Hematopoietic stem cell transplantation has been used in some cases of severe refractory LCH with complete remission, but death may occur from therapy (25).

Cutaneous LCH has been treated effectively with topical nitrogen mustard (26). Additional therapeutic modalities for cutaneous and mucosal disease have included topical steroids (15), PUVA (27), thalidomide (28), and α-interferon (29). Should disease resolution occur, clinical follow-up is advised because of potential for long-term complications, recurrence of disease, or the development of associated malignancy.

References

1. Farber S. The nature of "solitary or eosinophilic granuloma" of bone. *Am J Pathol* 1941; 17: 625–629.
2. Lichtenstein L. Histiocytosis X, integration of eosinophilic granuloma of bone, Letterer-Siwe disease and Schuller-Christian disease as related manifestations of a single nosologic entity. *Arch Pathol* 1953; 56: 84–102.
3. Birbeck MS, Breathnach AS, Everall JD. An electron microscopic study of basal melanocytes and high-level clear cells (Langerhans cells) in vitiligo. *J Invest Dermatol* 1961; 31: 51–64.
4. Writing Group of the Histiocyte Society. Histiocytosis syndromes in children. *Lancet* 1987; 1: 208–209.
5. Willman CL, Busque L, Griffith BB, et al. Langerhans'-cell histiocytosis (histiocytosis X): A clonal proliferative disease. *N Eng J Med* 1994; 331: 154–160.
6. Yu RC, Chu C, Buluwela L, Chu AC. Clonal proliferation of Langerhans cells in Langerhans cell histiocytosis. *Lancet* 1994; 343: 767–768.
7. Yousem SA, Colby TV, Chen YY, et al. Pulmonary Langerhans' cell histiocytosis: molecular analysis of clonality. *Am J Surg Pathol* 2001; 25: 630–636.
8. Egeler RM, Neglia JP, Puccetti DM, Brennan CA, Nesbit ME. Association of Langerhans cell histiocytosis with malignant neoplasms. *Cancer* 1993; 71: 865–873.
9. Richmond I, Eyden BP, Banerjee SS. Intranodal Langerhans' cell histiocytosis associated with malignant melanoma. *Histopathol* 1995; 26: 380–382.
10. Leahy MA, Krejci SM, Friednash M, et al. Human herpes virus 6 is present in lesions of Langerhans cell histiocytosis. *J Invest Dermatol* 1993; 101: 642–645.
11. McClain K, Jin H, Gresik V, Favara B. Langerhans cell histiocytosis: Lack of viral etiology. *Am J Hematol* 1994; 47: 16–20.
12. Arico M, Nichols K, Whitlock JA, et al. Familial clustering of Langerhans cell histiocytosis. *Br J Hematol* 1999; 107: 883–888.
13. Betts DR, Leibundgut KE, Feldges A, et al. Cytogenetic abnormalities in Langerhans cell histiocytosis. *Br J Cancer* 1998; 77: 552–555.
14. Hamre M, Hedberg J, Buckley J, et al. Langerhans cell histiocytosis: An exploratory epidemiologic study of 177 cases. *Med Pediatr Oncol* 1997; 28: 92–97.
15. Lieberman PH, Jones CR, Steinman RM, et al. Langerhans cell (eosinophilic) granulomatosis. *Am J Surg Pathol* 1996; 20: 519–552.
16. Howarth DM, Gilchrist GS, Mullan B, Wiseman GA, Edmonson JH, Schomberg PJ. Langerhans cell histiocytosis: Diagnosis, natural history, management, and outcome. *Cancer* 1999; 85: 2278–2290.
17. Helm KF, Lookingbill DP, Marks JG. A clinical and pathologic study of histiocytosis X in adults. *J Am Acad Dermatol* 1993; 29:166–170.
18. Emile JF, Wechsler J, Brousse N, et al. Langerhans' cell histiocytosis: Definitive diagnosis with the use of monoclonal antibody O10 on routinely paraffin-embedded samples. *Am J Surg Pathol* 1995; 19: 636–641.
19. Geissmann F, Lepelletier Y, Fraitag S, et al. Differentiation of Langerhans cells in Langerhans cell histiocytosis. *Blood* 2001; 97: 1241–1248.
20. Kissenpfennig A, Ait-Yahia S, Clair-Moninot V, et al. Disruption of the langerin/CD207 gene abolishes Birbeck

granules without a marked loss of Langerhans cell function. *Mol Cell Biol* 2005; 25: 88–99.
21. The French Langerhans' Cell Histiocytosis Study Group. A multicentre retrospective survey of Langerhans' cell histiocytosis: 348 cases observed between 1983 and 1993. *Arch Dis Child* 1996; 75: 17–24.
22. Arico M, Girschikofsky M, Genereau T, et al. Langerhans cell histiocytosis in adults: Report from the International Registry of the Histiocyte Society. *Eur J Cancer* 2003; 39: 2341–2348.
23. Donadieu J, Rolon MA, Thomas C, et al. Endocrine involvement in pediatric-onset Langerhans' cell histiocytosis: A population-based study. *J Pediatr* 2004; 144: 344–350.
24. Pardanani A, Phyliky RL, Li CY, Tefferi A. 2-Chlorodeoxyadenosine therapy for disseminated Langerhans cell histiocytosis. *Mayo Clin Proc* 2003; 78: 301–306.
25. Akkari V, Donadieu J, Piguet C, et al. Hematopoietic stem cell transplantation in patients with severe Langerhans cell histiocytosis and hematological dysfunction: Experience of the French Langerhans Cell Study Group. *Bone Marrow Transplant* 2003; 31: 1097–1103.
26. Sheehan MP, Atherton DJ, Broadbent V, et al. Topical nitrogen mustard: an effective treatment for cutaneous Langerhans' cell histiocytosis. *J Pediatr* 1991; 119: 317–321.
27. Iwatsuki K, Tsugiki M, Yoshizawa N, Tagikawa M, Yamada M, Shamoto M. The Effect of phototherapies on cutaneous lesions of Histiocytosis X in the elderly. *Cancer* 1986; 57: 1931–1936.
28. Thomas L, Ducros B, Secchi T, et al. Successful treatment of adult's Langerhans cell histiocytosis with thalidomide. *Arch Dermatol* 1993; 129: 1261–1264.
29. Kwong YL, Chan ACL, Chan TK. Widespread skin-limited Langerhans cell histiocytosis: Complete remission with interferon α. *J Am Acad Dermatol* 1997; 36: 628–629.

5 Leukemia Cutis

▪ Synonyms:	Cutaneous leukemia, extramedullary myeloid tumor
▪ Etiology:	Unknown
▪ Associations:	Systemic leukemia
▪ Clinical:	Erythematous patches, papules, nodules, hemorrhagic and purpuric lesions, blue-green nodules
▪ Histology:	Malignant immature hematopoietic precursor cells in dermis, diffusely or in patchy distribution
▪ IHC repertoire:	Lymphocyte surface markers and/or markers of specific granules rarely necessary
▪ Staging:	Systemic work-up required
▪ Prognosis:	Poor, except for CLL
▪ Adverse variables:	Histologic subtype of high-grade leukemias
▪ Treatment:	No local therapy; systemic chemotherapy

Leukemia cutis is an uncommon cutaneous eruption that may be difficult to diagnose. In the vast majority of patients, there is a known history of leukemia at the time of the skin manifestations. However, leukemia may have its initial manifestation in the skin, in some cases with simultaneous bone marrow involvement, or less commonly, in the absence of simultaneous marrow involvement. (In these cases, the cutaneous eruptions have been called extramedullary myeloid tumors (1)). In one series, approximately 38% of patients had cutaneous findings at the time of bone marrow diagnosis (2). In other series, anywhere from 3% to 7% of patients had cutaneous lesions prior to detection of marrow involvement (3). Patients with all types of leukemia may demonstrate cutaneous lesions. It has been reported in 2% to 3% of patients with acute myelogenous leukemia (4). Cutaneous involvement is less common in patients with acute lymphoblastic leukemia (5). Chronic myelogenous leukemia patients have skin manifestations in 6% to 20% of cases (6). The incidence ranges from 4% to 20% in patients with chronic lymphocytic leukemia (7).

The clinical manifestations of leukemia cutis are protean. In some cases, the disparate clinical appearances correlate with the subtypes of leukemia involved and the systemic complications caused by these types of leukemia. For instance, hemorrhagic lesions are commonly found in the subtypes of leukemia that are associated with coagulopathies (such as acute promyelocytic leukemia), but are rarely seen in patients with chronic lymphocytic leukemia. Tumor nodules may occur in patients with any subtype of leukemia, but are most commonly seen in those with chronic myelogenous leukemia (Figure 5.1). In other patients, diffuse erythematous papules and nodules correlate with diffuse infiltrates of neoplastic cells throughout the dermis. The etiology for bullae that have been reported in rare patients is less well understood. Some types of leukemia have more specific findings, such as gingival hyperplasia associated with acute myelomonocytic leukemia.

The histologic findings in leukemia cutis are varied. In most cases, there is a diffuse infiltrate of atypical hematopoietic cells throughout the dermis (Figure 5.2).

In some cases, the neoplastic cells appear in such density as to form dermal tumor nodules. More commonly, however, the cells are dispersed individually throughout the dermis. The cells show little tendency for cohesion and percolate between splayed collagen bundles. In some cases, there is a predilection for aggregates of leukemic cells surrounding the peri-eccrine vascular spaces (8).

The cytologic features of the infiltrating cells vary with the type of leukemia. In acute myeloid leukemias, large, immature precursor cells are present (Figure 5.3).

These cells are readily identified with routine sections in most cases. In some cases, a chloroacetate esterase stain or the use of an anti-myeloperoxidase antibody may be helpful in identifying characteristic cytoplasmic granules.

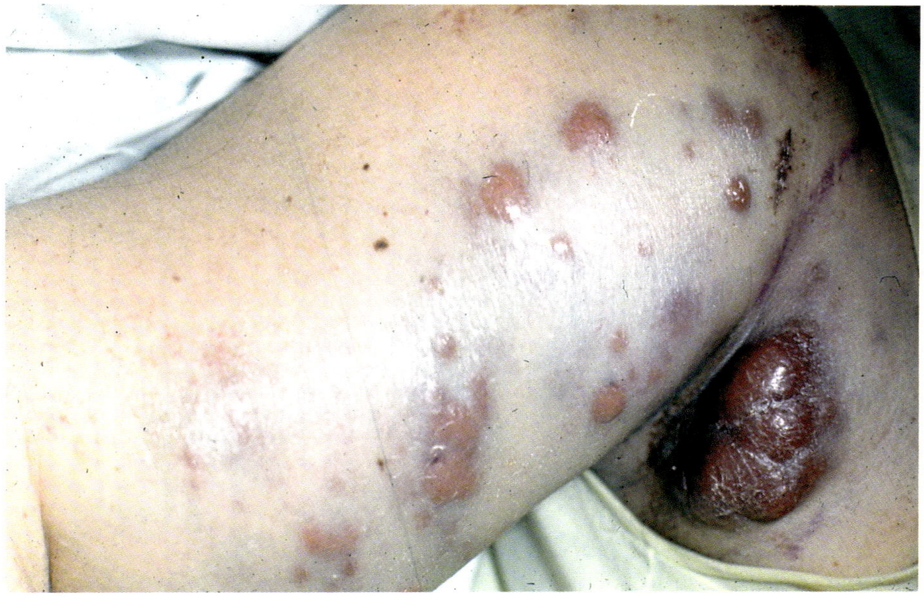

FIGURE 5.1. Widely scattered violaceous nodules of leukemia cutis.

Similarly, the chronic myeloid leukemias feature immature myeloid forms coursing throughout the dermis. In these types of leukemia, abundant mitoses and individual cell necrosis are common features. This subtype of leukemia is usually straightforward to recognize in the skin.

The lymphoid leukemias are more difficult to recognize as involving the skin. In acute lymphoblastic leukemia (ALL), large and atypical immature cells are present throughout the dermis. Abundant mitotic activity and individual cell necrosis are commonly seen. These cells are very difficult to classify based upon routine sections or special stains; however, correlation with cytometric studies is helpful, and in most cases, the patient's prior history makes the diagnosis straightforward. Chronic lymphocytic leukemia (CLL) may also occur in the skin, both in patients with long-standing disease, and as an initial manifestation. In these cases, a *de novo* diagnosis is difficult to make. The histologic findings include only a monomorphous population of relatively small and unremarkable lymphocytes within the dermis. The key observation is that the usual heterogeneity of cell type is absent, as is the usual variation in lymphocyte size and shape. Clonality can be ascertained in most cases, if the diagnosis is entertained based upon routine sectioning. Some investigators have noted a tendency for the neoplastic lymphocytes in CLL to comprise the immune response underlying primary keratinocytic neoplasms or infectious processes (9,10). This may be the first clue to the diagnosis in some patients.

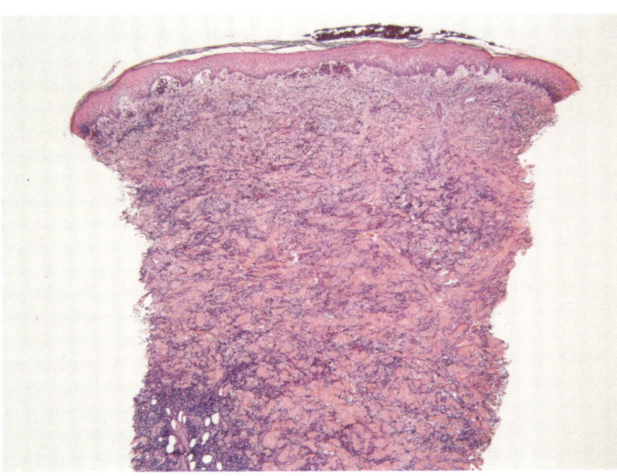

FIGURE 5.2. Low power photomicrograph of dense dermal infiltrate in leukemia cutis. Note the Grenz zone typical of this condition.

The prognosis for patients with cutaneous involvement by leukemia is generally poor. It suggests widely disseminated disease in most cases. However, for patients with CLL, there is no evidence that the presence of neoplastic lymphocytes within the dermis serves as any type of adverse marker and long-term survival has been seen in these patients.

There is no specific treatment for the cutaneous leukemia other than palliation and symptomatic relief. Aggres-

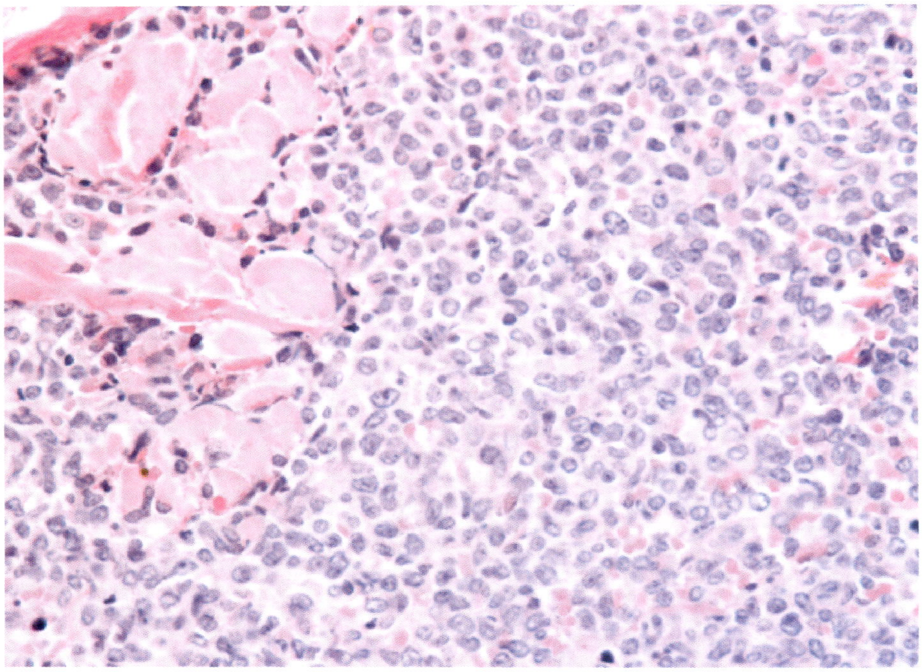

Figure 5.3. High power detail of neoplastic infiltrate. Note the large atypical cells with vesicular nuclei and surrounding myeloid precursors with eosinophilic cytoplasm.

sive and appropriate treatment of the bone marrow–derived process is the appropriate regimen. Even in patients with no evidence of leukemia on bone marrow biopsy, close clinical follow-up is essential and treatment is indicated in some patients.

References

1. Traweek ST, Arber DA, Rappaport H, Brynes RK. Extramedullary myeloid cell tumors: An immunohistochemical and morphologic study of 28 cases. *Am J Surg Pathol* 1993; 17: 1011–1019.
2. Su WPD, Buechner SA, Li C-Y. Clinicopathologic correlations in leukemia cutis. *J Am Acad Dermatol* 1984; 11: 121–128.
3. Stawiski MA. Skin manifestations of leukemias and lymphomas. *Cutis* 1978; 21: 814–818.
4. Baer MR, Barcos M, Farrell H, Raza A, Preisler HD. Acute myelogenous leukemia with leukemia cutis: Eighteen cases seen between 1969 and 1986. *Cancer* 1989; 2192–2200.
5. Forjaz de Lacerda J, do Carmo A, Guerra L, Soares de Almeida L, Fernandes A, Forjaz de Lacera JM. Leukemia cutis in acute lymphoblastic leukemia. *J Am Acad Dermatol* 1994; 30: 1041–1043.
6. Long JC, Mihm MC. Multiple granulocytic tumors of the skin: Report of six cases of myelogenous leukemia with initial manifestations in the skin. *Cancer* 1977; 39: 2004–2016.
7. Kaiserling E, Horny H-P, Geerts M-L, Schmid U. Skin involvement in myelogenous leukemia: Morphologic and immunophenotypic heterogeneity of skin infiltrates. *Mod Pathol* 1994; 7: 771–779.
8. Longacre TA, Smoller BR. Leukemia cutis: Analysis of 50 biopsy-proven cases with an emphasis on occurrence in myelodysplastic syndrome. *Am J Clin Pathol* 1993; 100: 276–284.
9. Cerroni L, Zenahlik P, Kerl H. Specific cutaneous infiltrates of B-cell chronic lymphocytic leukemia arising at the site of herpes zoster and herpes simplex scars. *Cancer* 1995; 76: 26–31.
10. Smoller BR, Warnke RA. Cutaneous infiltrate of chronic lymphocytic leukemia and relationship to primary cutaneous epithelial neoplasms. *J Cutan Pathol* 1998; 25: 160–164.

6
Mast Cell Disease (Urticaria Pigmentosa)

■ Synonyms:	Urticaria pigmentosa, telangiectasia macularis eruptive perstans, mastocytoma, mastocytosis
■ Etiology:	Unknown
■ Associations:	Nausea, vomiting, diarrhea, syncope, mast cell leukemia, other hematologic malignancies
■ Clinical:	Papules or nodules with or without associated hyperpigmentation and telangiectasia; positive Darier's sign
■ Histology:	Increased dermal mast cells perivascular or as tumor nodules, basilar hyperpigmentation, vascular ectasia
■ IHC repertoire:	CD117 (c-kit) and mast cell tryptase positive
■ Staging:	Bone marrow involvement conveys poor prognosis
■ Prognosis:	Varies with subtype of disease; benign in children
■ Adverse variables:	Bone marrow involvement
■ Treatment:	Chemotherapy including interferon alfa if bone marrow involvement; topical steroids; close clinical follow-up in patients with adult-onset disease

Cutaneous mast cell disease has several different manifestations. It can present during the neonatal period or throughout life. Different age populations generally develop different clinical manifestations and different associated conditions. It is the systemic form of mastocytosis in adults that has the most potentially severe complications. It has been estimated that from 15% to 50% of patients with adult-onset mast cell disease will have systemic involvement (1,2). However, for the sake of completeness, the other variants of this disease spectrum will also be considered. Urticaria pigmentosa is the global term for all conditions that are characterized by increased numbers of mast cells within the dermis. There is no gender predilection.

Mast cell disease in childhood is only rarely associated with systemic disease (less than 2% of the time in one series). About one-third of all patients with mast cell disease are less than 15 years old (3). The disease resolves spontaneously in two to three years in the vast majority of these patients, by adolescence in virtually all. Children with mast cell disease often have single or a few large, nodular lesions called mastocytomas (Figure 6.1). These most commonly appear within the first three years of life. These lesions urticate easily with stroking (Darier's sign). Bullous lesions may be present due to extensive papillary dermal edema secondary to histamine release from mast cells. Vesicles do not generally occur as part of cutaneous mast cell disease in patients older than 10 years of age. Rarely, children with diffuse mast cell disease may present with erythroderma (Figure 6.2). Despite the absence of systemic disease, these children are at risk for hypotension, shock, and even death.

Adults with mast cell disease are more likely to present with a widely scattered macular eruption. Individual lesions are often red-brown or hyperpigmented. The lesions are randomly distributed and generalized, but are accentuated on the chest. Petechiae and ecchymoses may occur. Depending upon the mast cell burden within each lesion, an urticarial reaction can be elicited by gently stroking these lesions. Pruritus is the most common symptom. Less commonly, nausea, vomiting, diarrhea, and abdominal pain may be reported. These symptoms occur in patients with limited cutaneous disease as frequently as those with systemic involvement. One type of adult-onset form of the disease is known as telangiectasia macularis eruptive perstans (TMEP). In this variant, abundant hyperpigmented 2–6-mm macules are present on the back and chest in concert with telangiectasias. Pru-

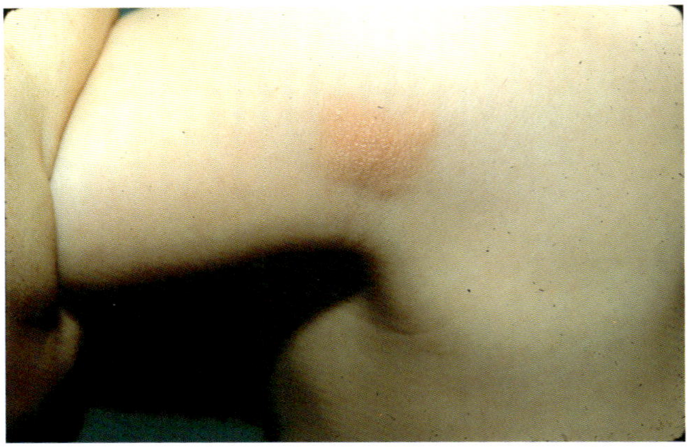

FIGURE 6.1. Erythematous/tan plaque of mastocytosis in a child.

ritis and urtication are not common. It is currently not possible to distinguish adult patients with disease limited to the skin from those with systemic disease based purely on the cutaneous disease. There is no difference in the age of presentation between those with and without systemic involvement. The mean age of presentation is in the fourth decade. Systemic disease presents much later, often with as much as 20 years separating these findings from the initial cutaneous presentation (3). Patients with systemic disease may remain alive with persistent disease for many years, or may succumb to their illness.

In adults with cutaneous mast cell disease, hepatosplenomegaly is often seen in addition to the macular, hyperpigmented eruption. Lymph node involvement is not uncommon. Osteoblastic lesions can be detected with radiographs. The bone marrow is the most frequently involved extracutaneous site. Eosinophilia is present in 15% of all patients with systemic disease. In these patients, pancytopenia may be present and a bone marrow biopsy and aspiration is necessary to eliminate the presence of mastocytosis or leukemia (mast cell leukemia or chronic myelogenous leukemia). Leukemia is reported to develop in 4%–5% of patients with systemic mastocytosis (4). Involvement of the gastrointestinal tract has been reported but is very uncommon. Increased serum tryptase and increased urinary levels of *t*-methyl histamine may also be detected in these patients (5).

The histologic findings in child-onset mast cell disease include a very dense dermal infiltrate of mast cells, often filling the entire dermis and extending into the subcutaneous fat. In some cases, prominent papillary dermal edema leads to a subepidermal bulla, correlating with the blisters encountered clinically.

The histologic findings in adult-onset mast cell disease fall into two general categories. Mast cells may be distributed in a perivascular pattern or diffusely (Figure 6.3A and 6.3B).

Neither pattern is predictive of systemic involvement, though the superficial perivascular pattern is more common (3). The number of perivascular mast cells varies widely, but in most cases is relatively slight, with only a minimal increase in cellularity over physiologic levels.

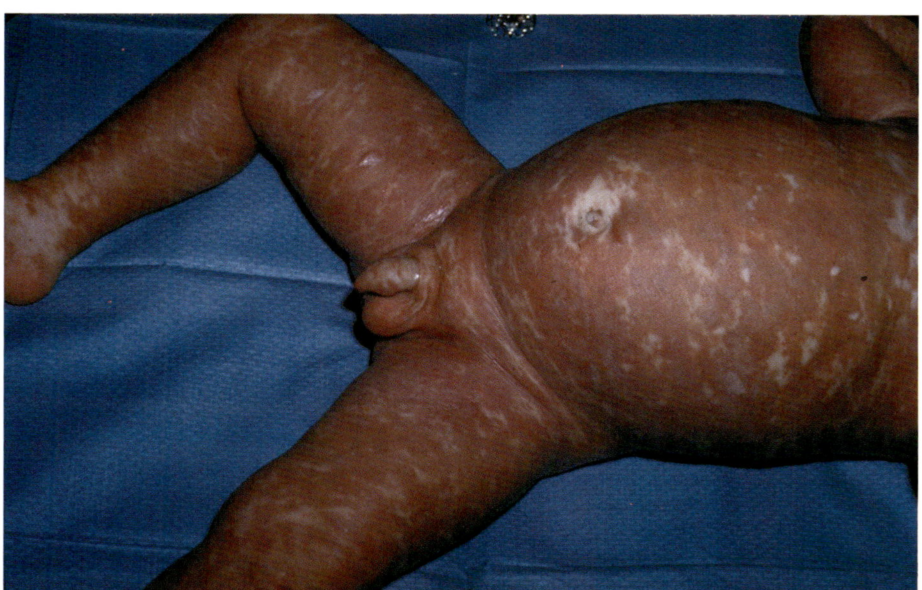

FIGURE 6.2. Erythroderma with islands of sparring and hepatosplenomegaly associated with parenchymal organ infiltration in systemic mastocytosis.

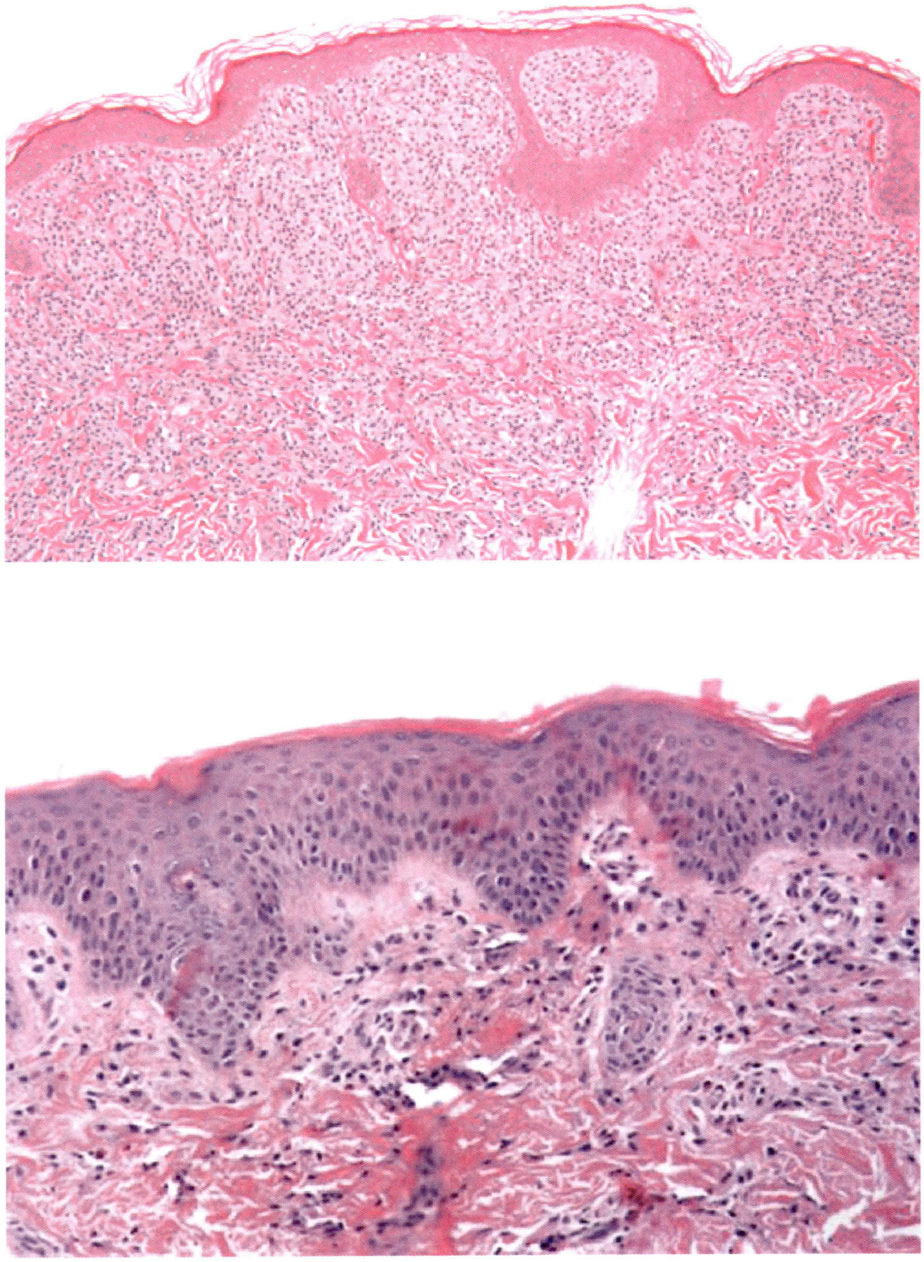

A

B

FIGURE 6.3. (A) Low power photomicrograph depicting superficial dermal infiltrate of mastocytosis. (B) Low power photomicrograph depicting superficial dermal infiltrate of mastocytosis in adult T.M.E.P.

Morphometric point counting has suggested that while the absolute numbers may be small, there is a nine-to-160-fold increase in numbers of mast cells in these cases compared with normal patients (6). Dense diffuse infiltrates within the papillary dermis are encountered less commonly (Figure 6.4).

In these cases, prominent nuclear atypia and presence of nucleoli and multinucleation may be present; however, these findings do not associate invariably with systemic involvement. Mitotic activity is rare in all cases of mast cell disease (Figure 6.5).

In one study, electron microscopy suggested that mast cells from patients with systemic disease are larger, and have more cytoplasm and larger cytoplasmic granules (7). In biopsies from both patterns, an admixture of lymphocytes and eosinophils are present within

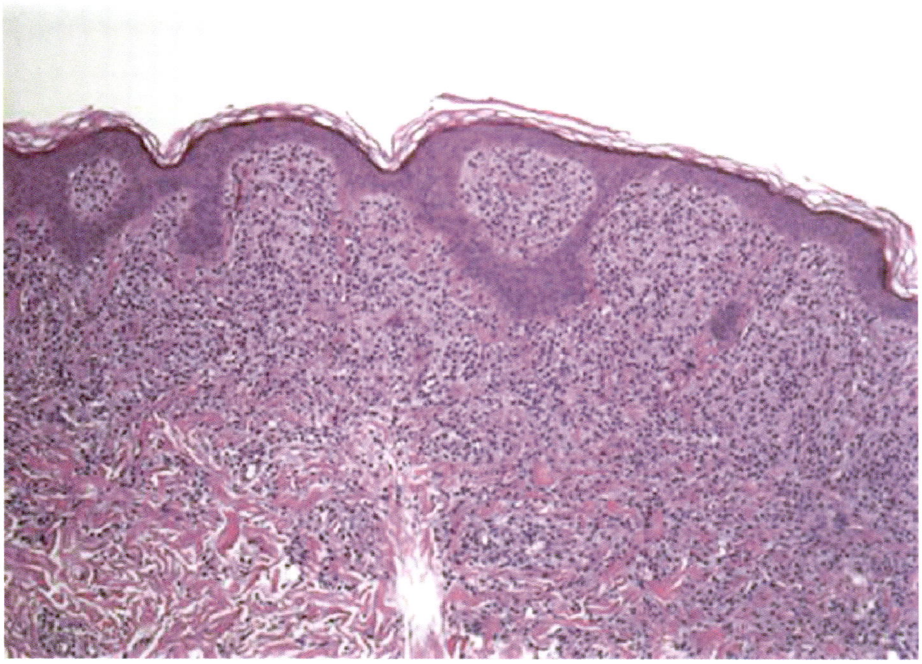

FIGURE 6.4. Medium power photomicrograph depicting uniform population of epithelioid cells within the superficial dermis.

the dermis. In more subtle cases, mast cell numbers can be better assessed with special stains such as toluidine blue or Giemsa's stains, or more specifically, staining with CD117 (c-kit) or mast cell tryptase (Figure 6.6).

Bone marrow involvement with mast cell disease may be very focal and a negative biopsy does not guarantee limited cutaneous disease (3). Conversely, skin involvement is not present in all cases of systemic mast cell disease (8,9).

Treatment options vary with the extent of disease. Cutaneous lesions can be watched or treated with topical steroids or even surgical excision of limited lesions. More extensive disease requires topical steroids, antihistamines, chemotherapy, interferon, and ultraviolet light therapy. None of these options are entirely effective.

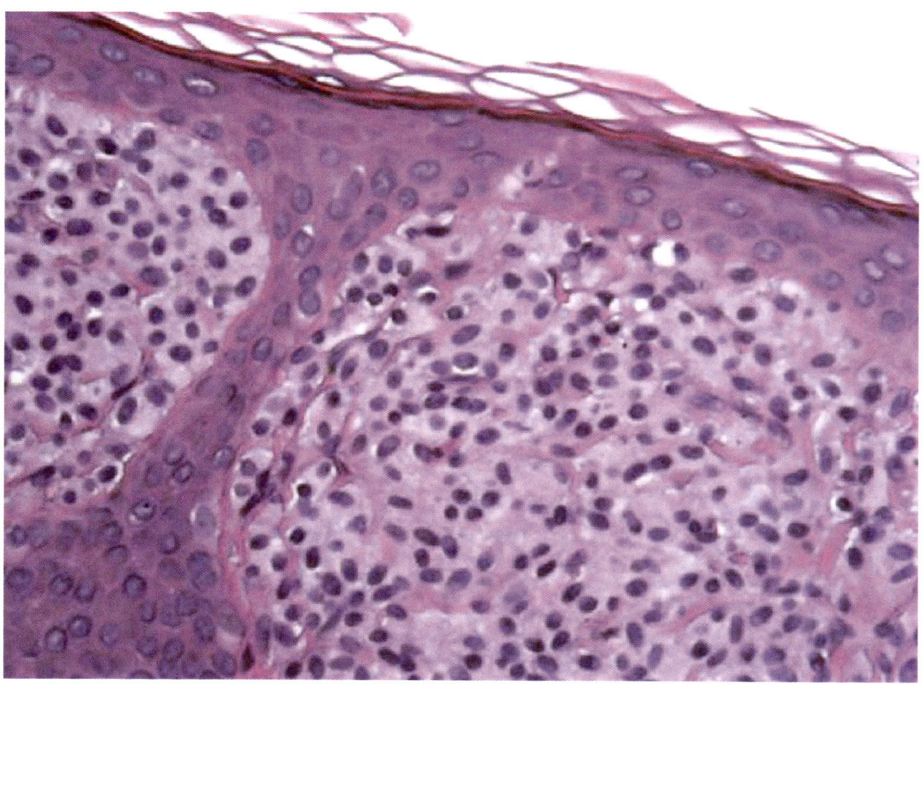

FIGURE 6.5. High power photomicrograph depicting uniform population of rounded cells possessing oval nuclei with amphophilic staining cytoplasm.

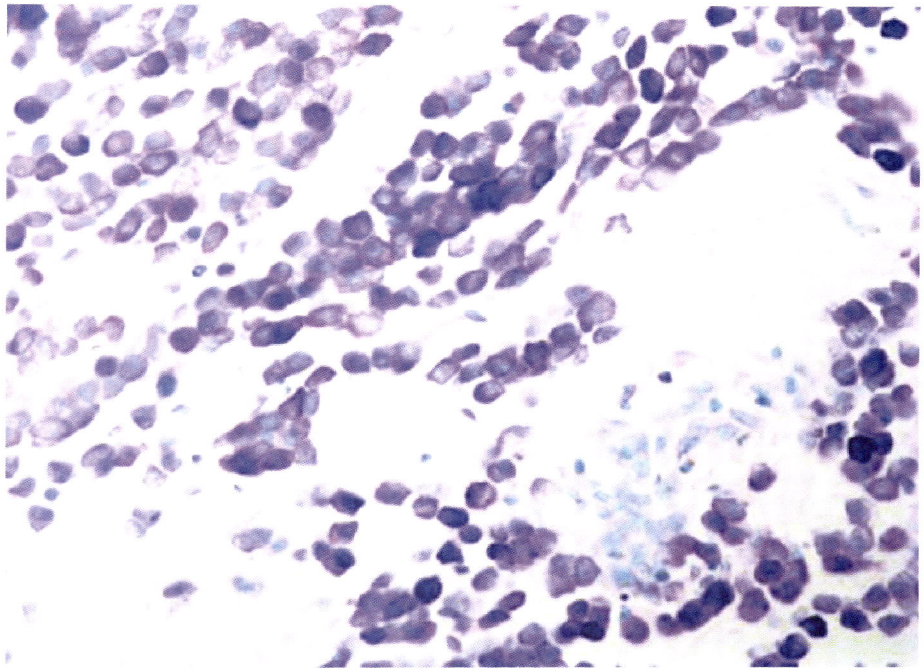

FIGURE 6.6. Giesma stains reveal metachromatic staining of cytoplasmic granules within mast cells.

References

1. Caplan RM. The natural course of urticaria pigmentosa. *Arch Dermatol* 1983; 87: 146–157.
2. Ridell B, Olafsson JH, Roupe G, Swolin B, Granerus G, Rodjer S, Enerback L. The bone marrow in urticaria pigmentosas and systemic mastocytosis. *Arch Dermatol* 1986; 122: 422–427.
3. Travis WD, Li C-Y, Su WPD. Adult-onset urticaria pigmentosa and systemic mast cell disease. *Am J Clin Pathol* 1985; 84: 710–714.
4. DiBacco RS, DeLeo VA. Mastocytosis and the mast cell. *J Am Acad Dermatol* 1982; 7: 709–722.
5. Asmis LM, Cirardet C. Systemic mast-cell disease (mastocytosis): Letter to the editor. *N Eng J Med* 2002; 346: 174.
6. Kaspar CS, Freeman RG, Tharp MD. Diagnosis of mastocytosis subsets using a morphometric point counting technique. *Arch Dermatol* 1987; 123: 1017–1021.
7. Soter NA. The skin in mastocytosis. *J Invest Dermatol* 1991; 96: 32S–39S.
8. Mutter RD, Tannenbaum M, Ultmann JE. Systemic mast cell disease. *Ann Int Med*. 1963: 59: 887–906.
9. Roberts LJ II, Fields JP, Oates JA. Mastocytosis without urticaria pigmentosa: A frequently unrecognized cause of recurrent syncope. *Trans Assoc Am Physicians* 1982; 85: 36–41.

7
Merkel Cell Carcinoma

■ Synonyms:	Trabecular carcinoma of skin, primary small cell carcinoma of skin, cutaneous APUDoma
■ Etiology:	Ultraviolet light, chromosome 1 abnormalities, p53, bcl-2, c-kit receptor
■ Associations:	Aging, immunosuppression, other cutaneous and visceral malignancies
■ Clinical:	Painless, solitary rapidly growing nodule on exposed cutaneous site
■ Histology:	Diffuse or aggregated dermal nests of small blue cells, numerous mitoses
■ IHC repertoire:	CK-20(+), synaptophysin (+), S-100 (+/−), Melan-A (−), CK-7 (−), CD-45 (−)
■ Staging:	I = localized disease, II = I and regional node(s) (+), III = extranodal metastases
■ Prognosis:	Overall 5-year ~60% survival
■ Adverse variables:	Male, head location, mitoses >10/HPF, vascular permeation, (+) lymph nodes
■ Treatment:	I = WLE/XRT, II = WLE/XRT/ELND, III = XRT/?CTX/ ?ABMT/limb perf HPF = high power fields, WLE = wide local excision, XRT = X-ray radiotherapy, CTX = chemotherapy, ABMT = autologous bone marrow transplantation

Merkel cell carcinoma, as first described by Toker, et al. (1) in 1972, and otherwise known as trabecular carcinoma of the skin, neuroendocrine carcinoma of the skin, cutaneous APUDoma, primary small cell carcinoma of the skin with endocrine differentiation, is an uncommon, aggressive cutaneous neoplasm. Friederich Merkel first discovered the Merkel cell in 1875. It is a large, clear, usually round or oval cell found in the basal layer of the epidermis. It is found in close association with terminal axons, and is joined to keratinocytes. They are found in highest concentrations in acral skin, namely the fingertips and nasal tip, as well as glabrous skin, hairy skin, and mucous membranes. The exact function of Merkel cells is unclear, but it is generally thought that they are a form of touch receptor (2–4). The origin of Merkel cell carcinoma is controversial as well. It may arise from epidermal Merkel cells, dermal neuroendocrine cells, or poorly differentiated epidermal stem cells.

The etiology of this tumor is unknown, although it is likely that a number of different factors play a role in its development. Merkel cell carcinoma is located primarily on the head and neck, areas that commonly receive actinic damage. Hence, it is thought that UV radiation may play a role in the development of these tumors. However, there have been many reports of tumors arising in non-sun-exposed regions as well, and thus other factors must play a role. Changes in chromosome 1 have been frequently identified in MCC, thus lending to the hypothesis that there may be a genetic predisposition in certain individuals to develop this tumor (5). More recent data have examined the role of bcl-2 and p53 genes in Merkel cell carcinoma. P53 and bcl-2 expression in MCC is variable, and either loss of function or excess function of either bcl-2 and/or p53 may promote tumor development (6). In one study by Su, et al., CD117 (KIT receptor) was found to be expressed in 95% of tumors (7). Merkel cell carci-

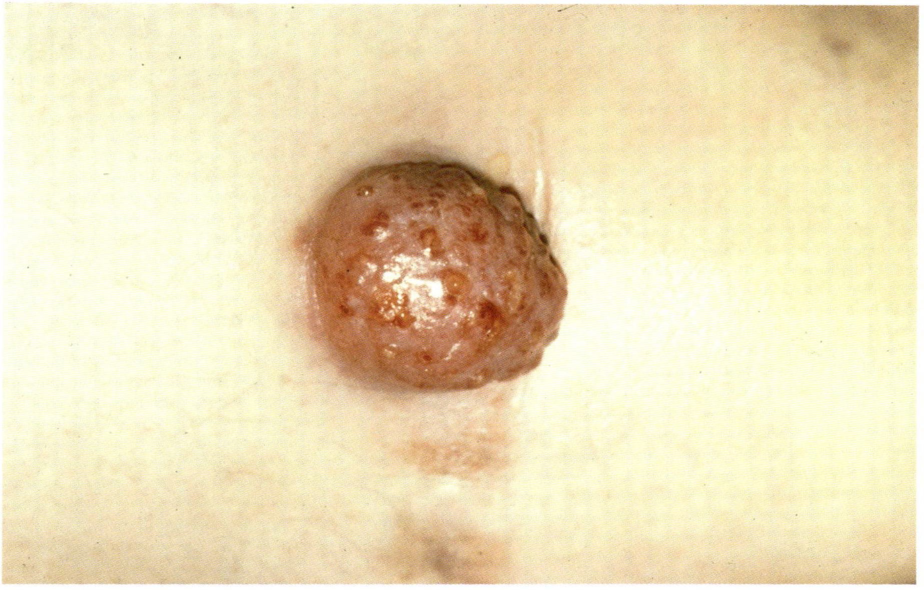

FIGURE 7.1. Erythematous glistening papule of merkel cell carcinoma.

noma is a very rare neuroendocrine cutaneous neoplasm, and as of the year 2000, approximately 1100 cases have been reported in the literature since first noted by Toker in 1972 (4). Herbst, et al. reported that approximately 400 new cases are diagnosed in the United States each year. It is most common in elderly individuals, primarily on the head and neck (44%–50%, 20% of which arise in the periocular region), followed by the extremities (40%–44%), the trunk (8%), and the buttocks (9%) (1–4). This tumor occurs primarily in Caucasians, with a few case reports in African Americans and Polynesians. Most patients are in their 60 s and 70 s at the time of diagnosis, with the average age being 65, but the literature cites cases documented on patients as young as 7 years of age and up to 97 years of age. The ratio of men to women varies among different reports, with some citing equal incidence of occurrence among both sexes, some reporting a slightly higher incidence in men (1.5:1), and others finding a slightly higher incidence in women. Merkel cell carcinoma has also been reported to arise in patients with other neoplasms, at a frequency higher than expected by chance alone (4). These include squamous cell carcinoma, basal cell carcinoma, and lentigo maligna. Other internal malignancies that have been documented to be associated with MCC are Hodgkin's lymphoma, breast carcinoma, endometrial carcinoma, colon carcinoma, prostate cancer, ovarian cancer, bladder transitional cell carcinoma, squamous cell carcinoma of the larynx, B-cell lymphoma, and chronic lymphocytic leukemia (CLL). Merkel cell carcinoma has also been reported to arise in sites of previous radiation therapy (2–4). Immunosuppressed patients have been found to be at an increased risk for many malignancies, including Merkel cell carcinoma. Immunosuppressed individuals tend to have tumors that behave more aggressively than those seen in the general population.

Merkel cell carcinoma can present in many different ways, but is most often a solitary, painless, pink to reddish-blue or brown dome-shaped nodule or plaque on sun-exposed skin of elderly individuals (Figure 7.1). The lesion may sometimes ulcerate, and can range in size from 0.2 cm to 5.0 cm, with the largest lesion reported as 23.0 cm in greatest diameter (2–4).

Merkel cell carcinoma is composed of small, monomorphic, basophilic tumor cells with round to oval-shaped nuclei and scanty cytoplasm. The nuclei have finely granular dispersed chromatin, and nucleoli are absent or few in number. The nuclear-to-cytoplasmic ratio is high, as is as the mitotic rate, and pyknotic nuclei and apoptotic bodies may be present. The tumor cells occupy the dermis, and may extend into the subcutaneous fat (Figures 7.2 and 7.3). The epidermis is generally spared, but there are reports of epidermotropism or "pagetoid" spread. In these instances, MCC may mimic melanoma, mammary and extramammary Paget's disease, mycosis fungoides, pagetoid Bowen's disease, and intraepidermal epithelioma (8–9). The association of Merkel cell carcinoma with the aforementioned tumors, and its propensity to develop both squamous and eccrine differentiation, support a link between MCC and the epithelium. A dense lymphocytic infiltrate is typically present within and surrounding the tumor. There may be involvement of the dermal lymphatics and blood vessels. Merkel cell carcinoma has been classified into 3 histologic subtypes. The intermediate cell type is considered the most common variant of MCC,

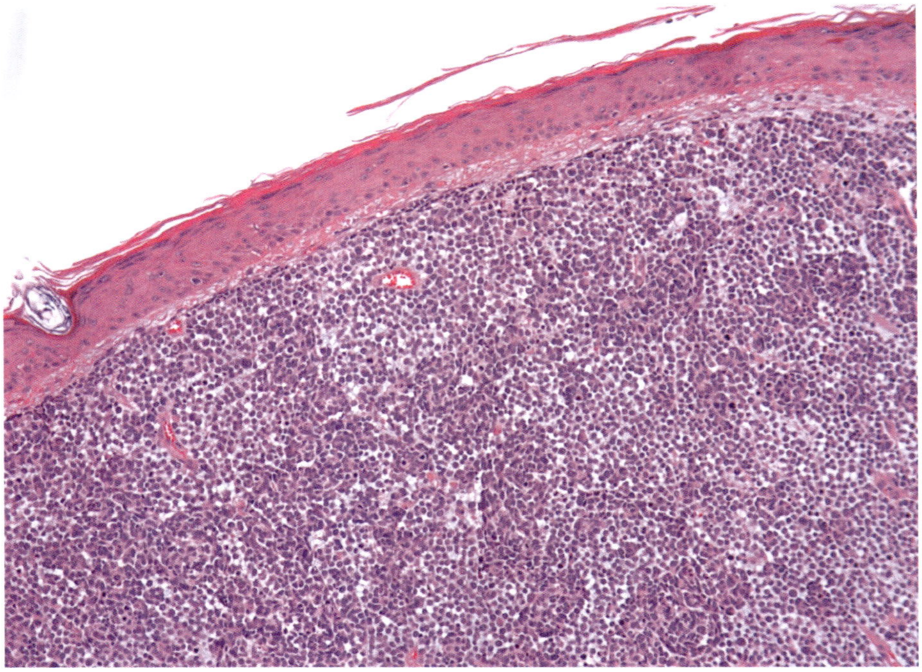

FIGURE 7.2. Low power photomicrograph depicting diffuse dermal permeation by neoplastic cells.

seen in approximately 50% of all Merkel cell carcinomas. It displays a solid, diffuse pattern made up of cells that are less compact, with focal areas of necrosis. Mitotic figures are conspicuous. There is a lymphocytic infiltrate within and around the tumor. The second histologic variant described by Gould, et al., the small cell variant, is composed of solid sheets and clusters of cells in the dermis, lacks glandular differentiation, and often has areas of necrosis. The trabecular pattern, considered to be the least common pattern, is characterized by round to polygonal cells arranged in organoid clusters and trabeculae, which may occasionally exhibit gland-like formations. This clas-

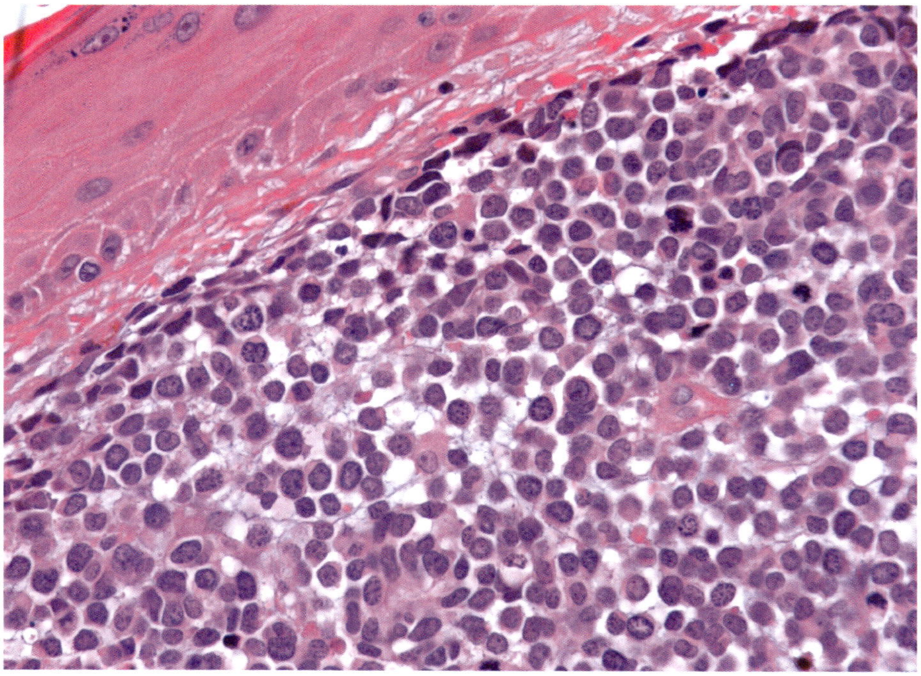

FIGURE 7.3. High power photomicrograph depicting small blue cells containing speckled nuclear chromatin. Note scattered mitotic figures.

sification scheme arranged by Gould, et al., is comprehensive; however, many tumors are composed of cells of different sizes and patterns, and not all tumors will fit exactly into one subtype. A triad of findings suggested to be virtually pathognomonic of MCC includes vesicular nuclei with small nucleoli, abundant mitoses, and apoptosis. The differential diagnosis includes other poorly differentiated small cell tumors. These include small cell carcinoma of the lung (oat cell carcinoma), cutaneous large cell lymphomas, neuroblastoma, metastatic carcinoid, amelanotic melanoma, sweat gland carcinoma, medullary carcinoma of the thyroid, Langerhans cell histiocytoses, plasmacytoma, Ewing's sarcoma, leukemias, and anaplastic carcinoma.

The definitive diagnosis of Merkel cell carcinoma requires the use of immunohistochemistry. The armamentarium of immunohistochemical stains that may be useful in diagnosing MCC is vast, and controversy exists as to which markers are best suited for this purpose. Anticytokeratin antibodies are the most sensitive markers for MCC, with various studies citing up to 100% positive reactivity to anti-keratin antibodies to low molecular weight cytokeratins (Figure 7.4). A perinuclear dot-like pattern of positivity is characteristic for MCC, and is a feature generally not observed in SCC (10–12). Keratin reactivity favors the diagnosis of MCC, and excludes melanoma and lymphoma. Diagnoses that MCC cannot be differentiated from with these markers include carcinoid and metastatic small cell lung cancer. Positive reactivity with anti-CK 8, 18, 19, and 20 also support an epithelial derived component of MCC. Among the anti-cytokeratin markers, most studies suggest than anti-CK 20 is highly specific for MCC, and is thought to be a strong predictor of MCC when determining the diagnosis of small cell carcinomas. The newest marker being investigated for use in identifying Merkel cell carcinomas is thyroid transcription factor 1 (TTF-1). It is a nuclear transcription factor expressed in thyroid and lung epithelial cells. TTF-1 belongs to a family of transcription factors that are expressed in the thyroid, lung, and certain regions of the brain. This marker is also found in pulmonary carcinomas, reacting with 72.5% of adenocarcinomas, 83%–100% of small cell carcinomas, 100% of atypical carcinoid tumors, and 75% of neuroendocrine carcinomas. It is not, however, expressed at all in MCC. TTF-1 is a sensitive and specific marker for small cell lung carcinoma, and CK 20 is a sensitive but not 100% specific marker for MCC. Thus, with the above information, it appears that a combination of TTF-1 and anti-CK 20 should provide the best sensitivity and specificity when needing to distinguish MCC from other small cell carcinomas.

Staging, based on the extent of local and systemic disease, is important in guiding treatment as well as determining prognosis. Stage I disease is local disease without lymph node or systemic involvement. Stage II disease refers to regional lymph node disease without evidence of systemic spread. Stage III refers to metastatic disease.

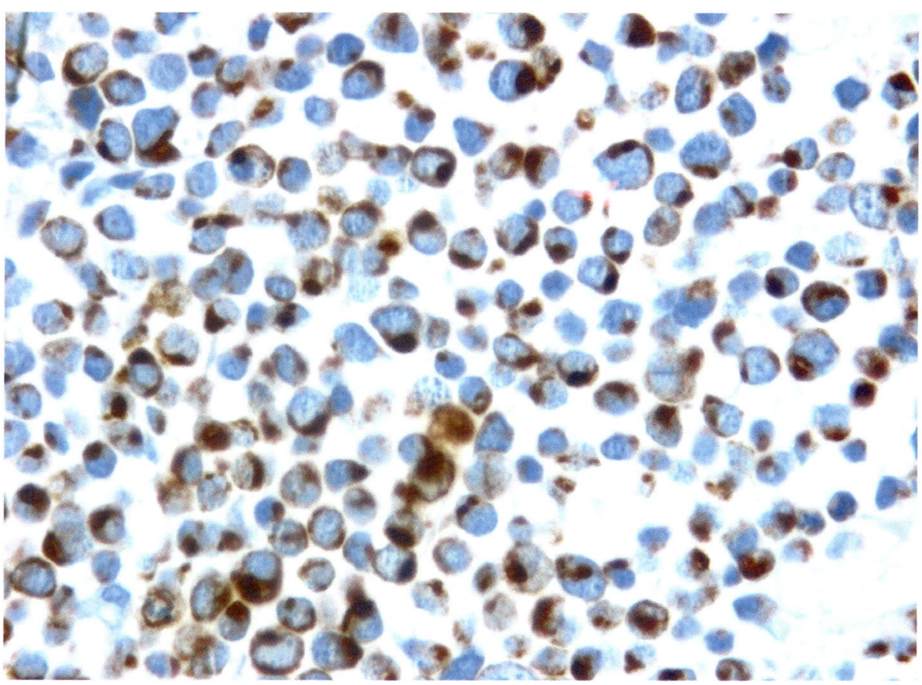

FIGURE 7.4. Dot-like paranuclear immunostaining with cytokeratin 20 in Merkel cell carcinoma.

Merkel cell carcinoma is a very aggressive malignancy in which metastatic disease is not uncommon. Survival rates vary, but the overall survival rate has been reported to range from 58% to 79% (13–27). It is considered to be the deadliest skin cancer, with a higher fatality rate than melanoma. Factors that have been found to be relevant to prognosis include tumor size and location, the sex and age of the patient, the stage of disease, and histologic characteristics. Tumors on the head and neck generally have the worst prognosis, followed by lesions on the trunk and extremities. Male sex has been reported to portend a worse prognosis, while age at diagnosis has been controversial. Histologic features associated with a poor prognosis include a mitotic rate of >10 per high power field, and evidence of vascular or lymphatic involvement.

Merkel cell carcinoma has been considered to follow a course similar to that of an intermediate or thick melanoma, but with a worse prognosis. Local recurrence usually occurs within 4 months of excision of the primary tumor, and is not uncommon, occurring in 20% to 44% of cases, with few reports citing up to 70%. Regional nodal metastases have been reported to occur in 31% to 80% of MCC; however, only 12% to 31% of these cases are present at the initial presentation. They are more common in tumors of the head and neck, and most nodal metastases are discovered within 7–24 months of initial treatment. Nodal involvement is a significant prognostic indicator, with a 5-year survival rate of 48% for patients with nodal disease, as compared to 88% for those without nodal involvement. Distant metastases indicate a very poor prognosis, and are the most important predictor of survival. They are found in 1/3 to 2/3 of patients with MCC, but are rarely present at initial presentation. The most common sites are lymph nodes, followed by liver, bone, brain, lung, skin, and GI tract. Distant metastases are diagnosed at a mean time of 18 months after initial diagnosis. The mortality rate of patients with systemic metastases ranges from 67% to 74%, with death usually occurring within 6 months of detection of the metastases. Spontaneous regression is a rare phenomenon that has been noted to occur in some cases of Merkel cell carcinoma. As of 2002, 10 cases in the literature have been reported.

Due to the rarity of this tumor, there are no widely adopted, standard treatment regimens. Early diagnosis and treatment are essential due to the aggressiveness of MCC and its propensity for local recurrence and metastases. Multimodality treatment is thought to offer the best overall survival rates, but specific treatments are controversial and their benefits debatable. The following are recommendations based on each stage of disease. Stage I disease should be treated with surgical excision, using wide local excision with 2–3-cm margins, dissecting to fascia. Excision may be followed by elective lymph node dissection or lymphoscintigraphy and sentinel node biopsy. Postoperative radiation may also be considered. The use of chemotherapy at this stage is not well defined and requires further investigation. Stage II disease requires re-excision of local recurrences, followed by postoperative radiation to the primary and regional nodal basins. Elective lymph node dissection or sentinel node biopsy should be considered. If regional nodal metastases have been detected, total lymphadenectomy and postoperative radiation provides the best management. Stage III disease most often requires systemic chemotherapy. Other investigational treatments, including bone marrow transplant, local hyperthermia, and hyperthermic limb perfusion therapy, have rarely been used, with disappointing results.

References

1. Toker C. Trabecular carcinoma of the skin. *Arch Dermatol* 1972; 105: 107–110.
2. Freedberg RM, Eisen AZ, Wolff K, Austem KF, Goldsmith LA, Katz SI, Fitzpatrick TB. *Fitzpatrick's Dermatology in General Medicine*, 5th ed., Vol. II. McGraw-Hill, 1999; 915–918, 1261, 2991.
3. Haag M, Glass LF, Fensek NA. Merkel cell carcinoma: Diagnosis and treatment. *Dermatol Surg* 1995; 21: 669–683.
4. Kennedy MM, Blessing D, King G, et al. Expression of bcl-2 and p53 in Merkel cell carcinoma: An immunohistochemical study. *Amer J Dermatopathol* 1996; 18 (3): 273–277.
5. Schlagbauer-Wadl H, Klosner G, Heere-Ress, et al. Bcl-2 antisense oligonucleotides (G3139) inhibit Merkel cell carcinoma growth in SCID mice. *J Invest Dermatol* 2000; 114 (4): 725–730.
6. Feinmesser M, Halpern M, Fenig E, et al. Expression of the apoptosis-related oncogenes bcl-2, bax, and p53 in Merkel cell carcinoma: Can they predict treatment response and clinical outcome? *Hum Pathol* 1999; 30 (11): 1367–1372.
7. Su LD, Fullen DR, Lowe L, Uherova P, Schnitzer B, Valdez R. CD 117 (KIT Receptor) expression in Merkel cell carcinoma. *Am J Dermatopathol* 2002; 24 (4): 289–293.
8. Gollard R, Weber R, Kosty M, et al. Merkel cell carcinoma: Review of 22 cases with surgical, pathologic, and therapeutic considerations. *Cancer* 2000; 88 (8): 1842–1851.
9. Walsh N. Primary neuroendocrine (Merkel cell) carcinoma of the skin: Morphologic diversity and implications thereof. *Hum Pathol* 2001; 32 (7): 680–689.
10. Leech SN, Kolar AJO, Barrett PD, et al. Merkel cell carcinoma can be distinguished from metastatic small cell carcinoma using antibodies to cytokeratin 20 and thyroid transcription factor 1. *J Clin Pathol* 2001; 54 (9): 727–729.
11. Kontochristopoulos GJ, Stavropoulos PG, Krasagakis K, et al. Differentiation between Merkel cell carcinoma and malignant melanoma: An immunohistochemical study. *Dermatol* 2000; 201 (2): 123–126.

12. Cheuk W, Kwan MY, Suster S, et al. Immunostaining for thyroid transcription factor 1 and cytokeratin 20 aids the distinction of small cell carcinoma from Merkel cell carcinoma, but not pulmonary from extrapulmonary small cell carcinomas. *Arch Pathol Lab Med* 2001; 125: 229–231.
13. Wasserberg N, Feinmesser M, Schachter J, et al. Sentinel-node guided lymph node dissection for Merkel cell carcinoma. *Eur J Surg Oncol* 1999; 25(4): 444–446.
14. Zeitouni N, Cheney R, Delacure M. Lymphoscintigraphy, sentinel lymph node biopsy, and Mohs micrographic surgery in the treatment of Merkel cell carcinoma. *Dermatol Surg* 2000; 26 (1): 12–18.
15. Rodrigues LKE, Leong SPL, Kashani-Sabet M, et al. Early experience with sentinel lymph node mapping for Merkel cell carcinoma. *J Am Acad Dermatol* 2001; 45 (2): 303–308.
16. Herbst A, Haynes HA, Nghiem P. The standard of care for Merkel cell carcinoma should include adjuvant radiation and lymph node surgery. *J Am Acad Dermatol* 2002; 46 (4): 640–642.
17. Ott M, Tanabe K, Gaad M, et al. Multimodality management of Merkel cell carcinoma. *Arch Surg* 1999; 134 (4): 388–393.
18. Brown TJ, Jackson BA, Macfarlane DF, et al. Merkel cell carcinoma: Spontaneous resolution and management of metastatic disease. *Dermatol Surg* 1999; 25 (1): 23–25.
19. Wasserberg N, Schachter J, Fenig E, et al. Applicability of the sentinel node technique to Merkel cell carcinoma. *Dermatol Surg* 2000; 26 (2): 138–141.
20. Boyer JD, Zitelli JA, Brodland DG, et al. Local control of primary Merkel cell carcinoma: Review of 45 cases treated with Mohs micrographic surgery with and without adjuvant radiation. *J Am Acad Dermatol* 2002; 47 (6): 885–892.
21. Gibbs P, Gonzalez R, Lee L, Walsh P. Medical management of cutaneous malignancies. *Clinics Dermatol* 2001; 19 (3): 298–304.
22. Yazijii H, Gown AM. Merkel cell carcinoma: Review of 22 cases with surgical, pathologic, and therapeutic considerations (letter; comment). *Cancer* 2000; 89 (8): 1866–1867.
23. Connelly TJ, Cribier B, Brown TJ, et al. Complete spontaneous regression of Merkel cell carcinoma: A review of the 10 reported cases. *Dermatol Surg* 2000; 26 (9): 853–856.
24. Duker I, Starz H, Bachter D, et al. Prognostic and therapeutic implications of sentinel lymphonodectomy and S-staging in Merkel cell carcinoma. *Dermatol* 2001; 202 (3): 225–229.
25. Messina JL, Reintgen DS, Cruse CW, et al. Selective lymphadenectomy in patients with Merkel cell (cutaneous neuroendocrine) carcinoma. *Ann Surg Oncol* 1997; 4(5): 389–395.
26. Waldmann V, Goldschmidt H, Jackel A, et al. Transient complete remission of metastasized Merkel cell carcinoma by high dose polychemotherapy and autologous peripheral blood stem cell transplantation. *Brit J Dermatol* 2000; 143 (4): 837–839.
27. Olieman A, Lienard D, Eggermont A, et al. Hyperthermic isolated limb perfusion with tumor necrosis factor alpha, interferon gamma, and melphalan for locally advanced nonmelanoma skin tumors of the extremities. *Arch Surg* 1999; 134 (3): 303–307.

8 Metastatic Carcinoma

■ Synonyms:	Cutaneous metastatic neoplasm, Sister Mary Joseph nodule
■ Etiology:	Hematogenous or lymphatic spread of primary tumor to umbilical skin
■ Associations:	Primary malignancies (most commonly gastrointestinal and genitourinary)
■ Clinical:	Nodule, occasionally ulcerated, scalp most common site
■ Histology:	Most commonly adenocarcinoma in dermis
■ IHC repertoire:	Cytokeratins 7, 20, carcinoembyronic antigen
■ Staging:	Implies widespread metastatic disease
■ Prognosis:	Less than 1-year survival in most cases
■ Adverse variables:	None (ovarian primary may be associated with slightly better prognosis)
■ Treatment:	Surgery, chemotherapy

Cutaneous metastases occur in approximately 10% of all cancer patients. The frequencies of cutaneous metastases correlate directly with the frequencies of primary malignancies. In women, breast carcinoma is the most common tumor to spread to the skin, followed by large intestine, melanoma, lung, and ovary. In men, primary tumors from the lung most commonly involve the skin, followed by tumors of the large intestine, melanoma, and squamous cell carcinomas of the oral cavity (1). Metastases can affect any part of the body, with a disproportionate number involving the scalp (presumably due to increased circulatory volume). Overall, skin metastases represent the presenting sign of underlying malignancy in about 8% of these patients (2). Umbilical metastases have been given the designation Sister Mary Joseph nodules, named for a nurse involved with the first surgical resection of such a lesion. Umbilical metastases involve from 5% to 10% of tumors involving the abdomen and may be the presenting sign of an internal malignancy in up to 45% of cases. In one study, 57% of tumor nodules located in the umbilicus were benign (3). Neoplasms originating in the gastrointestinal tract account for the great majority of the metastatic processes (Table 8.1) (1). Other primary neoplasms with umbilical metastases have been reported less commonly. These include adenocarcinomas of the gall bladder (4), renal cell carcinoma (5), and lymphoma (6).

Umbilical metastases most commonly present as firm nodules. A less common presentation is that of an indurated plaque. These growths rarely ulcerate and are not usually painful or tender. Hyperkeratosis is seen in some cases, but is unusual in this location (Figure 8.1A and 8.1B).

The tumor nodule with dermal sclerosis is apparent on the cut specimen. They are more common in women, in part due to the contribution of ovarian carcinomas to this clinical presentation (7).

The histologic features vary with the origin of the primary lesion. In about 75%–90% of cases, the primary tumor is an adenocarcinoma, and the resulting Sister Mary Joseph nodule has the histologic features of adenocarcinoma (3,7). Glandular structures course throughout the dermis, often surrounded by desmoplastic stroma. As with other metastatic neoplasms, the histologic features recapitulate the features of the primary tumor to different degrees. Metastases from colon carcinomas may demonstrate tall columnar epithelial lining to the glandular structures and may produce mucin. Ovarian metastases may be characterized by mucinous or serous type of glandular epithelia. In all cases, the better-differentiated neoplasms will recapitulate their sites of origin closely, while the less-differentiated ones are undifferentiated adenocarcinomas that may be difficult to further classify (Figures 8.2–8.5).

Table 8.1.

Site of Primary Tumor	% of Cases of Umbilical Metastasis
Stomach	28%
Pancreas	15%
Sigmoid colon	10%
Ovary	10%
Endometrium	3%
Cecum	3%
Transverse colon	3%
Penis	3%
Cervix	3%
Appendix	3%
Liver	3%

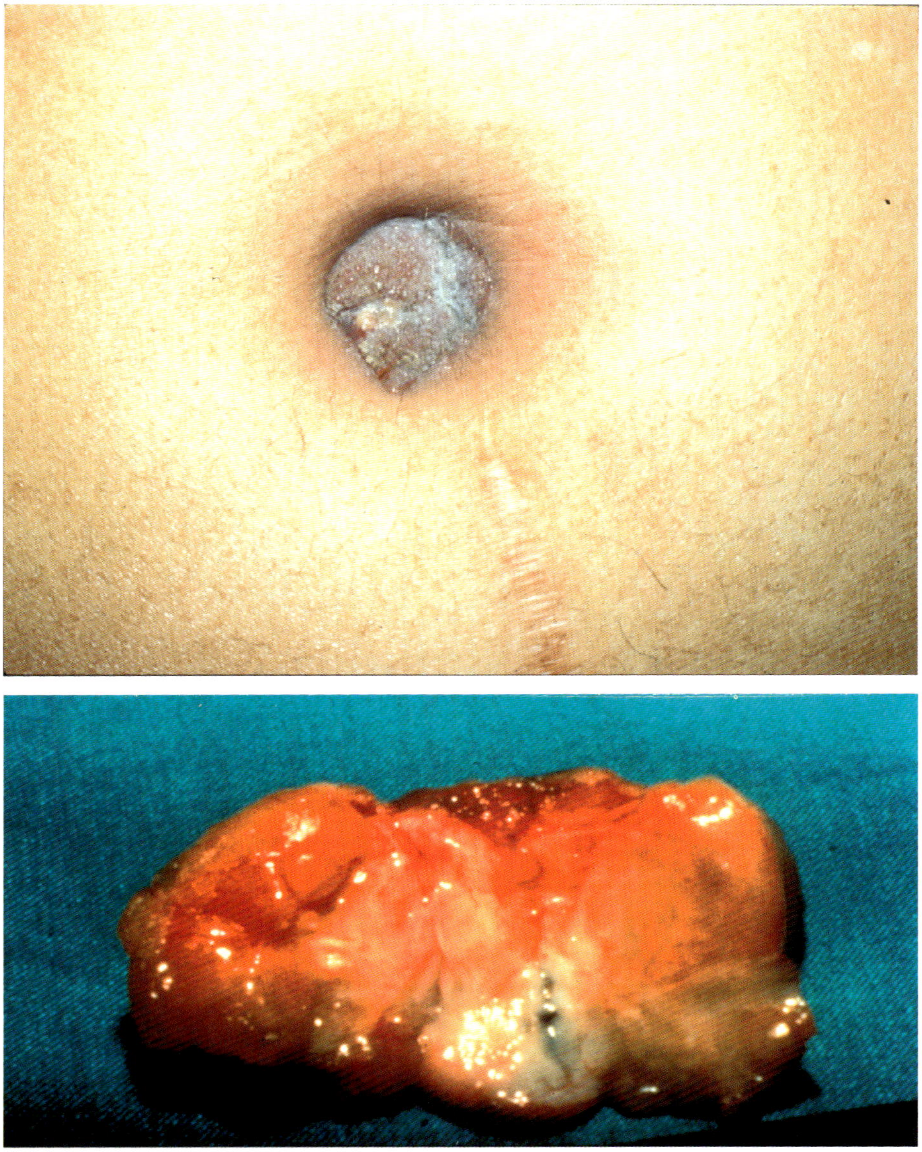

A

B

Figure 8.1. (A) Periumbilical nodule seen in Sister Mary Joseph nodule. (B) Gross specimen removed from umbilicus.

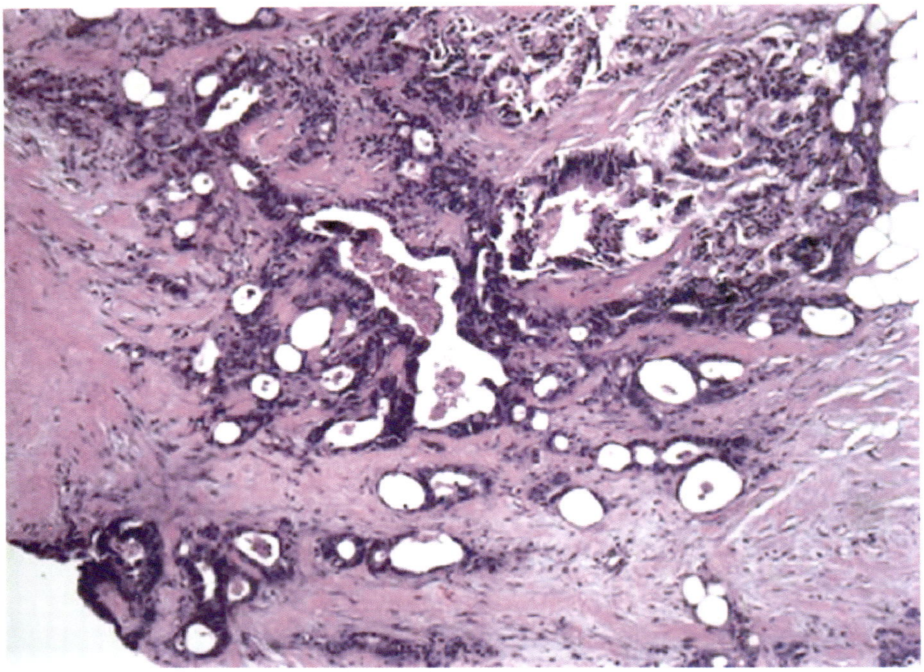

FIGURE 8.2. Medium power photomicrograph depicting metastatic colon cancer. Note ductular structures embedded in dense (desmoplastic) collagenous stroma.

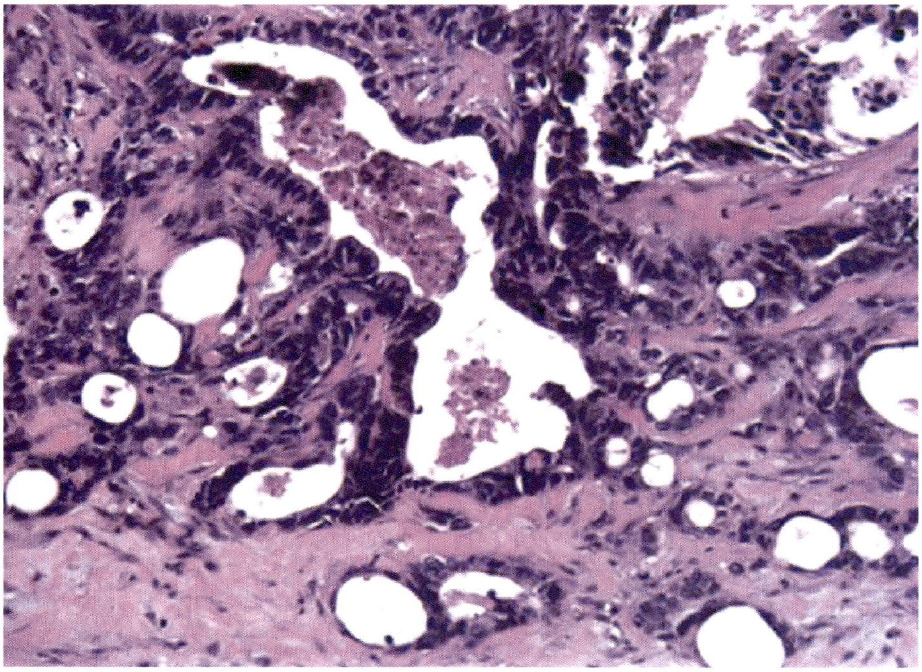

FIGURE 8.3. High power photomicrograph depicting glands with columnar lining and inspissated luminal secretions.

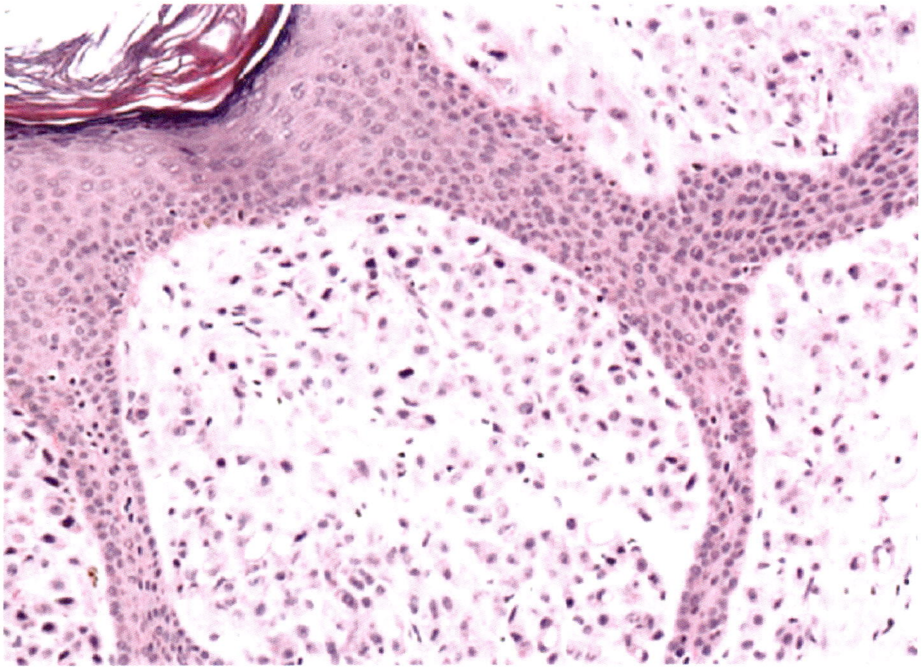

FIGURE 8.4. Medium power photomicrograph depicting metastatic gastric carcinoma. Note characteristic signet rings.

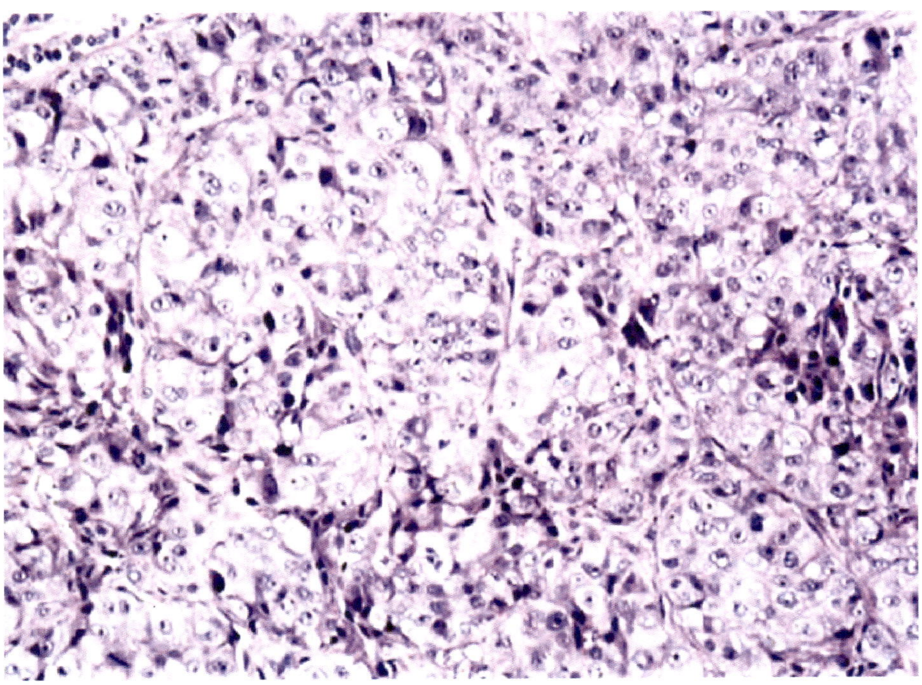

FIGURE 8.5. This undifferentiated neoplasm is a metastasis from the prostate, identified by staining with prostate-specific antigen.

Immunostains with antibodies directed against cytokeratins 7 and 20 may be helpful in aiding in making these distinctions, as might antibodies directed against CEA (carcinoembryonic antigen), estrogens and progesterones. Colon carcinomas often express cytokeratin 20 and carcinoembryonic antigen, but only rarely strongly express cytokeratin 7. In contrast, ovarian neoplasms often express cytokeratin 7 strongly and diffusely, along with staining with hormonal markers, but rarely express either cytokeratin 20 or CEA. Pancreatic tumors also express cytokeratin 7, and not usually cytokeratin 20, but do not contain estrogen or progesterone receptors. Biliary duct carcinomas may strongly express both cytokeratins 7 and 20 (7).

Sister Mary Joseph nodules portend an ominous prognosis. Surgery and chemotherapy have been used with some success, but in most cases, the patient succumbs to widespread metastatic disease within a year of diagnosing the umbilical nodule (8). Patients with primary ovarian carcinomas involving the umbilicus may have a slightly better prognosis than those with metastases from other sites (9).

References

1. Schwartz RA. Cutaneous metastatic disease. *J Am Acad Dermatol* 1995; 33: 161–182.
2. Lookingbill DP, Spangleer N, Helm KF. Cutaneous metastases in patients with metastatic carcinoma: a retrospective study of 4020 patients. *J Am Acad Dermatol* 1993; 29: 228–236.
3. Steck WD, Helwig EB. Tumors of the umbilicus. *Cancer* 1965; 18: 907–915.
4. Cosentini T, Tempesta R, Gentile F, Colavita N. Sister Mary Joseph nodule secondary to gallbladder carcinoma. *Radiol Med (Torino)* 2003; 105: 391–394.
5. Chen P, Middlebrook MR, Goldman SM, Sandler CM. Sister Mary Joseph nodule from metastatic renal cell carcinoma. *J Comput Assist Tomogr* 1998; 22: 756–757.
6. Dornier C, Reichert-Penetrat S, Barbaud A, Kaisse W, Schmutz JL. Lymphoma presenting as Sister Mary-Joseph's nodule. *Ann Dermatol Venereol* 2000; 127: 732–734.
7. Cabibi D, Licata A, Barresi E, Craxi A, Aragona F. Expression of cytokeratin 7 and 20 in pathological conditions of the bile tract. *Pathol Res Pract* 2003; 199: 65–70.
8. Touraud JP, Lentz N, Dutrone Y, Mercier E, Sagot P, Lambert D. Umbilical cutaneous metastasis (or Sister Mary Joseph's nodule) disclosing an ovarian adenocarcinoma. *Gynecol Obstet Fertil* 2000; 28: 719–721.
9. Majmudar B, Wiskind AK, Croft BN, Dudley AG. The Sister (Mary) Joseph nodule: Its significance in gynecology. *Gynecol Oncol* 1991; 40: 152–159.

9
Paget's Disease

■ Synonyms:	Extramammary Paget's disease, mammary Paget's disease
■ Etiology:	Ductular extension of carcinoma from breast genitourinary, gastrointestinal, or apocrine glands
■ Associations:	Underlying adenocarcinoma of breast (mammary) or genitourinary or gastrointestinal carcinoma (extramammary) or primary appendageal adenocarcinoma
■ Clinical:	Scaly, erythematous patch on nipple (mammary) or anogenital region (extramammary Paget's)
■ Histology:	Large, atypical cells at all levels of epidermis
■ IHC repertoire:	Cytokeratins 7, CEA, EMA
■ Staging:	Essential to workup for underlying adenocarcinoma
■ Prognosis:	Excellent if no underlying carcinoma; poor if internal carcinoma present
■ Adverse variables:	Dermal invasion by neoplastic cells; association with underlying malignancy
■ Treatment:	Surgery, (topical chemotherapy, radiation)

Mammary and extramammary Paget's disease represent two clinical conditions with potentially serious consequences for the patient. Mammary Paget's disease is associated with underlying carcinoma of the breast in virtually all cases. Exact incidence numbers vary, but with meticulous serial sections of major ducts entering into the nipple, foci of ductular carcinoma are identified in most cases (1). The disease has the same epidemiologic characteristics as breast carcinoma, independent of the presence of Paget's disease. It is most frequently encountered in middle-aged to elderly women and it may be unilateral or bilateral. Mammary Paget's disease presents as an erythematous, scaling patch on the nipple (Figure 9.1).

The clinical differential diagnosis usually includes squamous cell carcinoma *in situ*, and most commonly, eczematous processes.

Extramammary Paget's disease has an identical appearance, but is located in areas with abundant apocrine glands (Figure 9.2).

The most frequently involved site is the anogenital region, though cases have been reported in the axillae and within the external auditory canal. Extramammary Paget's disease is slightly more common in women and is more frequent in elderly patients (2). The relationship between underlying carcinoma is less strong with extramammary Paget's disease. Incidence estimates range from 0% to 54% of cases, depending upon series (3). In approximately 25% of these cases, the underlying tumor appears to arise from apocrine or (less commonly) eccrine glands (4). Another 10%–15% of these cases have underlying tumors of the genitourinary or gastrointestinal tracts (2). Cases of extramammary Paget's disease involving the anogenital region seem to have a higher association with underlying carcinoma.

The histologic features of Paget's disease of the nipple and extramammary Paget's disease are identical except for site-specific anatomic variations. Large cells with abundant pale cytoplasm are present at all levels of the affected epidermis (Figure 9.3).

The atypical cells may display vesicular nuclei, and nucleoli are often visible, though not usually as prominent as those seen in melanoma cells (Figure 9.4).

There is no tendency for nest formation by the atypical cells. In some cases, intracytoplasmic vacuoles may be present, suggesting early ductular differentiation. This finding can be accentuated with the use of a periodic acid-Schiff stain that demonstrates cytoplasmic acidic mucopolysaccharides. The background epidermis is often acanthotic and spongiotic, with overlying parakeratosis.

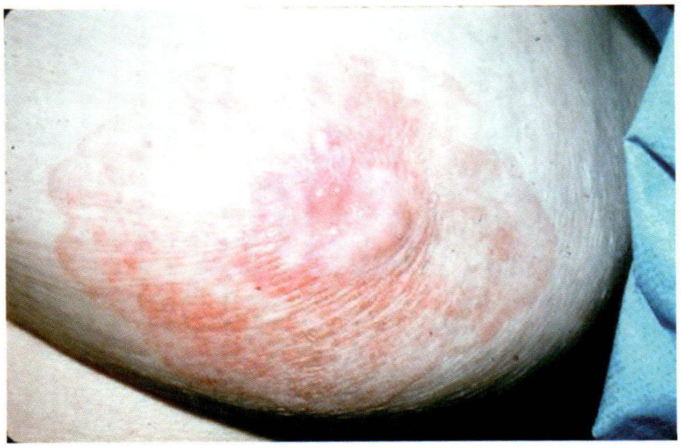

FIGURE 9.1. Scaly eruption centered on the nipple in Paget's disease.

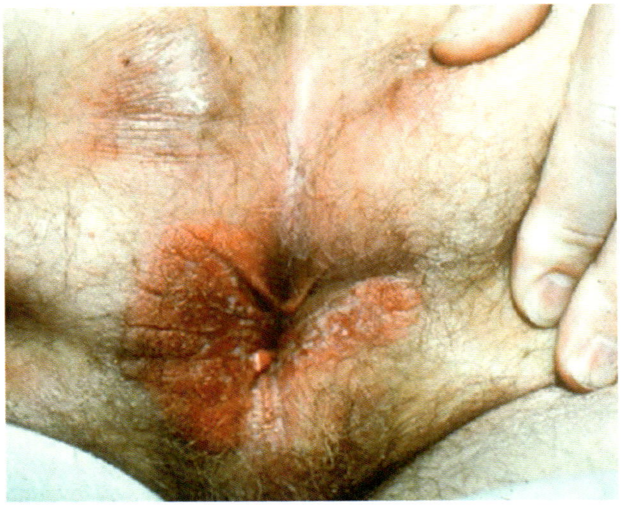

FIGURE 9.2. The anogenital region is a frequent site of involvement with extramammary paget's disease.

The histologic differential diagnosis includes entities characterized by individual, atypical intraepidermal cells. The major differential possibilities include malignant melanoma and squamous cell carcinoma in situ. In most cases, it is useful to make this distinction with the use of immunostains. Melanoma cells strongly express S100 protein, an antigen that is occasionally expressed weakly and focally by Paget's disease cells (especially when they are ductular breast carcinoma cells). Squamous cell carcinoma cells express some pan-cytokeratin markers, as do the cells in Paget's disease. The most useful distinguishing markers are cytokeratin 7 (Figure 9.5), which is expressed by neither the cells in malignant melanoma nor those in squamous cell carcinoma *in situ*, and epithelial membrane antigen, which has a similar staining profile (Figure 9.6).

CAM5.2 and carcinoembryonic antigen have also been used with good success in establishing the diagnosis. The use of an antibody panel using the reagents suggested makes the distinction between these entities very straightforward in most cases. It should be noted, however, that

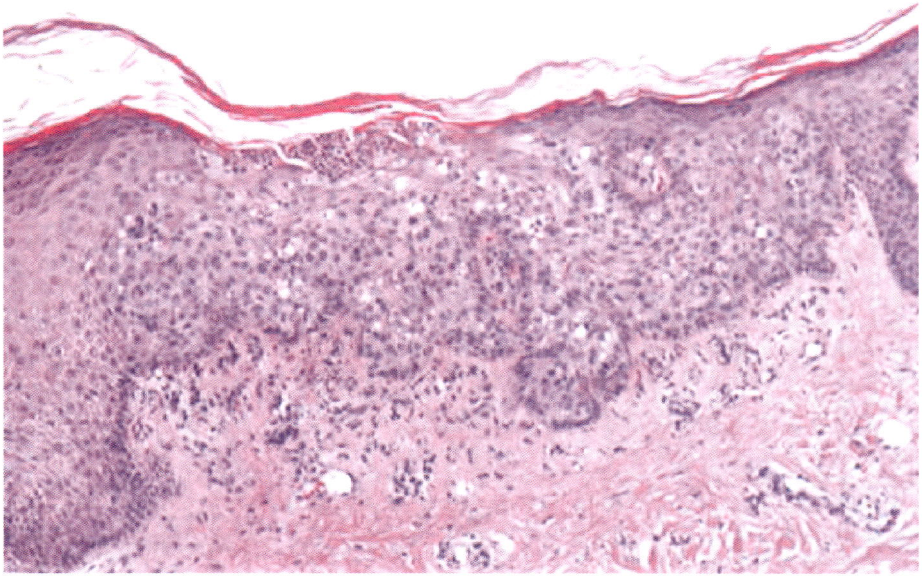

FIGURE 9.3. Medium power photomicrograph depicting scattered atypical clear cells, Paget's cells occupying all levels of the epithelium.

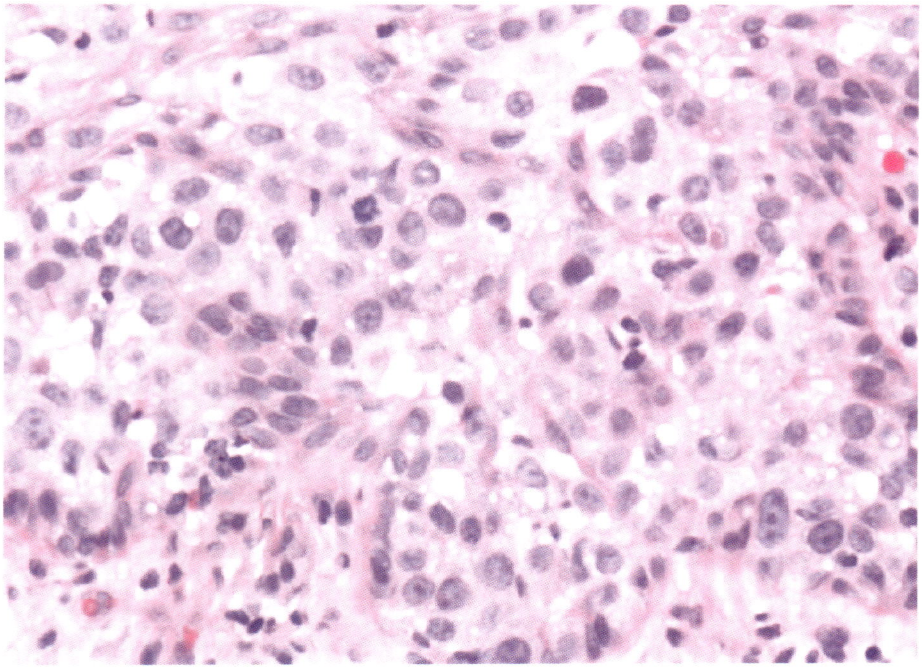

FIGURE 9.4. The neoplastic cells in Paget's disease have vesicular nuclei with prominent nucleoli.

melanoma is not usually in the clinical differential diagnosis of this process.

In cases of extramammary Paget's disease, the neoplastic cells within the epidermis may represent upward extension of malignant transformation of cutaneous appendages (i.e., apocrine or eccrine structures). In these cases, similar-appearing tumor cells are apparent within the glandular apparatus. In more advanced cases, the same tumor cells may violate the basement membrane, invading the dermis. Lymphatic involvement has also been reported. This portends a significantly worse prognosis (5). In other cases of extramammary Paget's disease, the tumor cells represent upward extension of underlying tumors arising within the genitourinary system (most commonly, bladder), or gastrointestinal tract (most commonly, colon). In these cases, invasion of the dermis

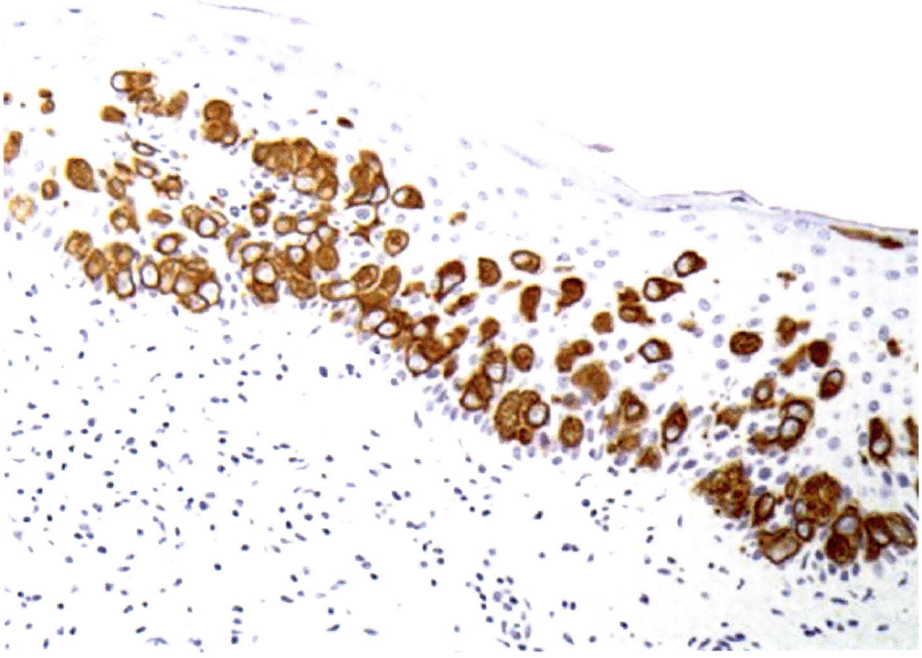

FIGURE 9.5. Cytokeratin 7 is strongly expressed by intraepithelial neoplastic cells , but not by the background keratinocytes within the epidermis.

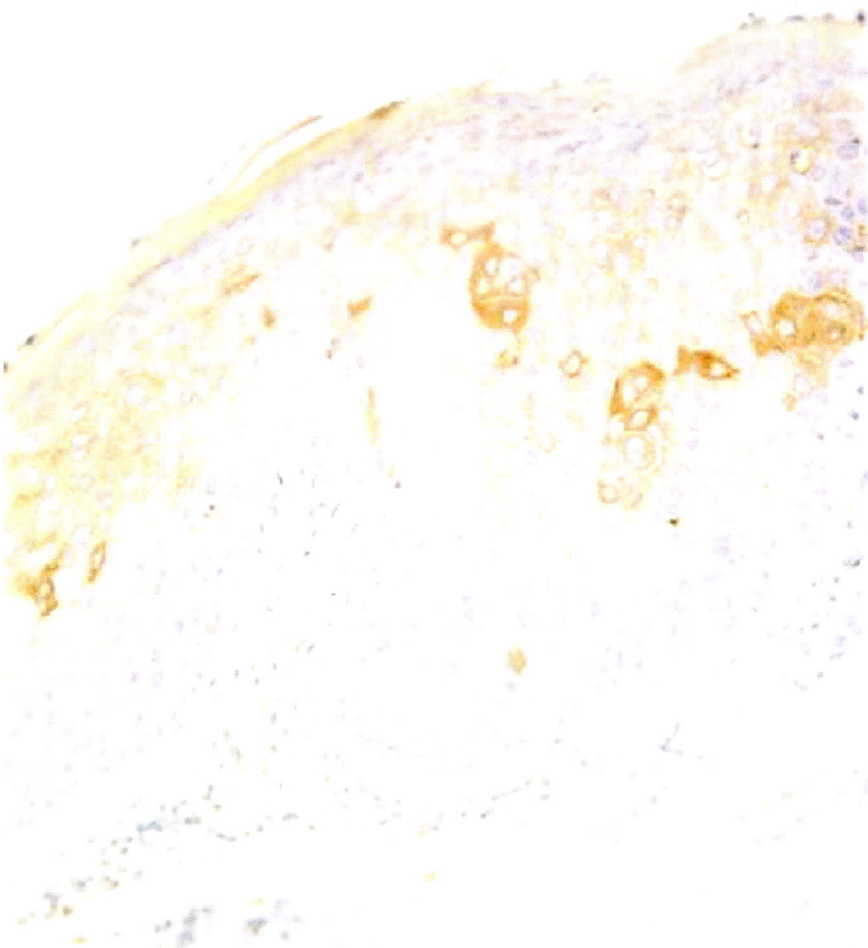

FIGURE 9.6. Epithelial membrane antigen is expressed by tumor cells in Paget's disease, but not by the background keratinocytes within the epithelium.

denotes a more aggressive neoplasm, but careful histologic evaluation of the primary tumor is necessary for determining accurate prognostic data.

Paget's disease (mammary and extramammary) is treated with locally destructive therapy. Complete surgical excision is usually the first line of treatment for suitable candidates. Prior to excision, a staging workup is performed in order to isolate any underlying malignancies. In Paget's disease of the nipple, the underlying ductular tissue is removed, as a minimum, in most cases in order to identify any associated breast carcinoma. In extramammary Paget's disease, screening procedures are initiated prior to the surgical procedure. For patients who are not candidates for surgery, radiation and topical chemotherapeutic agents have been used with some success.

References

1. Ashikari R, Park K, Huvos AG, Urban JA. Paget's disease of the breast. *Cancer* 1970; 26: 680–685.
2. Lee SC, Roth LM, Ehrlich C, Hall JA. Extramammary Paget's disease of the vulva: A clinicopathology study of 13 cases. *Cancer* 1977; 39: 2540–2549.
3. Chand JJ. Extramammary Paget's disease: Prognosis and relationship to internal malignancy. *J Am Acad Dermatol* 1985; 13: 1009–1014.
4. Piura B, Zirkin HJ. Vulvar Paget's disease with an underlying sweat gland adenocarcinoma. *J Dermatol Surg Oncol* 1988; 14: 533–537.
5. Murata Y, Kumano K, Tani M. Underpants pattern erythema: A previously unrecognized cutaneous manifestation of extramammary Paget's disease of the genitalia with advanced metastatic spread. *J Am Acad Dermatol* 1999; 40: 949–956.

10 Subcutaneous Panniculitis-like Lymphoma

■ Synonyms:	Subcutaneous lymphoma, cytophagic histiocytic panniculitis
■ Etiology:	Unknown
■ Associations:	Bleeding diathesis
■ Clinical:	Hemorrhagic plaques and nodules, abdomen and extremities
■ Histology:	Dense lymphoid infiltrate in subcutis with hemorrhage and necrosis
■ IHC repertoire:	CD3, CD4, CD8
■ Staging:	Systemic workup required to assess extent
■ Prognosis:	Bimodal; 5-year survival
■ Adverse variables:	Unknown
■ Treatment:	Systemic chemotherapy

Subcutaneous panniculitis-like lymphoma (SPL) occurs primarily in younger adults, but can arise in persons of any age. The usual presentation is that of an ulcerative and hemorrhagic panniculitis, presenting as multiple erythematous nodules often involving the lower extremities and abdomen (Figure 10.1). Coagulopathies are frequently observed in these patients. In addition, many of these patients display constitutional symptoms such as weight loss, fever, and fatigue. This disease may represent what was previously known as cytophagic histiocytic panniculitis, at least in some cases (1). The prognosis is ominous for some patients with the disease, while others tend to have a more indolent course (2). Fatal leukemic transformation has also been reported in these patients (3). While the parameters that affect the ultimate course of the disease and prognosis have not been fully elucidated, there have been preliminary attempts at developing criteria for those with a more favorable prognosis (4).

The epidermis and superficial dermis are unremarkable in most cases of SPL, so a deep biopsy is required to establish a diagnosis. An infiltrate of atypical lymphocytes is present within the deep reticular dermis and throughout the subcutis (Figure 10.2).

The infiltrate is present diffusely within the lobules of adipocytes, as well as within the fibrous septa, and may demonstrate transmural invasion of blood vessels. Atypical lymphocytes are admixed with eosinophils and large histiocytes, some of which demonstrate emperipolesis, appearing as "bean-bag" cells. The lymphocytes are slightly enlarged and hyperchromatic, but rarely display marked cytologic atypia (Figure 10.3).

In some cases, however, more vesicular, anaplastic lymphocytes are seen (2). Zonal necrosis is present in many cases, and individual cell necrosis of tumor cells is common (Figure 10.4).

Karyorrhectic debris is a common finding (3). Mitoses, including atypical forms, are commonly observed. Immunostains reveal SPL to be a T-cell lymphoma. In most cases, there is a predominance of CD8+ cells, but in some cases, a CD4+ proliferation has been reported. CD30 is also seen in some cases (2). Gene rearrangements can be detected in virtually all cases. T-cell gene rearrangements are reported in most cases (1,6). In some cases, the distinction from NK lymphoma can be made only on the basis of immunophenotyping (6,7).

The major differential diagnoses include reactive panniculitides such as erythema nodosum (EN) and erythema induratum (EI). In EN, the inflammatory infiltrate is largely confined to the fibrous septa with only slight spillage into the lobules. Zonal necrosis is not seen and the lymphocytes are not atypical. While giant cells and histiocytes may be present, large, "bean bag" cells are not present.

EI may be more difficult to separate from SPL. In EI, zonal necrosis is seen, but is usually surrounded by a palisading granulomatous response resembling tuberculosis.

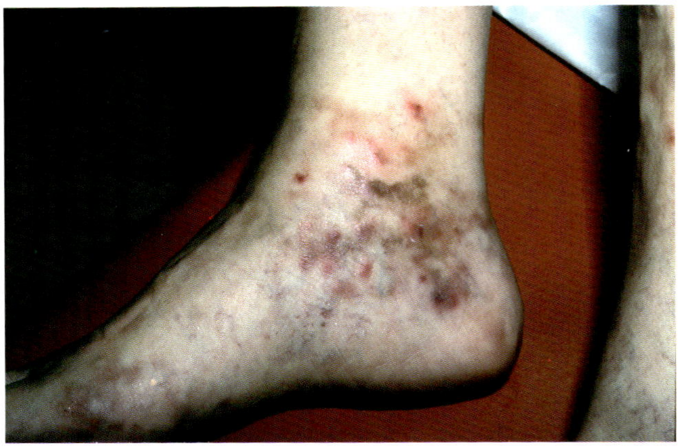

FIGURE 10.1. Erythematous and violaceous nodules with ecchymoses on lower extremity of patient with subcutaneous T-cell lymphoma.

Histiocytes, including multinucleated forms, are present, as is a neutrophilic infiltrate. Vasculitis may also be present. However, lymphocyte atypia is not present and an abundance of dying neoplastic cells is not a feature of this entity.

It may be difficult to distinguish SPL from angiocentric lymphoma. However, the clinical presentation is usually somewhat different. In addition, the neoplastic infiltrate in angiocentric lymphoma is usually centered more in the reticular dermis, extending into the subcutis, while in SPL, the infiltrate is centered within the subcutaneous fat, in some cases pushing into the deep reticular dermis. Further, the distinction may not be essential in terms of treatment options and prognosis.

Other cutaneous lymphomas also enter into the histologic (though not usually the clinical, differential) diagnosis. Mycosis fungoides in the tumor stage may involve the subcutaneous fat, but there is also usually a dense infiltrate of neoplastic lymphocytes within the dermis and these cells may extend into the epidermis or appendageal epithelium. Cutaneous B-cell lymphomas such as follicular lymphoma and marginal zone lymphoma may involve the subcutaneous fat; however, eosinophils are uncommon in these tumors. These B-cell lymphomas are usually centered primarily in the dermis and not in the subcutaneous fat. In addition, necrosis of the adipocytes is not commonly seen. The cytologic characteristics are also somewhat different between these B-cell lymphomas and the subcutaneous panniculitis-like T-cell lymphoma.

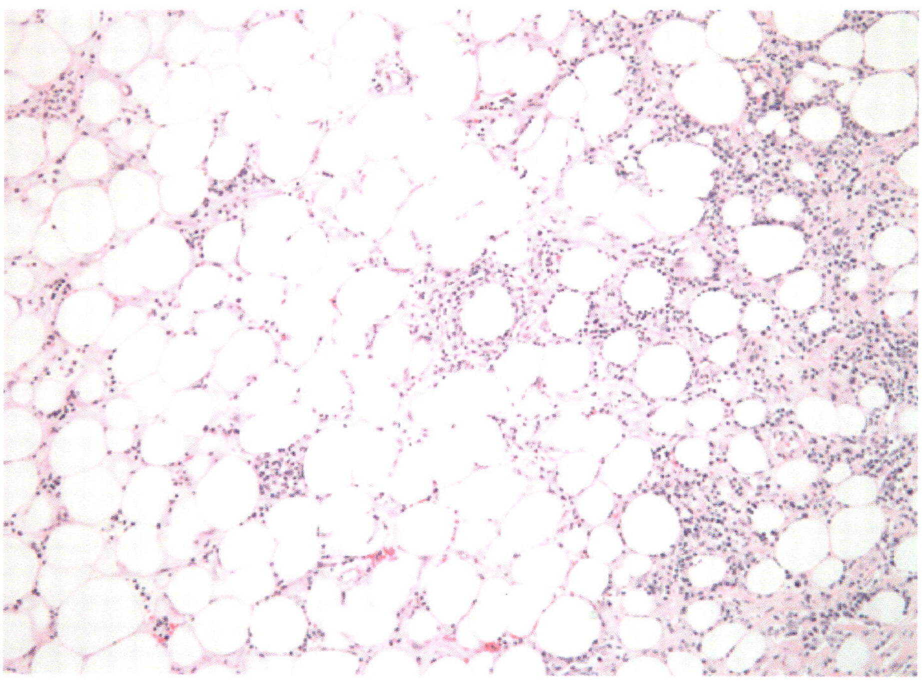

FIGURE 10.2. Low power photomicrograph depicting diffuse infiltration of the subcutaneous fat lobules by a dense lymphocytic infiltrate.

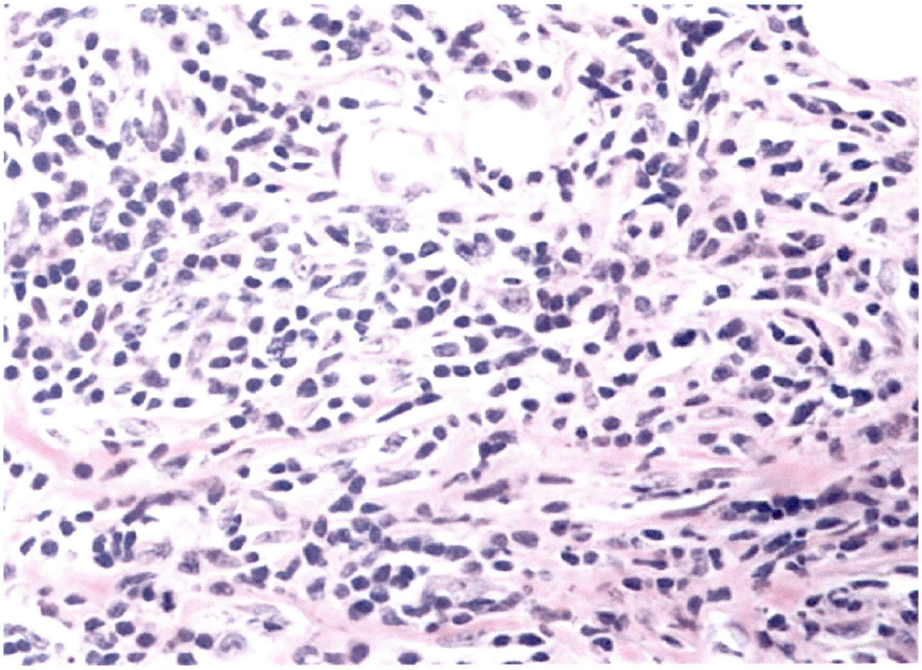

FIGURE 10.3. High power photomicrograph depicting small to medium-sized hyperchromatic lymphocytes located throughout the subcutaneous fat.

Lupus panniculitis may also demonstrate some histologic features in common with SPL. In lupus, zonal necrosis would be most unusual, as would the presence of atypical lymphocytes and eosinophils. Lupus panniculitis invariably demonstrates a plasmacellular infiltrate, often at the periphery of the inflammatory cells, and a characteristic homogenization of the adipose tissue within the lobules.

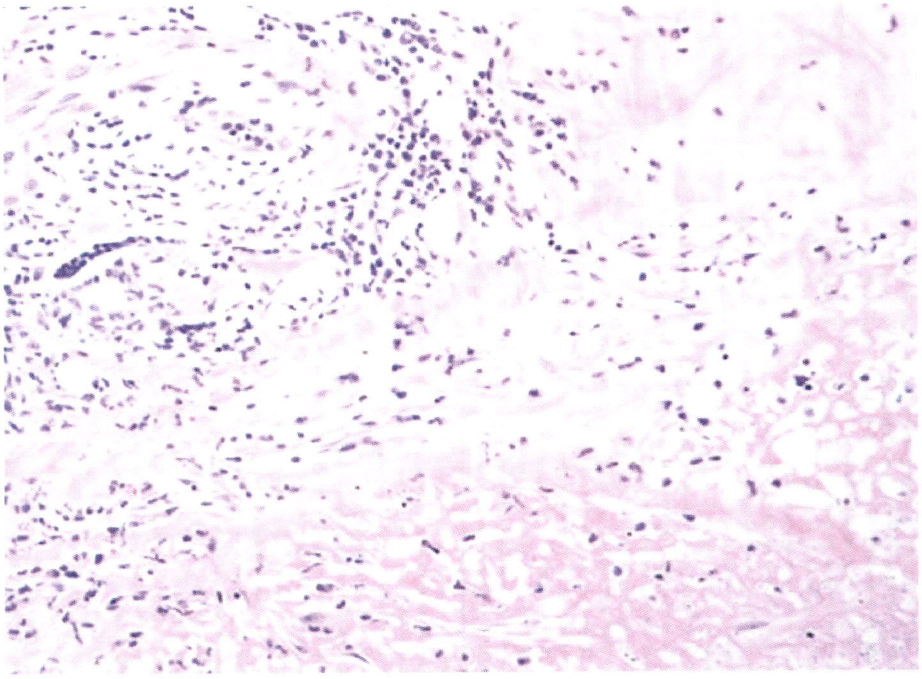

FIGURE 10.4. Zonal necrosis is a helpful feature in distinguishing subcutaneous T-cell lymphoma from reactive panniclitides.

References

1. Marzano AV, Berti E, Paulli M, Caputo R. Cytophagic histiocytic panniculitis and subcutaneous panniculitis-like T-cell lymphoma: Report of 7 cases. *Arch Dermatol* 2000; 136: 889–896.
2. Mehregan DA, Su WPD, Kurtin PJ. Subcutaneous T-cell lymphoma: A clinical, histopathologic, and immunohistochemical study of six cases. *J Cutan Pathol* 1994; 21: 110–117.
3. Romero LS, Goltz RW, Nagi C, Shin SS, Ho AD. Subcutaneous T-cell lymphoma with associated hemophagocytic syndrome and terminal leukemic transformation. *J Am Acad Dermatol* 1996; 34: 904–910.
4. Magro CM, Crowson AN, Bryd JC, Soleymani AD, Shendrik I. Atypical lymphocytic lobular panniculitis. *J Cutan Pathol* 2004; 31: 300–306.
5. Salhany KE, Macon WR, Choi JK, Elenitasa R, Lessin SR, Felgar RE, Wilson DM, Przybylski GK, Lister J, Wasik MA, Swerdlow SH. Subcutaneous panniculitis-like T-cell lymphoma: Clinicopathologic, immunophenotypic, and genotypic analysis of alpha-beta and gamma/delta subtypes. *Am J Surg Pathol* 1998; 22: 881–893.
6. Yamashita Y, Tsuzuki T, Nakayama A, Fujino M, Nori M. A case of natural killer/T cell lymphoma of the subcutis resembling subcutaneous panniculitis-like T cell lymphoma. *Pathol Int* 1999; 49: 241–246.
7. Takeshita M, Imayama S, Oshiro Y, Kurihara K, Okamoto S, Matsuki Y, Nakashima Y, Okamura T, Shiratsuchi M, Hayashi T, Kikuchi M. Clinicopathologic analysis of 22 cases of subcutaneous panniculitis-like CD56– or CD56+ lymphoma and review of 44 other reported cases. *Am J Clin Pathol* 2004: 121: 408–416.

Part II
Hereditary Cancer-Predisposition Syndromes and Paraneoplastic Disorders

11
Muir-Torre Syndrome

■ Synonyms:	None
■ Etiology:	Mutations in MLH1 and/or MSH2
■ Associations:	Visceral malignancies (mainly gastrointestinal)
■ Clinical:	Asymptomatic yellow papule/nodule
■ Histology:	Lobules of sebocytes surrounded by basaloid keratinocytes
■ IHC repertoire:	EMA+
■ Staging:	N/A
■ Prognosis:	100% benign
■ Adverse variables:	Visceral malignancies
■ Treatment:	Careful screening

Sebaceous adenomas are benign adnexal tumors that have no malignant potential. They are of no clinical significance in isolation, but may be indicators of internal malignancy when occurring as part of the Muir-Torre syndrome. Sebaceous adenomas grow as exophytic, yellowish papules and nodules. In most cases, these lesions are less than 1 cm in diameter (1). While they may occur at any body site, they are most common on the face. They usually appear in middle age. Ulceration is not a common feature.

Muir-Torre is inherited in an autosomal dominant manner (2). It has a high degree of penetrance and variable expression. The syndrome is twice as common in men as in women. It usually manifests in middle age, with the sixth decade the most common time of onset. In some studies, as many as 61% of afflicted families will have a family history of visceral malignancy (3). The syndrome is defined as the presence of at least one sebaceous neoplasm (excluding sebaceous hyperplasia and nevus sebaceous of Jadassohn) or keratoacanthoma with sebaceous differentiation, and one visceral cancer. Alternatively, a patient with multiple keratoacanthomas, multiple visceral malignancies and a family history of Muir-Torre syndrome can be so classified (2). In most cases, however, multiple cutaneous neoplasms are present (Figure 11.1). In one review, the cutaneous tumors preceded the development of the visceral cancers in 22% of cases, occurred concurrently in an additional 6%, and presented after the internal malignancy in 56%. No temporal relationship was established in the other cases (4).

An inherited mutation of the mismatch DNA repair gene MSH2 has been reported in many patients with Muir-Torre syndrome (5). Others have reported germline mutations in the MLH1 mismatch repair gene (6).

Sebaceous adenomas may occur as part of the Muir-Torre syndrome. Multiple sebaceous neoplasms, keratoacanthomas, and visceral carcinomas characterize this syndrome (Table 11.1) (2). The sebaceous tumors include sebaceous adenomas, epitheliomas, sebaceomas, and sebaceous carcinomas. Most investigators do not include sebaceous hyperplasia as a criterion for the syndrome, as the vast majority of these lesions are unrelated to a systemic process. The cutaneous neoplasms tend to be indolent. Even the sebaceous carcinomas, which can behave aggressively when isolated, do not usually metastasize in patients with the Muir-Torre syndrome. Keratoacanthomas also occur most frequently outside of the syndrome, but when multipled, may suggest visceral malignancy. Gastrointestinal, and more specifically, colonic adenocarcinomas are the most common visceral malignancies experienced by patients with the Muir Torre syndrome (Table 11.2). The colonic adenocarcinomas occur a decade earlier than in the general population and are more frequently located proximal to the splenic flexure. They tend to behave in a relatively indolent fashion.

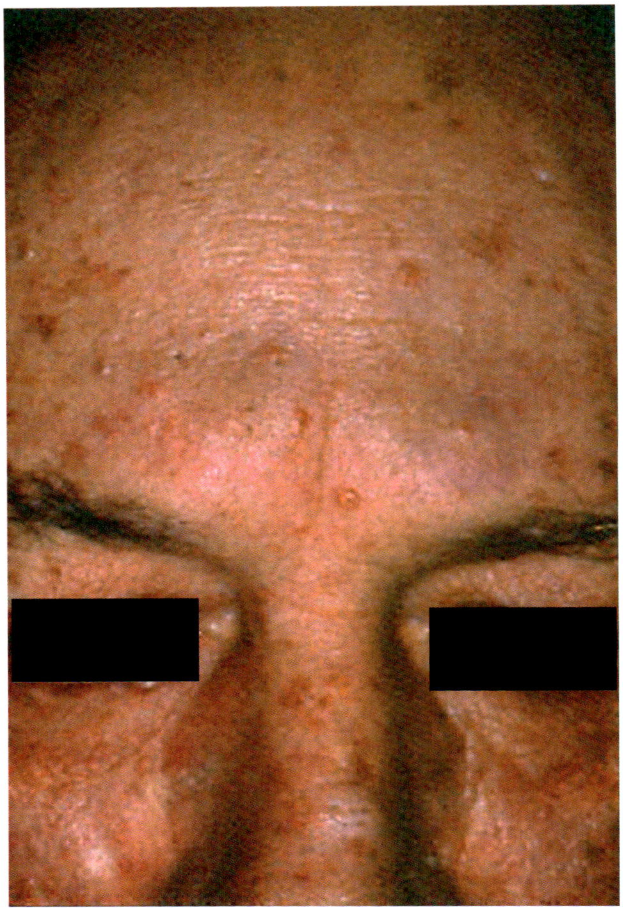

FIGURE 11.1. Multiple tan umbilicated papules representing sebaceous adenoma and sebaceous hyperplasia in patient with Muir-Torre syndrome.

TABLE 11.1. Tumors Associated with Muir-Torre Syndrome (Expressed as Percentage of Affected Patients)

Tumor	Percentage of Patients with MTS
Sebaceous adenoma	>90
Sebaceous carcinoma	24
Other sebaceous neoplasms	
Keratoacanthoma	22
Colonic polyps	48
2–3 Visceral neoplasms	37
>3 Visceral neoplasms	10

Sebaceous adenomas are neoplasms that are centered in the mid-reticular dermis. In some cases, they arise from follicular epithelium that is connected to the epidermis, while in other cases, the epidermal connection may not be apparent. Lobules of mature sebocytes with abundant clear cytoplasm are surrounded by a collarette of more basaloid-appearing cells. The basal layer palisades around the outside of the lobules and the cells within demonstrate progressive maturation as they move toward the middle of the lobules (Figures 11.2A and 11.2B). Mitoses may be seen in small numbers, but no atypical forms are present. Cytologic atypia is minimal and necrosis is not a common feature.

Sebaceous epitheliomas differ from sebaceous adenomas in having a larger percentage of basaloid cells and smaller percentage of mature sebocytes (Figure 11.3). Some investigators believe these to be indistinguishable from basal cell carcinomas with sebaceous differentiation. There is some overlap between sebaceous epithelioma and the more recently described tumor known as sebaceoma (7). The distinction from sebaceous adenoma is academic, as the prognosis for each of these neoplasms is invariably benign.

Sebaceous carcinomas are most prevalent, arising from the meibomian glands in the eyelids. However, they can occur in any hair-bearing body site. Eyelid lesions occur primarily in elderly patients, whereas extraocular neoplasms are more common in middle-aged men. Sebaceous carcinomas unassociated with the Muir Torre syndrome have a relatively high rate of metastasis, but this appears to be much lower when occurring in conjunction with the syndrome. These tumors demonstrate the characteristics of malignant neoplasms (Figure 11.4A and 11.4B). They are characterized by cells with greatly increased nucleus: cytoplasm ratios, high mitotic activity, abundant individual cell necrosis, and marked nuclear pleomorphism. Sebaceous differentiation may be difficult to detect. Immunostains with epithelial

TABLE 11.2. Visceral Tumors Associated with Muir-Torre Syndrome (Expressed as Percentage of Total Tumors)

Colonic Adenocarcinoma	50
Genitourinary carcinoma	24
Breast	5
Non-Hodgkin's lymphoma	2
Head and neck squamous cell carcinoma	3.9
Small intestinal adenocarcinoma	3.9
Lung carcinoma	1.5

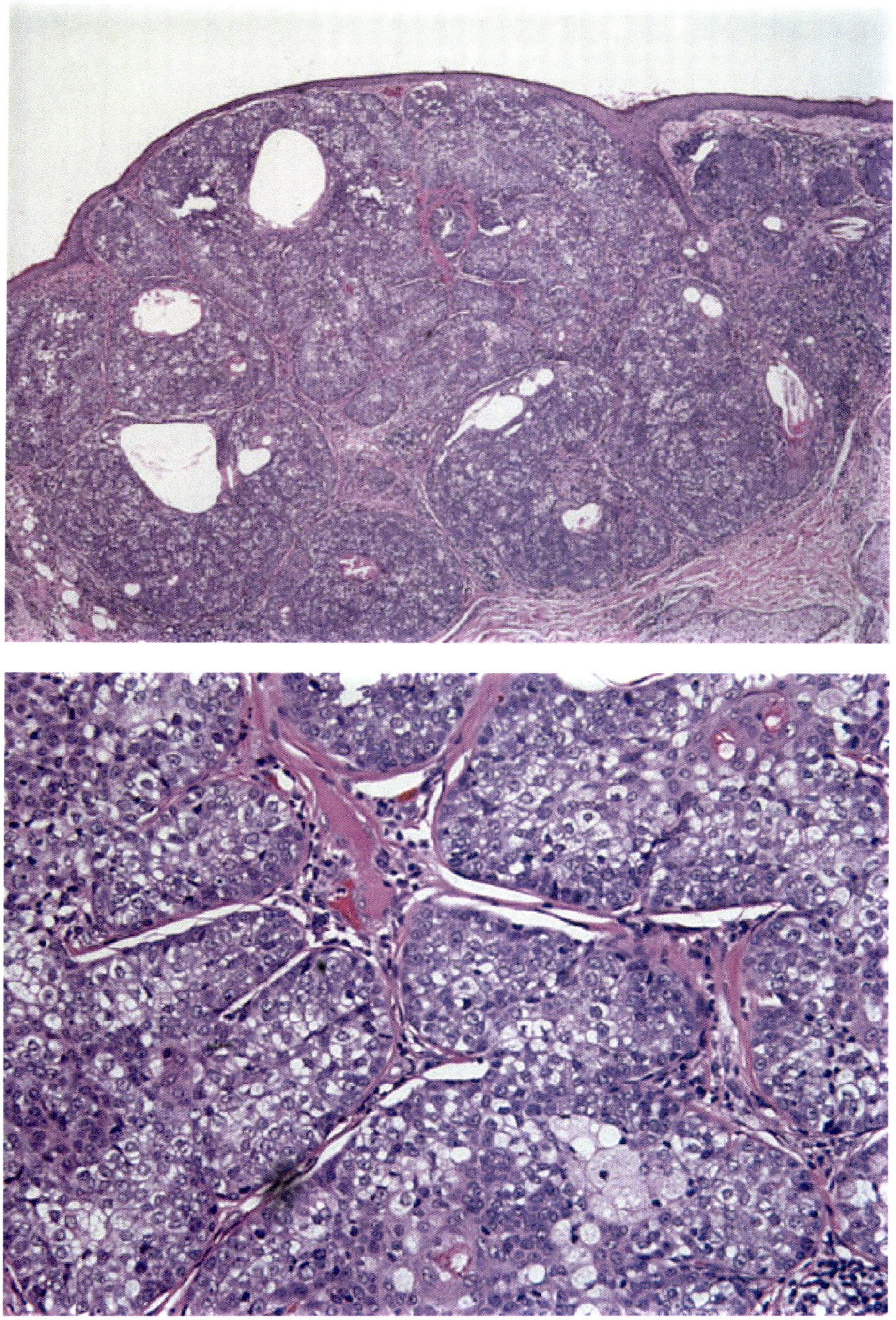

A

B

Figure 11.2. (A) Low power photomicrograph depicting lobular architecture of sebaceous adenoma. (B) High power photomicrograph depicting lobules of sebocytes. Note central mature sebocytes with clear-foamy cytoplasm and more immature basaloid cells at periphery.

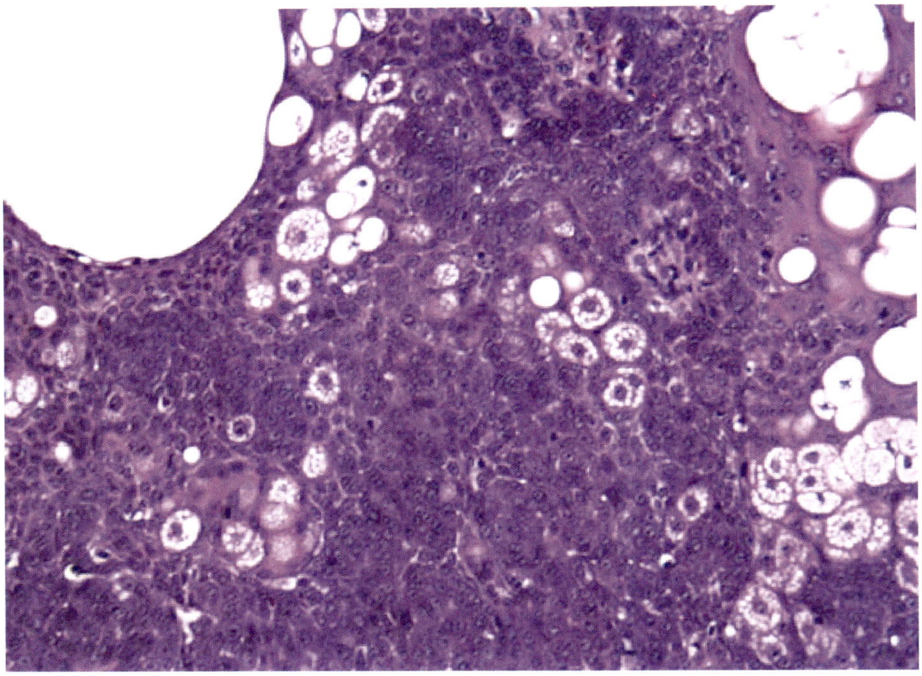

FIGURE 11.3. Predominance of basaloid cells in sebaceous epithelioma.

membrane antigen may be helpful in isolating the intracytoplasmic microvesiculation frequently seen in sebocytic differentiation.

Keratoacanthoma is a controversial entity that is considered by many to represent a rapidly growing yet indolent variant of cutaneous squamous cell carcinoma (8). The discussion of the etiology of these neoplasms is outside the purview of this volume. The histologic features of keratoacanthoma are best detected at low magnification. These tumors demonstrate a cup-shaped, invaginated

A

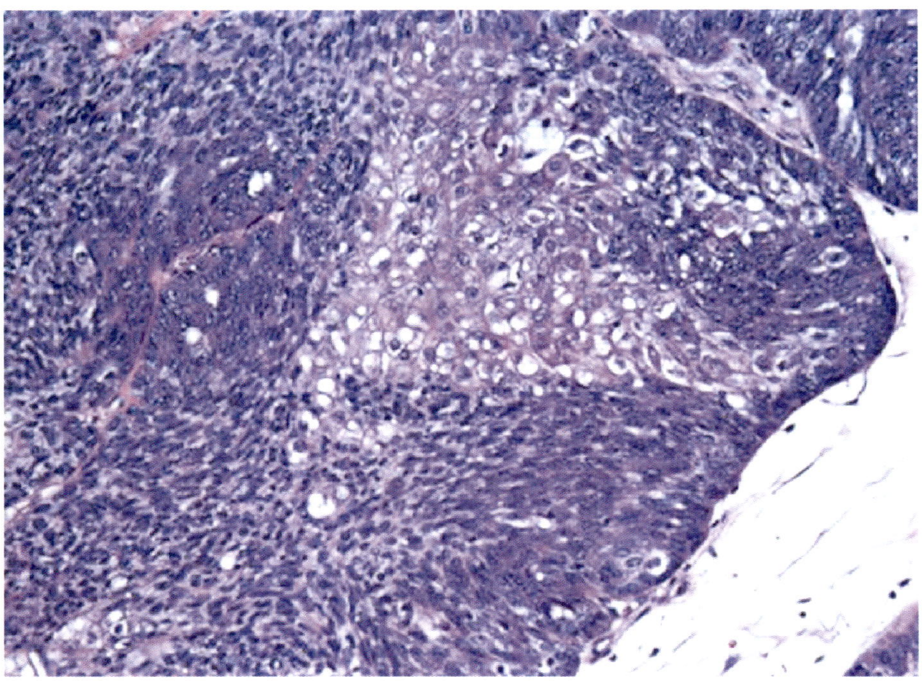

FIGURE 11.4. (A) Medium power photomicrograph of sebaceous carcinoma. Note the predominance of basaloid cells and the cellularity of the neoplasm.

FIGURE 11.4. (B) High power photomicrograph depicting the close apposition of the cells producing the cellularity of sebaceous carcinoma. Note the hyperchromatic nuclei of sebaceous carcinoma.

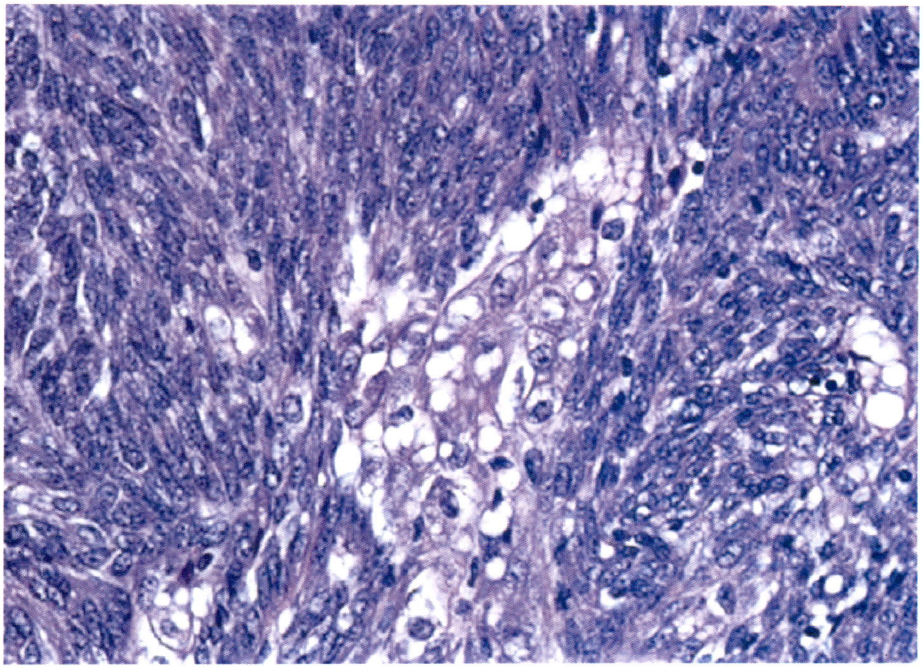

B

growth pattern. The central dell is filled with abundant keratin that is often orthokeratotic. Beneath the invagination, sheets of keratinocytes with abundant, often pale-staining cytoplasm extend into the dermis. These cells may demonstrate nuclear atypia, pleomorphism, and a high mitotic rate (Figure 11.5A and 11.5B). In many cases, there is a brisk underlying host response and in resolving lesions, dermal fibrosis may signify the regressing phase of the lesion.

Distinction between keratoacanthoma and other types of cutaneous squamous cell carcinoma is not always possible.

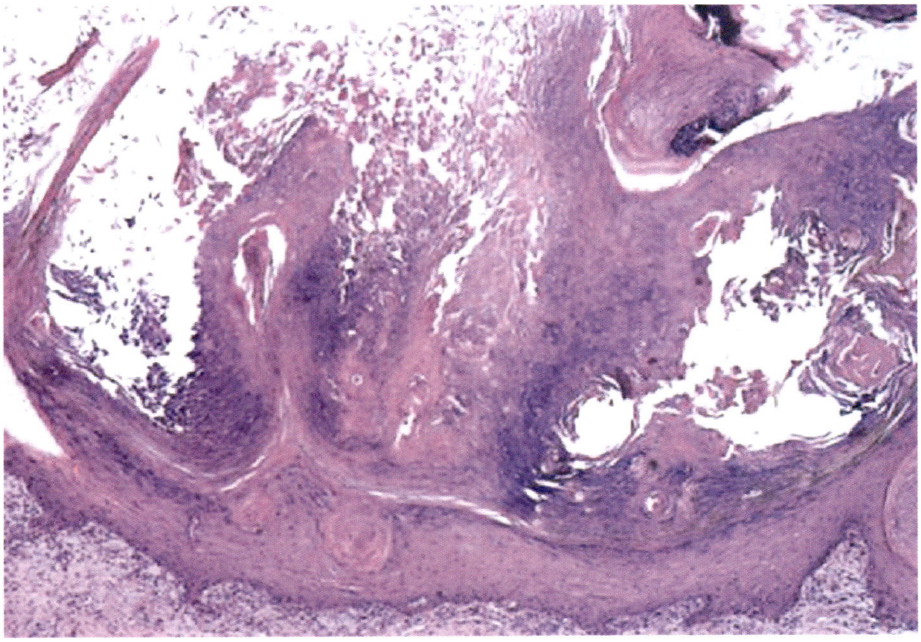

A

FIGURE 11.5. (A) Low power photomicrograph depicting the cup-shaped architecture of keratoacanthoma.

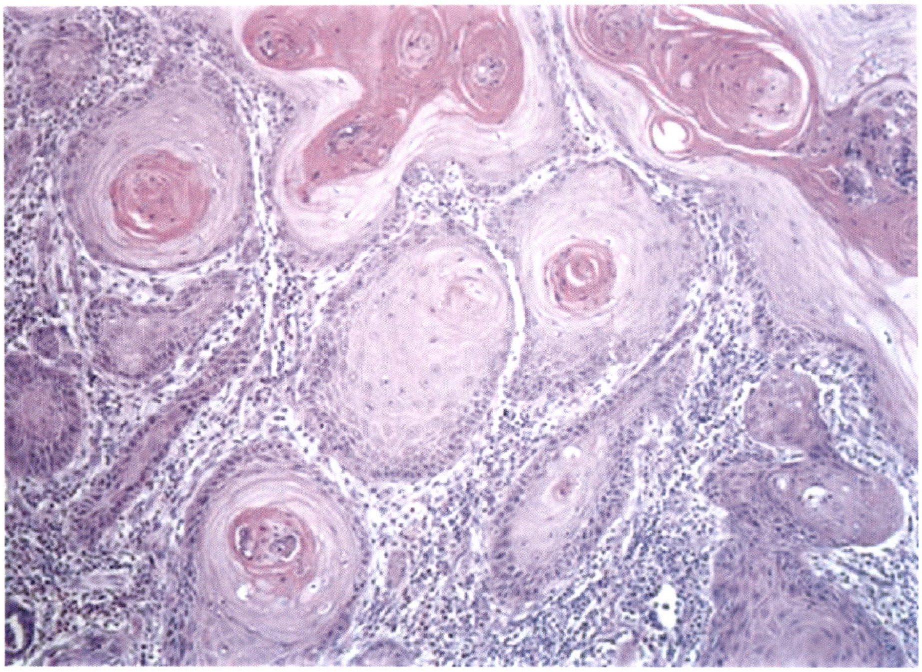

B

FIGURE 11.5. (B) Medium power photomicrograph depicting the irregular infiltrating islands of neoplastic keratinocytes typical of invasive well-differentiated squamous cell carcinoma.

References

1. Rulon DB, Helwig EB. Cutaneous sebaceous neoplasms. *Cancer* 1974; 33: 82–102.
2. Schartz RA. The Muir-Torre syndrome: A 25-year retrospective. *J Am Acad Dermatol* 1995; 33: 90–104.
3. Cohen PR, Kohn SR, Kurzrock R. Association of sebaceous gland tumors and internal malignancy: The Muir-Torre syndrome. *Am J Med* 1991; 90: 606–613.
4. Akhtar S, Oza KK, Khan SA, Wright J. Muir-Torre syndrome: Case report of a patient with concurrent jejunal and ureteral cancer and a review of the literature. *J Am Acad Dermatol* 1999; 41: 681–686.
5. Nystrom-Lahti M, Parsons R, Sistonen P, Pylkkanen L, Aaltonen LA, Leach FS, Hamilton SR, Watson P, Bronsen E., Fusar, R, et al. Mismatch repair genes on chromosomes 2p and 3p account for a major share of hereditary nonpolyposis colorectal cancer families evaluable by linkage. *Am J Human Genet* 1994; 55: 659–665.
6. Mathiak M, Rutten A, Mangold E, Fischer H-P, Ruzicka T, Friedl W, Propping P, Kruse R. Loss of DNA mismatch repair proteins in skin tumors from patients with Muir-Torre syndrome and MSH2 or MLH1 germline mutations: Establishment of immunohistochemical analysis as a screening test. *Am J Surg Pathol* 2002; 26: 338–343.
7. Troy JL, Ackerman AB. Sebaceoma. A distinctive benign neoplasm of adnexal epithelium differentiating toward sebaceous cells. *Am J Dermatopathol* 1984; 6: 7–13.
8. Hodek E, Jones RE, Ackerman AB. Solitary keratoacanthoma is a squamous-cell carcinoma: Three examples with metastases. *Am J Dermatopathol* 1993; 15: 332–342.

12
Acquired Ichthyosis, Acanthosis Nigricans, Palmar Hyperkeratosis

■ Synonyms:	AI—Pityriasis rotunda AN—None PH—Tylosis, Howel-Evans Syndrome, tripe palms, acrokeratosis of Bazex
■ Etiology:	Unknown
■ Associations:	AI—Lymphoma AN—Gastric carcinoma PH—Esophageal carcinoma
■ Clinical:	AI—Diffuse xerosis AN—Axillary pigmentation PH—Palmar/plantar hyperkeratosis
■ Histology:	AI—Hypogranulosis with hyperkeratosis AN—Acanthosis with hyperkeratosis PH—Acanthosis with hyperkeratosis and hypergranulosis
■ IHC repertoire:	N/A
■ Staging:	N/A
■ Prognosis:	Generally poor, associated with advanced internal malignancy
■ Adverse variables:	Dependent upon underlying malignancy type and stage of disease
■ Treatment:	Dependent upon tumor type and stage

Serious systemic diseases, including visceral cancer, may be indirectly signaled by the development of distinctive cutaneous eruptions. Important aspects of these eruptions include development of the rash concurrent with the diagnosis of the neoplasm and the fact that the two entities, though individually uncommon, are commonly seen together and pursue a similar clinical course. The more important, albeit uncommon, dermatoses that develop in conjunction with visceral cancer involve disorders of the epithelium and entail alterations in keratinization. This chapter will deal with the clinical and pathologic attributes of acquired ichthyosis, acanthosis nigricans, and paraneoplastic palmar/plantar keratoderma as they relate to underlying malignancy.

Ichthyosis refers to the presence of fish-like (Lat. *ikhthus*) or scaly skin. The characteristic clinical appearance is due to an inherited defect in keratinization involving the epithelium that with rare exception represents little more than a lifelong cosmetic nuisance. Acquired ichthyosis, however, referring to the sudden development of scaly-dry skin in the adult, may herald the presence of a serious underlying malignancy. The eruption usually develops over the extensor aspects of the extremities and scalp resembling the appearance of the most common autosomal dominant form, *ichthyosis vulgaris* (1). The rash typically spares the flexural folds. Erythema may be seen between the scaly fissures. The most common underlying malignancy is Hodgkin's and non-Hodgkin's lymphoma and the stage of the disease is often quite advanced. The rash may, however, presage the malignancy by many years. Important systemic illnesses that may also produce or be associated with acquired ichthyosis include malnutrition, HIV disease, hypothyroidism, leprosy, sarcoidosis, lupus erythematosus, dermatomyositis, bone marrow transplant in the setting of graft-versus-host disease, eosinophilic fascitis, and may follow exposure to certain medications such as nicotinic acid, triparanol, butyrophenone, dixyrazine, nafoxidine, clofazimine, and cetrimide (2,3). Among HIV-positive individuals, its development may be a marker for concomitant infection by the *human T-cell leukemia/lymphoma virus (HTLV-II)* (4). In dark-skinned races, the rash may produce sharply demarcated round-to-oval scaly patches termed *pityriasis rotunda* (5). The histopathology is distinctive and consists of a normally thickened epithelium with compacted hyperkeratosis. The epidermal granular layer is characteristically absent. The altered keratin layer may also extend down adjacent follicular ostia (acrotrichia). Supportive therapy is directed toward hydration of the skin (bathing, high ambient humidity) and the application of lubricants (creams and ointments). Investigation for the possibility of underlying malignancy, particularly hematologic cancer, with appropriate imaging studies and consideration for bone marrow examination is indicated.

Acanthosis nigricans (AN) is a common cutaneous malady associated with myriad unrelated systemic diseases including underlying cancer (6). The most common association involves obesity with or without insulin resistance and hyperinsulinemia. In most instances, the eruption begins as gray-black thickening of the flexural areas, and in particular, the axillae (Figure 12.1). Palpation of the involved areas yields a textural change likened to velvet. The eruption may rarely spread to involve the non-flexural areas and even the oral and anogenital mucosa. Certain demographic groups are overrepresented, including Hispanics and African-Americans. Rare familial tendencies have also been identified, suggestive of an underlying genetic predisposition. The pathogenesis is thought to involve a patterned response of the skin to increased serum levels of trophic epithelial hormones and cytokines, presumably released in conjunction with the underlying endocrinologic or neoplastic dyscrasia. In the setting of hyperinsulinemia and diabetes mellitus, it has been shown that excess binding of insulin to IGF receptors located on keratinocytes and fibroblasts results in increased proliferation. Similarly, increased transforming growth factor (TGF) released by neoplastic cells has been shown to increase keratinocyte proliferation via surface epidermal growth factor receptors. Other important disease associations include *h*yper*a*ndrogen states with *i*nsulin *r*esistance and *a*canthosis *n*igricans (*HAIR-AN syndrome*). Certain medications including nicotinic acid, glucocorticoids, triazinate, and the sex hormones including estrogen have also been implicated in its development. AN associated with underlying malignancy, alternatively referred to as *malignant* AN, is morphologically similar yet characterized by rapid onset and progression (7–9). It more commonly is associated with keratoderma or rugose-like thickening of the palms in which there is accentuation of the fingerprints, otherwise known as pachydermatoglyphy (or *tripe palm*) (10). Other important associations include oral involvement and the presence of multiple eruptive seborrheic keratosis (the sign of *Leser-Trelat*) (Figure 12.2). The most common internal malignancy is visceral adenocarcinoma of the stomach, intestines, or lung. Bladder, renal, and esophageal carcinoma, and lymphoma have also been reported as well. In most instances, the lesions are discovered in conjunction with internal malignancy diagnosis. The eruption, however, may precede or follow diagnosis of internal malignancy. The histopathology yields slight epidermal acanthosis with papillomatosis and hyperkeratosis (Figure 12.3). Although the basilar layer keratinocytes may show increased amounts of cytoplasmic melanin, the clinical appearance of hyperpigmentation is largely due to the epidermal hyperkeratosis.

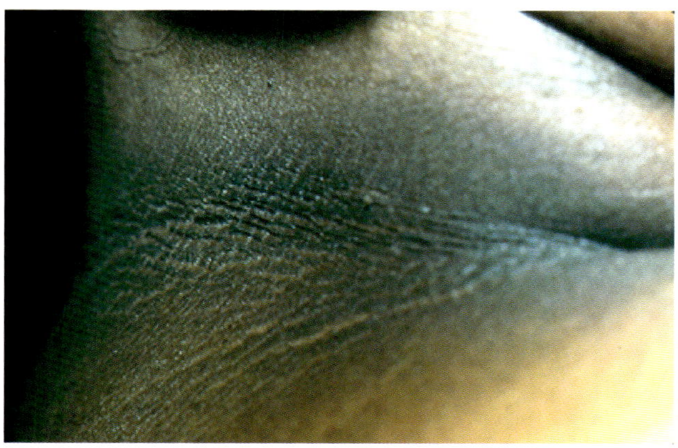

FIGURE 12.1. Velvety hyperpigmented intertriginous plaque in acanthosis nigricans.

The acquired *palmar/plantar keratodermas* comprise a heterogeneous group of keratinizing disorders characterized by thickening of the palms and soles that in many instances are associated with the development of visceral cancer (Figure 12.4) (11). These conditions are distinct from the more common forms of inherited palmoplantar keratoderma that typically manifest in children and are associated with inherited defects in keratinization. The acquired keratodermas can be broadly separated into three categories that involve diffuse thickening, punctate areas of thickening, or additional areas of the non-acral skin. The most well-documented form of diffuse acquired keratoderma was described by Dr. Howel-Evans in 1958 among two kindreds afflicted with esophageal carcinoma (12,13). This condition, alternatively referred to as *tylosis* or *Howel-Evans* syndrome, involves the development of

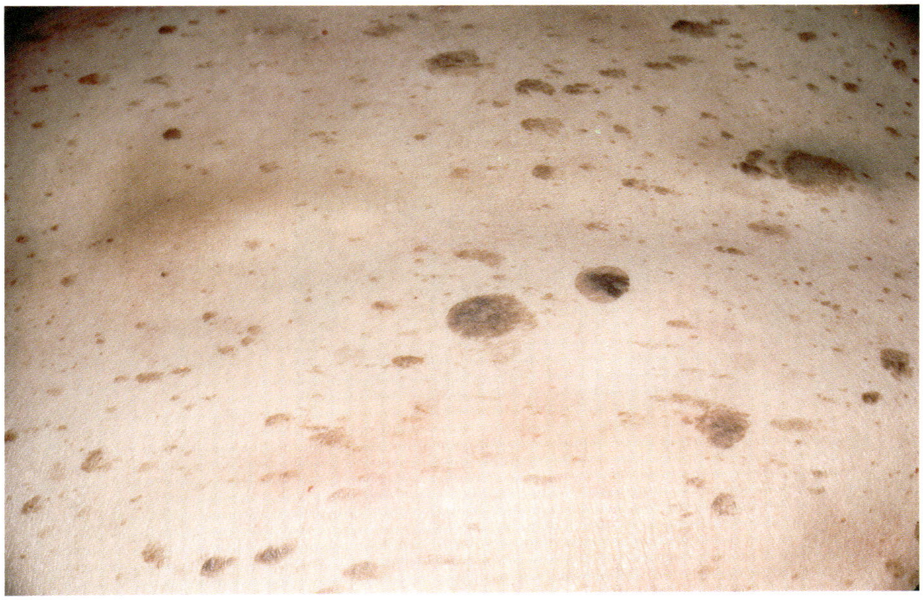

FIGURE 12.2. Sign of Leser-Trelat. Multiple seborrheic keratosis on trunk of patient with metastatic colorectal carcinoma.

poorly demarcated and irregular areas of palmar or plantar thickening in children who later develop esophageal carcinoma as adults. The gene responsible for this condition has been linked adjacent to the keratin type I gene cluster (17q24) (14). The punctate form of acquired keratoderma is associated with the development of breast and gynecologic malignancies. Finally, acquired keratoderma may be associated with an erythematous and psoriasiform dermatitis involving the non-acral skin. Referred to as *acrokeratosis of Bazex*, patients with this entity are typically male and are predisposed to develop carcinoma of the upper and lower aerodigestive tracts (15). The thickened areas of the palms and soles often appear erythematous or violaceous. Keratoderma has also been described among patients with hematologic malignancies including multiple myeloma, lymphoma, and mycosis fungoides.

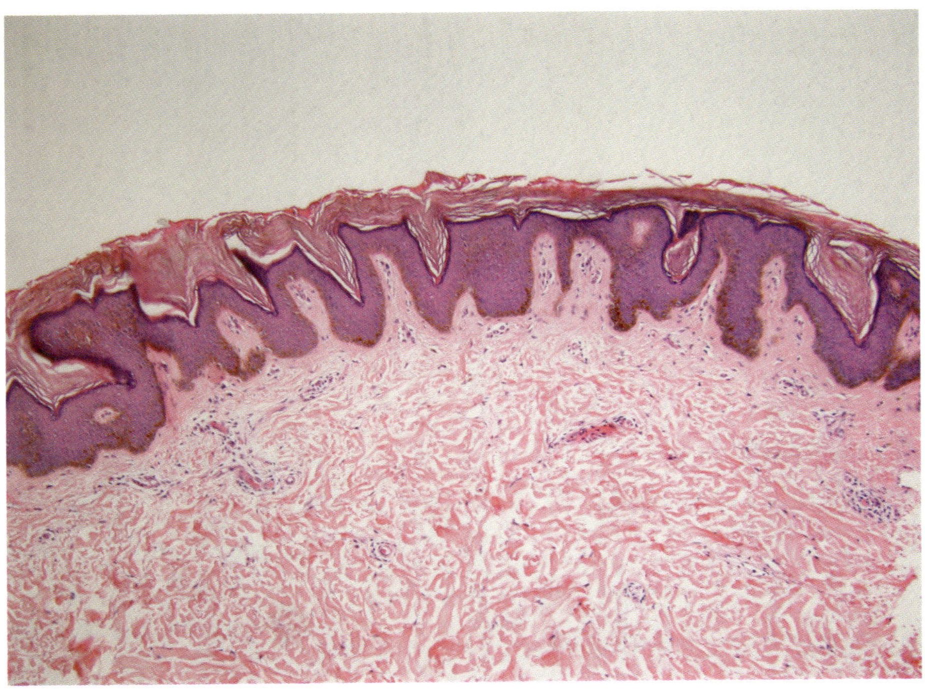

FIGURE 12.3. Medium power photomicrograph depicting domelike epidermal acanthosis with hyperpigmented basilar layer keratinocytes, seen in acanthosis nigricans.

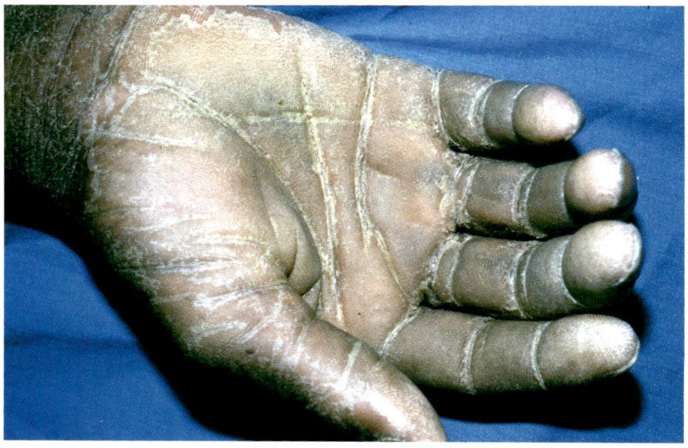

FIGURE 12.4. Hyperkeratosis of the palmar skin seen in the keratodermas. Note the accentuated palmar creases.

Non-neoplastic conditions including myxedema, arsenic exposure, menopause (*keratoderma climactericum*), water exposure (*aquagenic keratoderma*), and following ingestion of certain medications including glucan, tegafur, and fluoruracil, have been shown to also produce acquired keratoderma (11). The diffuse form of keratoderma histologically shows epidermal acanthosis and orthokeratotic hyperkeratosis with occasional epidermolytic hyperkeratosis. The punctate form shows a dense keratin plug of the stratum corneum with underlying depression of the stratum malpighii and adjacent pitting of the stratum corneum (Figure 12.5). Biopsy changes observed in conjunction with acrokeratosis of Bazex include acanthosis, hyperkeratosis, and exocytosis of lymphocytes with accompanying spongiosis and epidermal dyskeratosis.

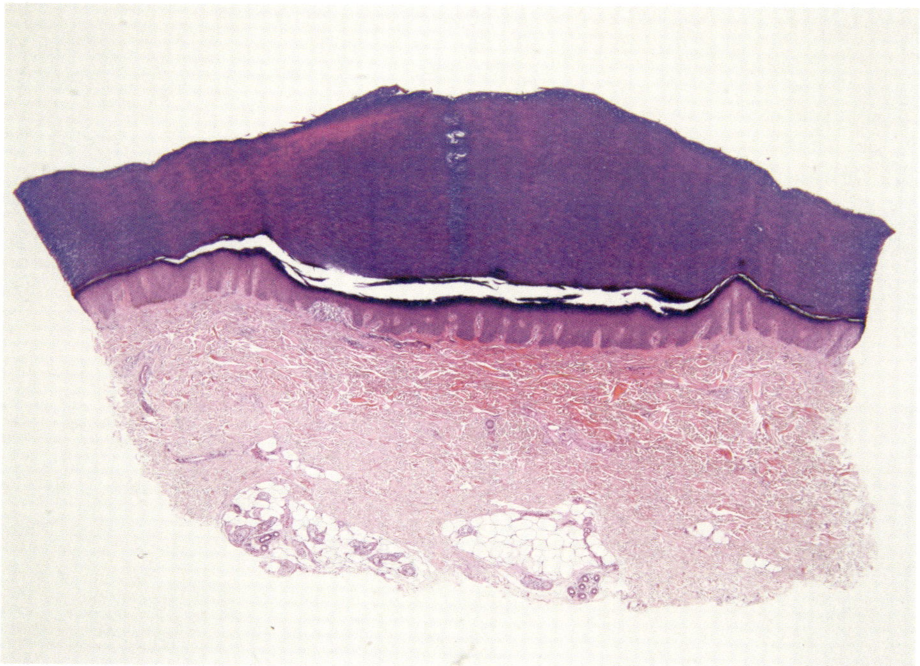

FIGURE 12.5. Low power photomicrograph depicting the exaggerated hyperkeratosis with central swelling observed in punctate keratoderma.

References

Acquired Ichthyosis

1. Aram H. Acquired ichthyosis and related conditions. *Int J Dermatol* 1984; 23: 458.
2. Dykes P, Marks R. Acquired ichthyosis: Multiple causes for an acquired generalized disturbance in desquamation. *Br J Dermatol* 1977; 97: 327.
3. Spleman L, Strutton G, Robertson I, et al. Acquired ichthyosis in bone marrow transplant recipients. *J Am Acad Dermatol* 1996; 35: 17.
4. Kaplan M, Sadick N, McNutt N, et al. Acquired ichthyosis in concomitant HIV-1 and HTLV-11 infection: A new association with intravenous drug abuse. *J Am Acad Dermatol* 1993; 29: 701.
5. Aste N, Pau M, Aste N, et al. Pityriasis rotunda: A survey of 42 cases observed in Sardinia, Italy. *Dermatology* 1997; 194: 32.

Acanthosis Nigricans

6. Schwartz R. Acanthosis nigricans. *J Am Acad Dermatol* 1994; 31:1.

7. Andreev V. Malignant acanthosis nigricans. *Semin Dermatol* 1984; 3: 265.
8. Rigel D, Jacobs M. Malignant acanthosis nigricans: A review. *J Dermatol Surg Oncol* 1980; 6: 923.
9. Brown J, Winkelman R. Acanthosis nigricans: A study of 90 cases. *Medicine* 1968; 47: 33.
10. Breathnach S, Wells G. Acanthosis palmaris: Tripe palms. *Clin Exp Dermatol* 1980; 5: 181.

Palmoplantar Keratoderma

11. Zemtsov A, Veitschegger M. Keratodermas. *Int J Dermatol* 1993; 32: 493.
12. Howel-Evans W, McConnell R, Clarke C, et al. Carcinoma of the oesophagus with keratosis palmaris et plantaris (tylosis). *Q J Med* 1958; 27: 413.
13. Marger R, Marger D. Carcinoma of the esophagus and tylosis. A lethal genetic combination. *Cancer* 1993; 72: 17.
14. Stevens H, Kelsell D, Bryant S, et al. Linkage of an American pedigree with palmoplantar keratoderma and malignancy (palmoplantar ectodermal dysplasia type III) to 17q24. *Arch Dermatol* 1996; 132: 640.
15. Bazex A, Griffiths A. Acrokeratosis paraneoplastica: A new cutaneous marker of malignancy? *Br J Dermatol* 1980; 102: 301.

13
Amyloidosis: Systemic, Nodular, and Epidermal Derived

■ Synonyms:	S—Primary, AL type, myeloma-associated N—None ED—Macular, lichenoid
■ Etiology:	S—Plasma-cell-derived light chains N—Plasma-cell-derived light chains ED—Epidermal keratins
■ Associations:	S—Multiple myeloma in 1/3 pts. N—10% with systemic amyloidosis ED—None
■ Clinical:	S—Hemorrhagic papules/plaques N—Waxy nodules ED—Hyperpigmented macules and lichenoid papules
■ Histology:	S—Fissured hyaline deposits, perivascular deposits N—Hyaline deposits c/ plasma cells ED—Hyaline dermal globules
■ IHC:	S—Monoclonal kappa or lambda light chain N—Monoclonal kappa or lambda light chain ED—Keratins
■ Staging:	N/A
■ Prognosis:	S—Poor in myeloma patients N—Dependent upon systemic status ED—Excellent
■ Adverse outcome:	S—Myeloma, cardiac disease N—Systemic amyloidosis ED—None
■ Treatment:	S—Chemotherapy N—Excision, laser, crythotherapy ED—Topical retinoids

The amyloidoses encompass a broad category of cutaneous and systemic disorders with important pathogenic consequences. These derive from the direct deposition of abnormal proteins or indirectly relate to potentially deadly systemic disorders that produce such deposits. Each of the amyloidoses can be defined by certain histomorphologic and chemical properties that permit their identification and inclusion into disease categories (1). These designations can be loosely grouped into systemic and cutaneous delimited forms.

The term *amyloidosis* historically derives from the gross starch-like deposits seen in conjunction with systemic amyloidosis. Despite the appellation, the chemical constituency of amyloid is either protein or glycoprotein. Each of the 16 chemical types possess similar histomorphologic and chemical properties including a predominantly extracellular location, an amorphous eosinophilic appearance on hematoxylin and eosin staining, and a meshwork of hollow 7.5- to 10-nanometer linear nonbranched fibrils on ultrastructural examination (2). The fibrils often align into a three-dimensional beta-pleated sheet configuration that is held responsible for their birefringence properties on diagnostic polaroscopic examination. Amyloid fibrils often associate with certain disease defining non-amyloid glycoproteins including *Protein P* (systemic disease) and *apolipoprotein E* (Alzheimer's disease). Among the various types of amyloid, only a few are commonly observed in the skin and thus merit discussion. The two most important responsible for the bulk of dermatologic disease derive from plasma-cell-produced immunoglobulin kappa or lambda light chains or from epidermal keratinocyte keratins. The former are seen in conjunction with primary or systemic amyloidosis and *nodular amyloidosis*, whereas the latter are seen in *macular* and *lichenoid amyloidosis*. The light chains may be monoclonal and systemically produced from abnormal collections of bone marrow or reticuloendothelial-associated plasma cells in multiple myeloma or lymphoma, or monoclonal and produced locally within the skin from associated plasma cells. The keratins deposited in macular/lichenoid amyloidosis derive from degenerated epidermal keratinocytes and as such are typically seen as aggregates in the superficial dermis juxtaposed to the overlying epithelium.

Primary and *myeloma-associated amyloidosis* involves the skin in approximately one-third of patients (3). Typical patients are in their sixties with a slight male predominance. There is no known ethnic predilection. Although the dermatologic manifestations may be overshadowed by the systemic stigmata of macroglossia, bilateral or unilateral carpal tunnel syndrome, or hepatosplenomegaly, distinctive cutaneous changes are often present. Waxy papules and nodules are typically seen on the flexural folds of the face, trunk, and extremities. The papules may undergo secondary hemorrhage and are rarely ulcerated. Mucocutaneous nodules may assume a warty appearance reminiscent of condyloma or a flattened plaque-like configuration suggestive of xanthoma. Non-vasculitic purpuric macules, petechiae, and ecchymoses are common, particularly in flexural fold areas such as the eyelids. Purpuric lesions may be elicited with trauma (*pinch purpura*) (Figure 13.1) or following a precipitous increase in intrathoracic pressure (Valsalva maneuver). Less common manifestations include diffuse involvement of the scalp (cutis verticis gyrata) and alopecia, scleroderma-like induration of the extremities, bullous lesions, nail dystrophy, cutis laxa, and cord-like thickening of the blood vessels. Important systemic signs and complications stemming from visceral organ involvement include the heart, reticuloendothelial system, blood vessels, and peripheral and autonomic nervous system. Cardiac disease is the most important cause of mortality with most cases resulting in arrythmias, congestive heart failure, or ischemic heart disease. Hepatosplenomegaly is seen in approximately one-half of patients and is an important cause of morbidity. Amyloid infiltration of the blood vessels may produce ischemic claudication of the gastrointestinal tract, extremities, or heart. Peripheral and autonomic neuropathy is common, with the latter often producing orthostatic hypotension. Massive amyloid deposits within the soft tissues of the wrist or when located around the shoulders (providing the *shoulder pad sign*) may result in carpal tunnel syndrome.

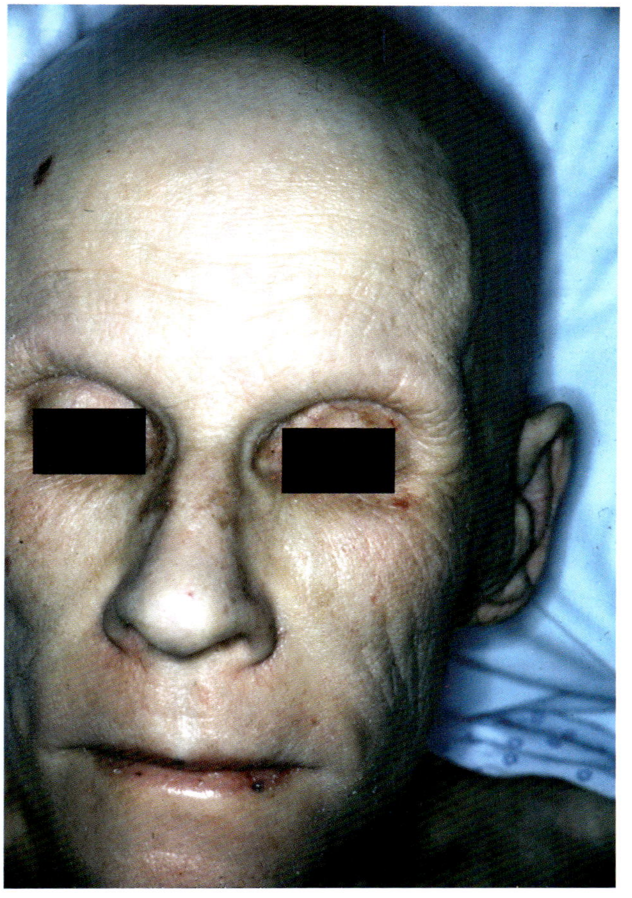

FIGURE 13.1. Periorbital purpura seen in systemic amyloidosis.

Other less common forms of systemic amyloidosis that rarely manifest in the skin include *secondary* or inflammatory-associated amyloidosis, and the extremely rare heredofamilial syndromes of *familial Mediterranean fever* (urticaria, vasculitic purpura, fever, serositis, and renal amyloid) and *Muckle-Wells* syndrome (urticaria, fever, deafness, and renal amyloidosis) (1).

The lesions of *nodular* or *localized amyloidosis* tend to be less numerous and individually larger than systemic amyloidosis. Demographically, most patients are in their sixties and there tends to be a male predominance. Lesions may occur on the extremities as well as the face or trunk. Although most lesions are asymptomatic, they tend to gradually enlarge in time. Approximately 10% of patients are found to have or subsequently develop systemic amyloidosis.

The epithelial-derived forms of cutaneous *lichenoid* and *macular amyloidosis* have distinctive demographic and clinical attributes (4). Both forms may coexist and likely represent a spectrum of disease with similar etiologic origins. Often pruritic, many believe that the lesions follow excoriation and represent the turnover of epithelial-derived keratinocytes. The lesions are more commonly encountered among races of darker skin color including individuals of Asian or Latin-American ancestry and consist of hyperpigmented macules or lichenoid papules. The former tend to occur over the trunk, in particular the interscapular area, with the lichenoid lesions typically seen over the extensor aspects of the lower extremities and penis. Less common forms of cutaneous limited amyloidosis include *anosacral amyloidosis*, consisting of lichenified plaques located on the buttocks of Chinese persons; *familial primary cutaneous amyloidosis*, a rare autosomal dominant genodermatoses consisting of amyloid-containing keratotic papules and swirled areas of cutaneous hypo/hyperpigmentation; and *poikilodermatous amyloidosis*, in which typical patients possess a short stature and show photosensitivity and palmoplantar keratoderma (5). Keratinocyte-derived amyloid may also be seen as part of a degenerative phenomenon permeating and surrounding the stroma of epithelial-derived tumors such as basal cell carcinoma, squamous cell carcinoma, and various adnexal tumors.

Biopsy of skin lesions, blind abdominal fat pad, or rectal aspiration are the most reliable means to establish a diagnosis (6). The latter techniques have a high diagnostic yield in systemic and myeloma-associated forms of the disease only. The histomorphologic features of amyloid are identical regardless of the type examined or clinical context and consist of amorphous aggregates of slightly eosinophilic extracellular material. Larger aggregates may contain internal artifactual clefts or fissures and may be associated with chronic inflammatory cells including plasma cells. The systemic and myeloma-associated forms of disease are more often characterized by larger aggregates of amyloid deposition located throughout the dermis and subcutaneous fat (Figures 13.2 and 13.3). Furthermore, the deposits are found within and surrounding vascular structures associated with purpura and may similarly outline the cell membranes of adipocytes within the panniculus, producing *amyloid rings*. Localized forms of the disease are characterized by smaller aggregates of amyloid usually located in the superficial dermis adjacent to the epithelium. The exception to this is the nodular localized form of disease in which large amyloid deposits are observed with abundant associated plasma cells (7). The deposits are accentuated surrounding the blood vessels and adnexal structures. In the lichenoid form, the overlying epithelium usually shows slight acanthosis. In both the macular and lichenoid forms, the overlying epithelial keratinocytes are hyperpigmented and scattered dyskera-

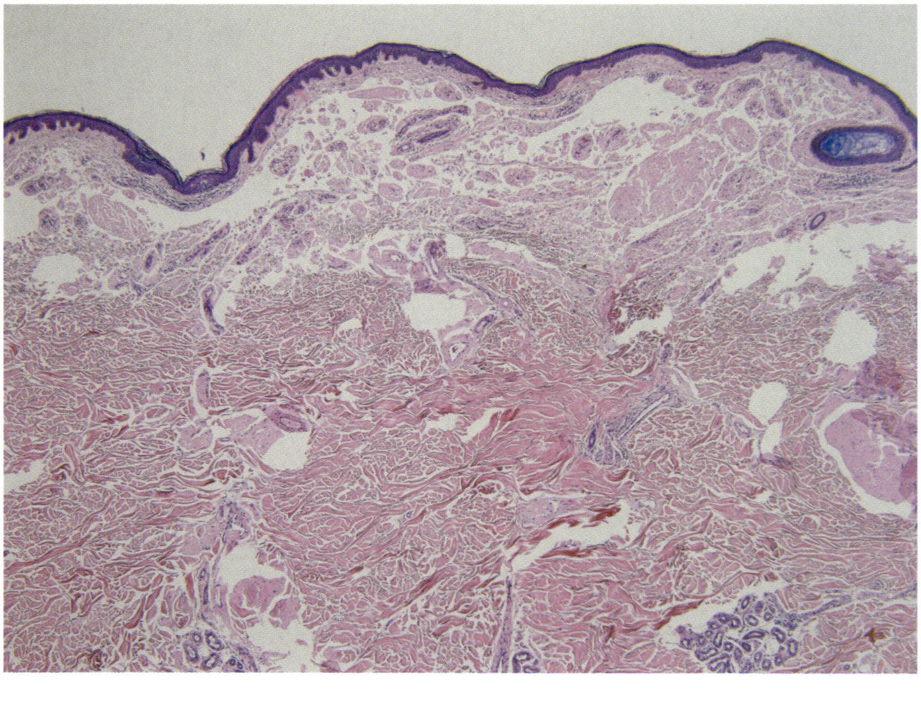

FIGURE 13.2. Low power photomicrograph depicting superficial dermal eosinophilic (amyloid) deposits.

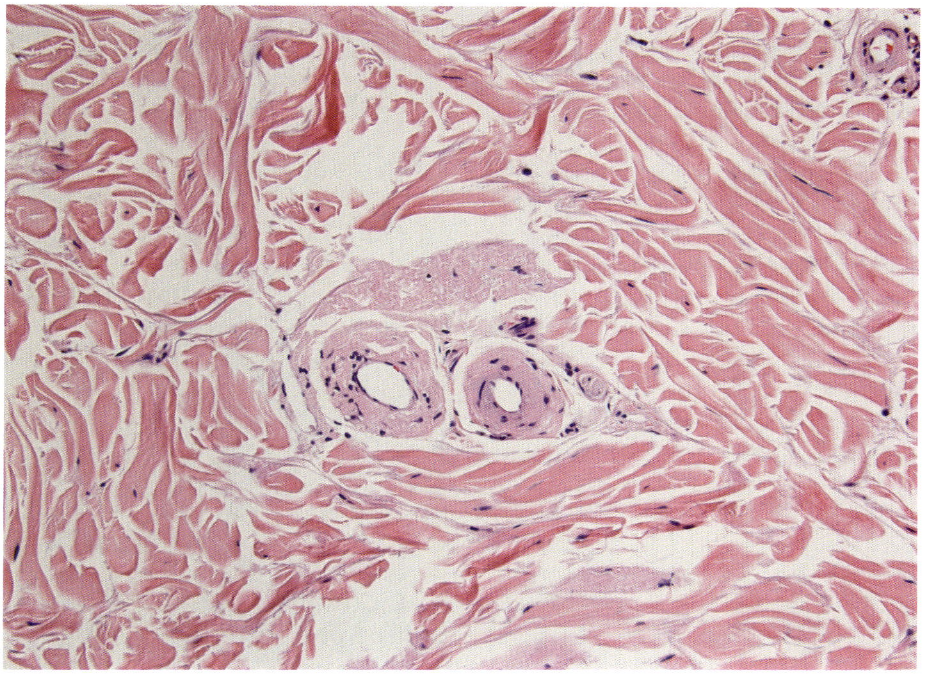

FIGURE 13.3. High power photomicrograph depicting amyloid deposits within the wall of the dermal blood vessels and perivascular stroma.

totic or apoptotic basilar keratinocytes are observed (Figure 13.4). Dermal incontinence of melanin and a sparse interface or superficial dermal perivascular lymphocytic infiltrate may be seen.

Several diagnostic adjuncts may be employed to confirm the diagnosis and establish the subtype of amyloidosis. Special stains may be employed that metachromatically stain the deposits (crystal or methyl violet) or that when exposed to polarized light produce birefringence (green with congo red and yellow with thioflavine T). It is important to realize that all forms of amyloid stain, as do nonamyloid deposits including elastin, colloid millium, and the deposits of lipoid proteinosis. Specificity of the staining can be improved with the addition of immunohisto-

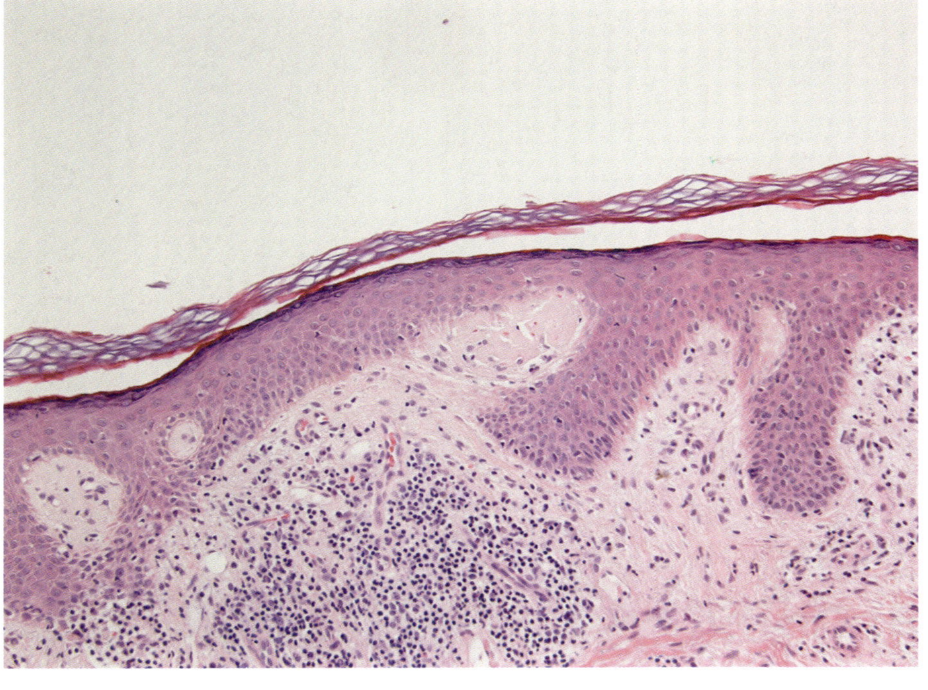

FIGURE 13.4. High power photomicrograph depicting fissured amyloid deposits at the dermoepidermal junction. Note additional changes of interface dermatitis.

chemical antibodies including to amyloid P protein, the immunoglobulin light chains, and keratins (8,9). Immunolabeling for P protein is found in all forms of amyloidosis. Monoclonal light chain restriction is typically observed within the plasma cell-associated forms of nodular and systemic/myeloma amyloidosis. Keratin antibodies are positive in the cutaneous derived forms of amyloidosis and are negative in the remainder (10). The specific types of amyloid may be determined through mass spectroscopy or amino acid sequencing. Electron microscopy can also be employed to identify the characteristic filaments.

The treatment is type-dependent (4). Patients with systemic and myeloma-associated forms of the disorder are usually administered systemic chemotherapy with or without autologous bone marrow transplantation. Organ transplantation of severely affected organs, most often the liver, heart, or kidney, can be performed but amyloid may reaccumulate in the transplanted organ. Localized nodular amyloidosis may be removed surgically or ablated with laser or cryotherapy. Lichenoid/macular amyloidosis is difficult to treat, although some have reported variable success with topical retinoids, calcipotriol, and dermabrasion.

The prognosis is similarly impacted by the type and stage of disease (1). The mean survival of patients with myeloma-associated disease is 5 months with most patients succumbing to complications stemming from cardiac or renal failure. The prognosis is slightly better for patients with systemic non-myeloma associated disease with a mean survival of 2 years. Response to chemotherapy and single-organ limited forms of the disease (i.e., neuropathy) fare better than most patients. Cardiac disease usually indicates a very poor overall prognosis.

References

1. Breathnach S. Amyloid and amyloidosis. *JAAD* 1988; 18: 1.
2. Tan S, Pepys M. The amyloidosis. *Histopathology* 1994; 25: 403.
3. Wright J. Clinico-pathologic differentiation of common amyloid syndromes. *Medicine* 1981; 69: 429.
4. Brownstein M, Helwig E. The cutaneous amyloidoses: localized forms. *Arch Dermatol* 1970; 102: 8.
5. Ratz J, Bailin P. Cutaneous amyloidosis. *JAAD* 1981; 4: 21.
6. Hashimoto K. Diseases of amyloid, colloid, and hyaline. *J Cutan Pathol* 1985; 12: 322.
7. Lee D, Huang C, Wong C. Dermatopathologic findings in 20 cases of systemic amyloidosis. *Am J Dermatopathol* 1998; 20: 438.
8. Noren P, Westermark P, Cornwell G, et al. Immunofluorescence and histochemical studies of localized cutaneous amyloidosis. *Br J Dermatol* 1983; 108: 277.
9. Breathnach S, Bhogal B, Dyck R, et al. Immunohistochemical demonstration of amyloid P component in skin of normal subjects and patients with cutaneous amyloidosis. *Br J Dermatol* 1981; 105: 115.
10. Kobayashi H, Hashimoto K. Amyloidogenesis in organ-limited cutaneous amyloidosis: An antigenic identity between epidermal keratin and skin amyloid. *J Invest Dermatol* 1983; 80: 66.

14
Birt-Hogg-Dubé Syndrome

■ Synonyms:	None
■ Etiology:	Mutation in the folliculin gene, chromosome 17p11.2
■ Associations:	Fibrofolliculomas, trichodiscomas, acrochordons, pulmonary cysts with spontaneous pneumothorax, renal carcinoma, and colorectal carcinoma in some kindreds
■ Clinical:	Skin-colored papules of face, neck, ears, and upper trunk, with intertriginous soft papules
■ Histology:	Trichodiscoma—interfollicular ovoid nodule with spindled cells in loose fibrillary stroma Fibrofolliculoma—central follicle with extension of irregular epithelial strands into surrounding well-defined cellular fibrous stroma
■ IHC:	CD34+, S100–
■ Evaluation:	Abdominal and chest CT
■ Treatment:	Early tumor excision, laser resurfacing of facial lesions for cosmetic improvement
■ Prognosis:	Excellent with early diagnosis and vigilant monitoring

In 1977, Birt, Hogg, and Dubé described a kindred of 70 individuals, some of whom presented with small skin-colored papules, predominantly of the face. These developed in early adulthood, and were noted to be inherited in a dominant pattern (1). The histomorphology of the papules was described as "abnormal hair follicles with epithelial strands extending out from the infundibulum of the hair follicle into a hyperplastic mantle of specialized fibrous tissue." The authors applied the term *fibrofolliculoma* to these lesions. Also described in these patients were trichodiscomas and acrochordons. Trichodiscoma is a benign tumor of perifollicular mesenchyme. It is thought to represent a proliferation of the *haarscheibe* (hair disk), a perifollicular "richly vascularized dermal pad covered with thick epidermis containing Merkel cells and supplied by a thick myelinated nerve the branches of which end at the lower epidermal surface and on the blood vessels of the dermal pad" (2). It is composed of a dermal interfollicular proliferation of spindle cells in a loose connective tissue matrix with varying amounts of mucin. It may have an orientation parallel to the skin surface. The *haarscheibe* is thought to represent a mechanoreceptor in animal skin. Its significance in humans is uncertain. The acrochordons reported in the original description of the syndrome were reported to have histologic findings typical of acrochordons (1). However, a subsequent study suggests that they have pathologic features of fibrofolliculoma and trichodiscoma (3).

The original kindred described by Birt, Hogg, and Dubé had several individuals who developed hereditary medullary carcinoma of the thyroid. This tumor susceptibility was apparently inherited from an individual without the syndrome. Subsequent series have confirmed that thyroid carcinoma is not a part of the syndrome. While there were no internal manifestations of the syndrome in the original report, there have been subsequent descriptions of renal tumors. These include chromophobe renal cell carcinomas, hybrid tumors with features of chromophobe carcinoma and oncocytoma, oncocytoma, clear cell renal cell carcinoma, and rarely, papillary carcinoma (4). Additional associations include pulmonary cysts with spontaneous pneumothorax (5), collagenomas (6), lipomas (7), angiolipomas (7), oral fibromas (8), parathyroid adenomas (7) including oncocytoma (9), and flecked chorioretinopathy (10). Colonic polyps and adenocarcinoma have been reported, but appear to occur in only some affected families (11,12). In the largest series of BHD kindreds, with 152 patients, no such cases were reported (5).

The Birt-Hogg-Dubé (BHD) gene has been mapped to chromosome 17p11.2 (13,14). It encodes a novel protein, folliculin, which is highly conserved across species (15). Mutations in the BHD gene result in formation of a truncated protein. Expression of BHD gene mRNA occurs in a wide variety of normal and neoplastic human tissue, but is markedly reduced in BHD renal tumors, suggesting that the BHD gene product may serve as a tumor suppressor gene (16). Based on studies in a rat model of inherited renal carcinoma, a germ line mutation is likely transmitted as a heterozygote, with the homozygous form being lethal in fetal life. A "second hit" in the normal gene copy is required for tumorigenesis. This second hit causes loss of heterozygosity. In this scenario, only the abnormal gene product is expressed, and there is a loss of expression of the normal gene copy. This causes a lack of production of a functional protein product that would aid in tumor suppression. The second hit can be caused by a somatic mutation in the normal gene copy, which would result in loss of the normal gene product (17). Alternatively, expression of the normal gene copy may be suppressed by methylation of the gene promoter region. Somatic inactivation of the BHD gene in sporadic renal cell carcinoma and colorectal carcinoma has been reported, implicating its role in the development of a subset of these tumors (18). A deletion in exon 4 of the BHD gene causes primary spontaneous pneumothorax without other features of BHD syndrome (19).

The fibrofolliculomas (FF) and trichodiscomas (TD) of Birt-Hogg-Dubé syndrome usually develop in early adulthood. These patients present with small skin-colored or white papules that have a predilection for the face, neck, ears, and upper trunk (Figure 14.1A and 14.1B). Acrochordons typically develop in intertriginous areas. The clinical

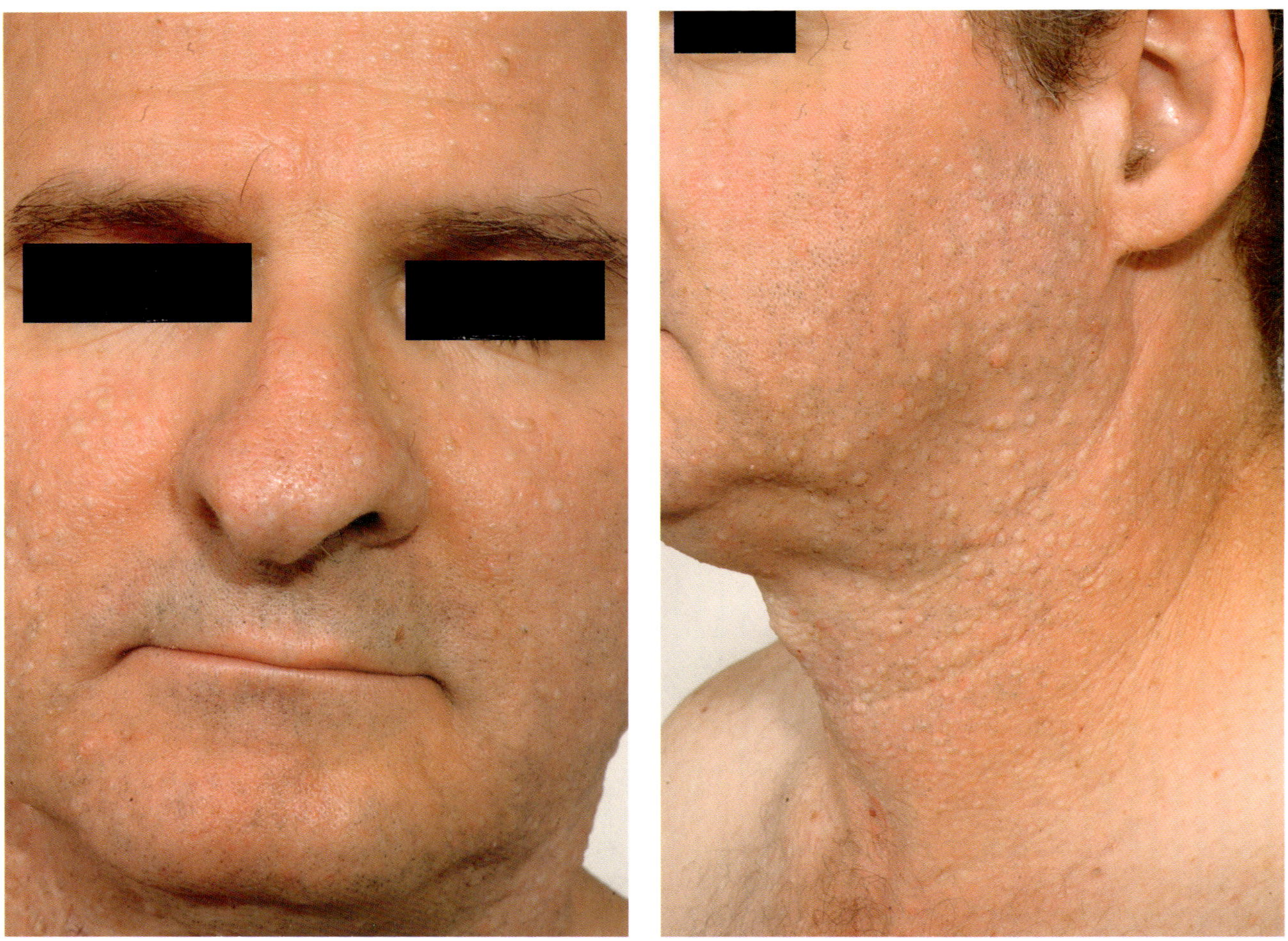

A B

FIGURE 14.1. (A and B) Trichodiscomas and fibrofolliculomas: dome-shaped skin-colored papules.

TABLE 14.1. Clinical Differential Diagnosis of Facial Papules

	Distribution	Onset	Associated Features/Syndrome
Trichodiscoma fibrofolliculoma	Diffuse involvement of face, extrafacial involvement	Adulthood	**Birt-Hogg-Dubé syndrome** +/− Oral papules
Syringoma	Periocular prominence	Adulthood	Yellow hue
Basaloid follicular hamartoma	Diffuse involvement of face, may have extrafacial involvement	Variable	+/− Pigment, comedos, +/−alopecia
Angiofibroma	Central face	Childhood	**Tuberous sclerosis** Red hue, periungual fibromas, Shagreen patch
Trichoepithelioma	Central face	Adolescence	Skin-colored, varied lesion size
Tricholemmoma	Nose, cheeks	Adulthood	**Cowden's syndrome** Tendency for epidermal change, cobblestone mucosa, acral keratoses

differential diagnosis of the facial papules includes trichoepithelioma, angiofibroma, tricholemmoma, basaloid follicular hamartoma, and syringoma. There are several clinical features that may help distinguish these entities (Table 14.1), but histopathologic evaluation is required for definitive diagnosis.

Trichodiscoma is an ovoid superficial dermal nodule filling an interfollicular space (Figure 14.2). There is generally epidermal flattening, with interwoven fascicles of fibrillar collagen with spindled cells in a loose stroma that contains varying amounts of mucin and vascularity. Fibrofolliculoma may contain a similar mesenchymal component, but has a central distorted follicle from which thin epithelial strands extend in a sometimes retiform configuration, invested within a well-defined cellular fibrous stroma with spindled cells (Figure 14.3). Much of the spindle cell component of both lesions is highlighted by antibodies to CD34, supporting perifollicular mesenchyme as the histogenic origin of both lesions (20). The histomorphology of fibrofolliculoma is specific, but that of trichodiscoma is not. The differential diagnosis includes neurofibroma, to which it may show considerable similarity. Neurofibroma and trichodiscoma both display immunoreactivity with antibodies to CD34, but elements of neurofibroma will also label with antibodies to S100 protein. Clinical presentation also helps distinguish these two entities.

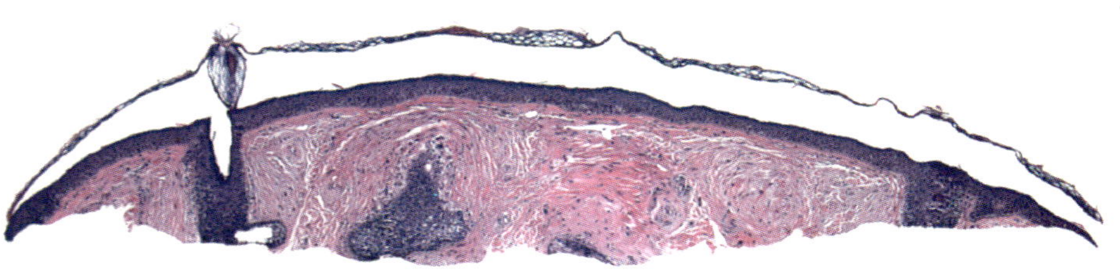

FIGURE 14.2. Trichodiscoma: periadnexal collagen is arranged in lamellae, with spindle cells and increased mucin.

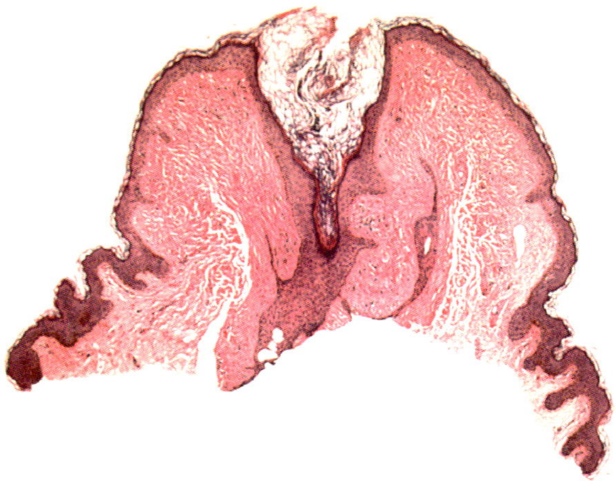

FIGURE 14.3. Fibrofolliculoma, perifollicular dense collagen within which are embedded thin follicular epithelial strands.

Once the diagnosis of multiple fibrofolliculomas and trichodiscomas has been made, a workup for underlying disease is mandatory, particularly because of the association of the syndrome with renal carcinoma. A suggested evaluation is given in Table 14.2.

Management of the Birt-Hogg-Dubé syndrome is aimed at early detection and treatment of tumors and pneumothorax. Treatment of cutaneous lesions is principally of cosmetic importance. Laser skin resurfacing of the face may result in significant improvement in appearance (21).

Birt-Hogg-Dubé syndrome is a more recently recognized cancer-susceptibility syndrome that is of particular importance because of the potential for early recognition based on typical cutaneous findings. The benefits of diagnosis may be life-saving not only for the index patient, but also for entire kindreds.

TABLE 14.2. Evaluation/management of the patient with Birt-Hogg-Dubé syndrome

1. Abdominal CT with contrast with attention to kidneys
2. Chest CT to evaluate for pulmonary cysts
3. Lower gastrointestinal tract evaluation for polyps/carcinoma age appropriate or as otherwise warranted based on family history
4. Patient education regarding informing relatives of disease with attendant risks

References

1. Birt AR, Hogg GR, Dubé J. Hereditary multiple fibrofolliculomas with trichodiscomas and acrochordons. *Arch Dermatol* 1977; 113: 1674–1677.
2. Pinkus H, Coskey R, Burgess GH. Trichodiscoma: A benign tumor related to *haarscheibe* (hair disk). *J Invest Dermatol* 1974; 63: 212–218.
3. De la Torre C, Ocampo C, Doval IG, Losada A, Cruces MJ. Acrochordons are not a component of the Birt-Hogg-Dubé syndrome: Does this syndrome exist? Case reports and review of the literature. *Am J Dermatopathol* 1999; 21: 369–374.
4. Pavlovich CP, Walther MM, Eyler RA, et al. Renal tumors in the Birt-Hogg-Dubé syndrome. *Am J Surg Pathol* 2002; 26: 1542–1552.
5. Toro JR, Glenn G, Duray P, et al. Birt-Hogg-Dubé syndrome: A novel marker for kidney neoplasia. *Arch Dermatol* 1999; 135: 1195–1202.
6. Weintraub R, Pinkus H. Multiple fibrofolliculomas (Birt-Hogg-Dubé) associated with a large connective tissue nevus. *J Cutan Pathol* 1977; 4: 289–299.
7. Chung JY, Ramos-Caro FA, Beers B, Ford MJ, Flowers F. Multiple lipomas, angiolipomas, and parathyroid adenomas in a patient with Birt-Hogg-Dubé syndrome. *Int J Dermatol* 1996; 35: 365–367.
8. Nadershahi NA, Wescott WB, Egbert B. Birt-Hogg-Dubé syndrome: A review and presentation of the first case with oral lesions. *Oral Surg Oral Med Oral Pathol Oral Radiol Endod* 1997; 83: 496–500.
9. Liu V, Kwan T, Page EH. Parotid oncocytoma in the Birt-Hogg-Dubé syndrome. *J Am Acad Dermatol* 2000; 43: 1120–1122.

10. Walter P, Kirchhof B, Korge B, Heimann K. Flecked chorioretinopathy associated with Birt-Hogg-Dubé syndrome. *Graefes Arch Clin Exp Ophthalmol* 1997; 235: 359–361.
11. Rongioletti F, Hazini R, Gianotti G, Rebora A. Fibrofolliculomas, trichodiscomas, and acrochordons (Birt-Hogg-Dubé) associated with intestinal polyposis. *Clin Exp Dermatol* 1989; 14: 72–74.
12. Khoo SK, Giraud S, Khanoski K, et al. Clinical and genetic studies of Birt-Hogg-Dubé syndrome. *J Med Genet* 2002; 39: 906–912.
13. Khoo SK, Bradley M, Wong FK, Hedblad MA, Nordenskjold M, Teh BT. Birt-Hogg-Dubé syndrome: Mapping of a novel hereditary neoplasia gene to chromosome 17p12-q11.2. *Oncogene* 2001; 20: 5239–5242.
14. Schmidt LS, Warren MB, Nickerson ML, et al. Birt-Hogg-Dubé syndrome: A genodermatosis associated with spontaneous pneumothorax and kidney neoplasia, maps to chromosome 17p11.2. *Am J Hum Genet* 2001; 69: 876–882.
15. Nickerson ML, Warren MB, Toro JR, et al. Mutations in a novel gene lead to kidney tumors, lung wall defects, and benign tumors of the hair follicle in patients with the Birt-Hogg-Dubé syndrome. *Cancer Cell* 2002; 2: 157–164.
16. Warren MB, Torres-Cabala CA, Turner ML, et al. Expression of Birt-Hogg-Dubé gene mRNA in normal and neoplastic human tissues. *Mod Pathoi* 2004; 17: 998–1011.
17. Okimoto K, Sakurai J, Kobayashi T, et al. A germ-line insertion in the Birt-Hogg-Dubé (BHD) gene gives rise to the Nihon rat model of inherited renal cancer. *Proc Nat Acad Sci* 2004; 101: 2023–2027.
18. da Silva NF, Gentle D, Hesson LB, Morton DG, Latif F, Maher ER. Analysis of the Birt-Hogg-Dubé (BHD) tumour suppressor gene in sporadic renal cell carcinoma and colorectal cancer. *J Med Genet* 2003; 40: 820–824.
19. Painter JN, Tapanainen H, Somer M, Tukiainen P, Aittomaki K. A 4-bp deletion in the Birt-Hogg-Dubé gene (FLCN) causes dominantly inherited spontaneous pneumothorax. *Am J Hum Genet* 2005; 76: 522–527.
20. Collins GL, Somach S, Morgan MB. Histomorphologic and immunophenotypic analysis of fibrofolliculomas and trichodiscomas in Birt-Hogg-Dubé syndrome and sporadic disease. *J Cutan Pathol* 2002; 29: 529–533.
21. Jacob CI, Dover JS. Birt-Hogg-Dubé syndrome: Treatment of cutaneous manifestations with laser skin resurfacing. *Arch Dermatol* 2001; 137: 98–99.

15
Cowden's Syndrome

▪ Synonyms:	None
▪ Etiology:	pTEN mutation
▪ Associations:	Multiple hamartomas, keratoacanthomas, neoplasms
▪ Clinical:	Hyperkeratotic folliculocentric papules
▪ Histology:	Proliferations of pale staining keratinocytes from epidermis
▪ IHC repertoire:	N/A
▪ Staging:	N/A
▪ Prognosis:	100% survival
▪ Adverse variables:	Visceral neoplasms
▪ Treatment:	Careful screening

Trichilemmomas are benign epidermal neoplasms that may serve as an indicator of underlying malignancy. Trichilemmomas appear, largely on the head and neck, as exophytic, small, hyperkeratotic papules (Figure 15.1). There is no particular gender predilection and they usually arise during the second decade. When occurring as isolated lesions, these tumors are invariably benign and are of no clinical significance.

Multiple trichilemmomas may occur as part of the multiple hamartoma or Cowden syndrome (1). This syndrome has an autosomal dominant inheritance pattern (2) and is associated with mutations in the pTEN gene located at 10q22–23 (3). Table 15.1 summarizes the systemic conditions associated with the syndrome (4–7). These patients develop many hamartomatous lesions, fibrocystic changes in the breast, and breast and thyroid carcinomas. The neoplastic proliferations tend to be relatively indolent and confer a good prognosis for afflicted patients. The gastrointestinal polyps do not appear to harbor malignant potential. There are isolated reports of many other neoplasms occurring in patients with the syndrome (8).

Cowden syndrome displays other cutaneous manifestations. These include cobblestone-like fibromas on the tongue and within the oral mucosa, sclerotic fibromas (9), lipomas, and hyperkeratotic plaques on the dorsa of the hands. While less common and less specific than trichilemmomas, these other processes can also be valuable clues in establishing the diagnosis.

Trichilemmomas have a characteristic histologic appearance. Keratinocytes proliferate down from the surface of the epidermis as an expansile plaque (Figure 15.2). There is frequently overlying parakeratosis, focal diminution of the granular layer, and clumped keratohyalin granules in other sections of the epidermis. In some cases, a central hair follicle may be present. The keratinocytes within the tumor have abundant, pale staining cytoplasm, resembling the appearance of the outer root sheath of follicular epithelium (Figure 15.3). The bottom of the lesion may have a lobulated configuration. Inward turning rete ridges may be seen at the periphery of the lesion. One characteristic finding is the presence of a thickened, PASD positive basement membrane immediately beneath the intraepidermal proliferation (Figure 15.4). This membrane is refractile. Squamous eddies are present. Some authors have contended that these lesions represent human papilloma virus infections involving hair follicles, but the scientific evidence for that position is lacking (10, 11).

Desmoplastic trichilemmoma is a histologic variant that may be confused with squamous cell carcinoma or basal cell carcinoma on microscopic examination. The overall architecture of the lesion is preserved; however, in

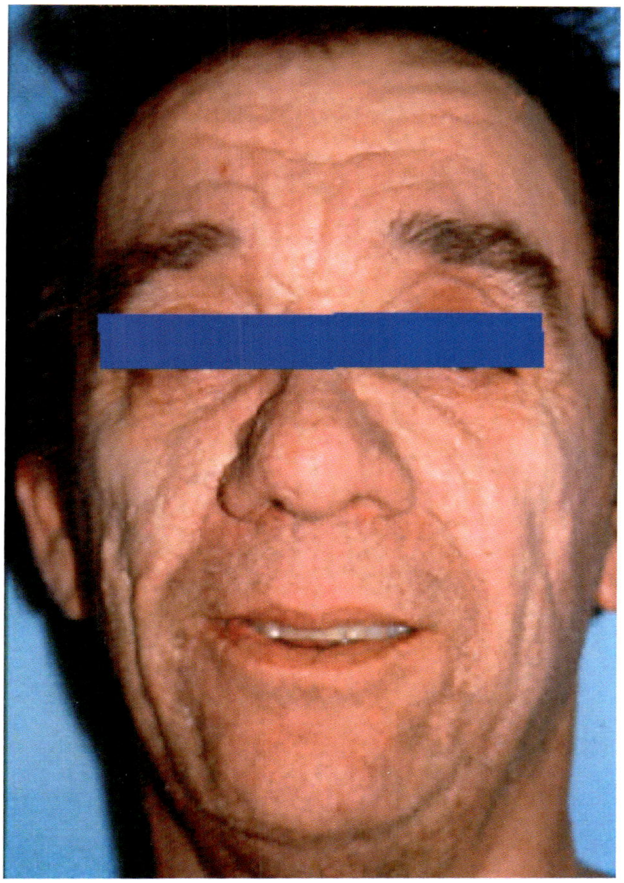

FIGURE 15.1. Multiple skin-toned papules distributed on the face of a patient with Cowden's disease.

TABLE 15.1. Cowden Syndrome

Abnormality	Incidence (Percentage) in Patients with Cowden Syndrome
Breast carcinoma	25–36
Fibrocystic changes of breast	53
Thyroid adenomas	68
Follicular carcinoma, thyroid	3
Gastrointestinal polyps and fibromas	35–60
Lipoma	31
Neuroma	5
Angiod streaks, eyes	13
Acanthosis nigricans	11
Enlarged head circumference	70–80
Adenocarcinoma, uterus	6
Trichilemmomas	>80
Bone cysts	
Hepatic hamartomas	
Meningiomas	
Ovarian cysts	
Retinal gliomas	
Sclerotic fibromas	76
Oral cobblestone fibromas	>50
Palmoplantar hyperkatoses	>50
Hemangioma	18

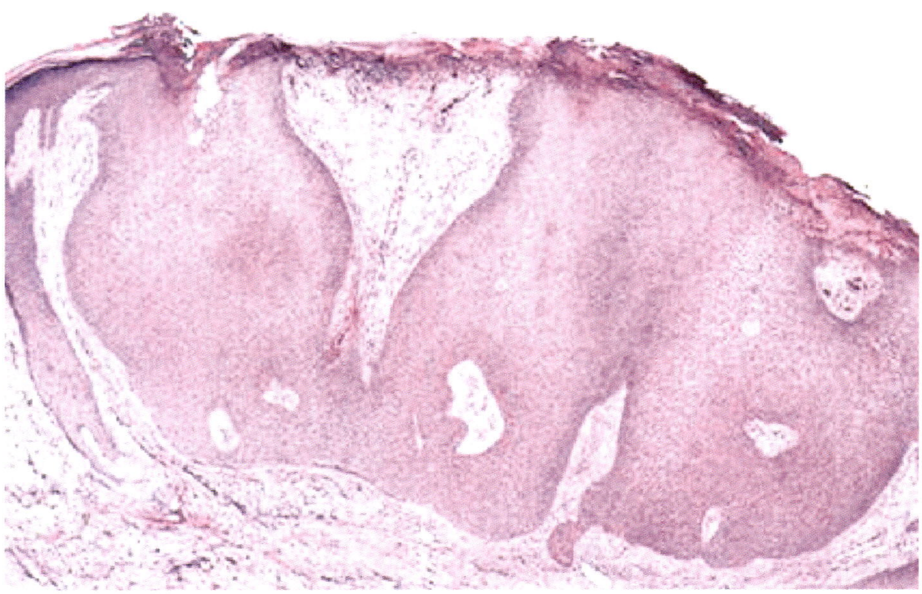

FIGURE 15.2. Low power photomicrograph depicting plate-like growth of the epithelium observed in tricholemmoma.

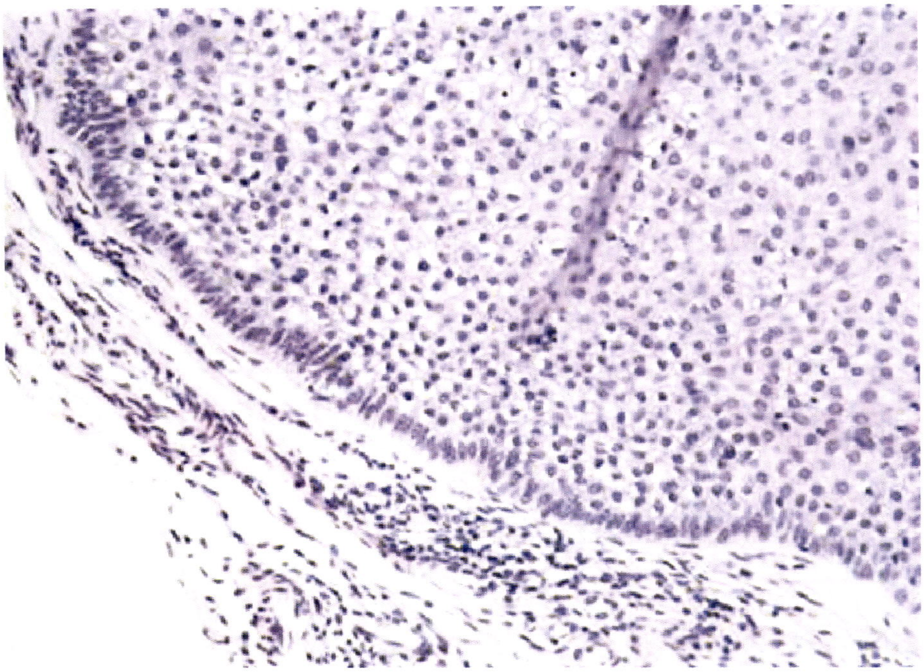

FIGURE 15.3. High power photomicrograph depicting pale staining keratinocytes with basilar palisading resembling the outer root sheath of the follicle.

the center of the growth, islands of proliferating keratinocytes are separated by a desmoplastic stromal response, mimicking an invasive growth pattern. Mitoses may be present. Careful attention to the overall growth pattern should prevent misdiagnosis.

There is a very rare malignant variant known as trichilemmal carcinoma. This neoplasm invades the dermis and is characterized by abundant mitoses, including atypical variants, zonal necrosis, and marked cytologic atypia.

Sclerotic fibroma, also known as storiform collagenoma and plywood fibroma, grows as nodular dermal proliferations. The epidermis is often atrophic, with effacement of rete ridges (Figure 15.5). Within the dermis, there is a

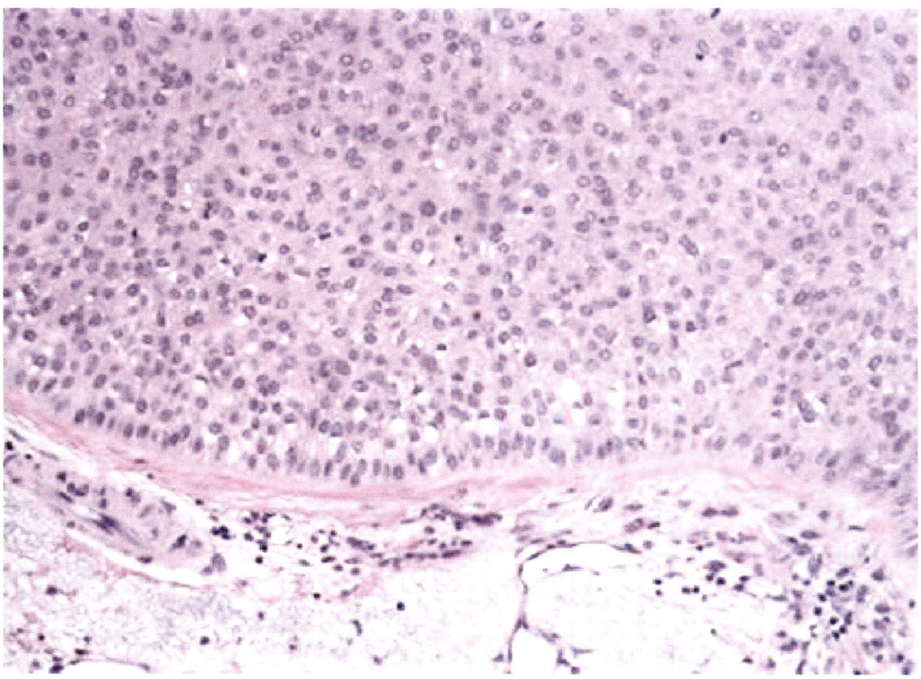

FIGURE 15.4. High power photomicrograph depicting the prominent eosinophilic basement membrane surrounding the tumor periphery.

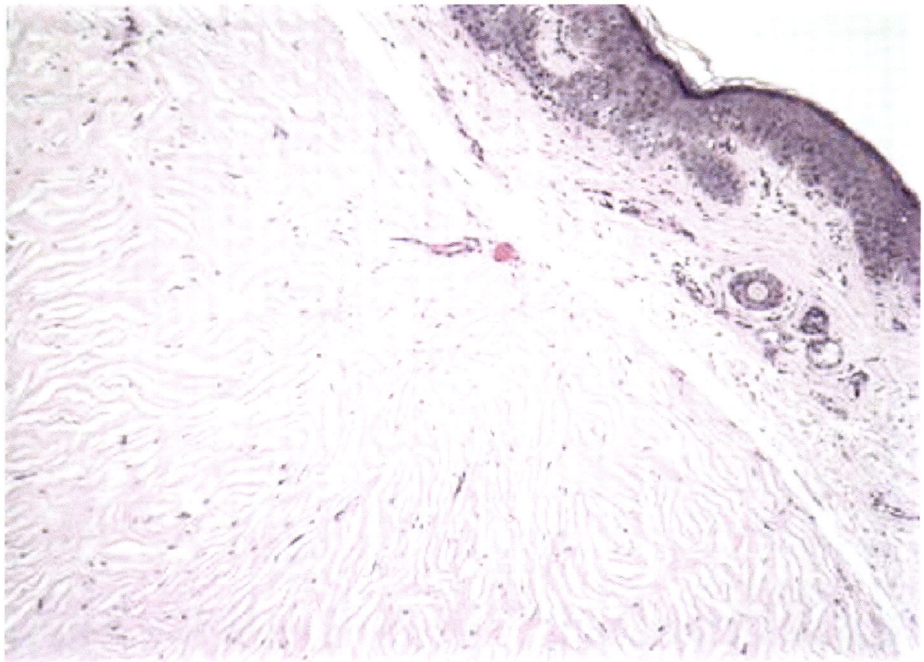

FIGURE 15.5. Low power photomicrograph depicting well-circumscribed laminated appearance of sclerotic fibroma.

sparse proliferation of spindle-shaped cells that grow in a storiform pattern. Dense, keloidal collagen is present between these cells in a pattern that has been described as resembling plywood (Figure 15.6). The exact nature of this process and the dermal cells is not fully established. Some investigators believe these lesions to represent end-stage lesions of dermatofibromas (12), while others maintain that they represent *de novo* growths (13). Sclerotic fibromas may occur as sporadic lesions unassociated with Cowden syndrome (14).

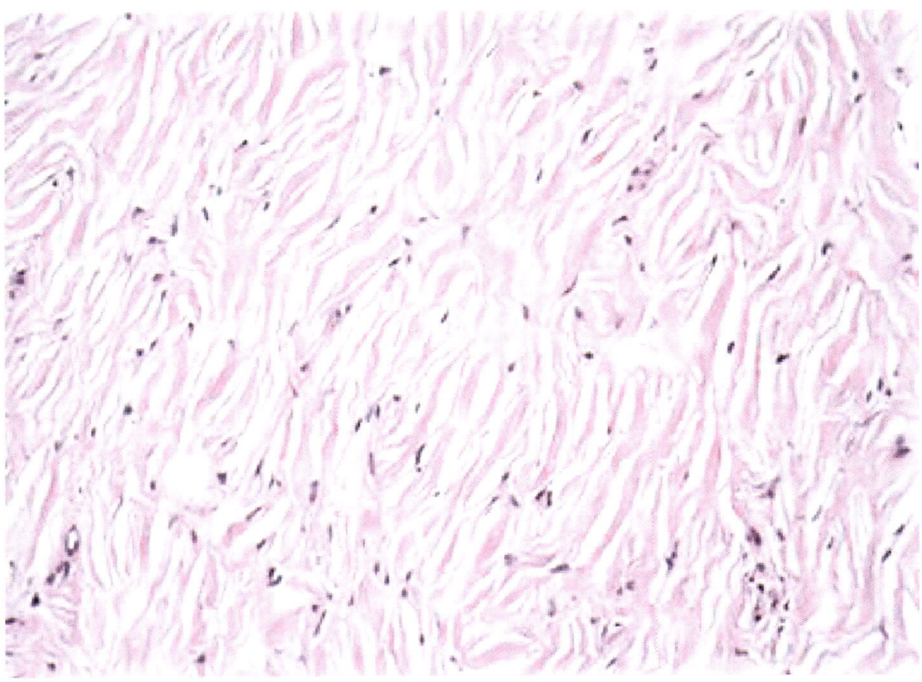

FIGURE 15.6. High power detail of the sclerotic fibroma.

References

1. Lloyd KM, Dennis M. Cowden's disease: A possible new symptom complex with multiple system involvement. *Ann Int Med* 1963; 58: 136–142.
2. Barax CN, Lebwohl M, Phelps RG. Multiple hamartoma syndrome. *J Am Acad Dermatol* 1987; 17: 342–346.
3. Eng C. Genetics of Cowden syndrome: Through the looking glass of oncology. *Int J Oncol* 1998; 12: 701–701.
4. Starink TM, van derVeen JPW, Arwert F, de Waal LP, de Langer GG, Gille JJ, Eriksson AW. The Cowden syndrome: A clinical and genetic study in 21 patients. *Clin Genet* 1986; 29: 222–233.
5. Elston DM, James WD, Rodman OG, Graham GF. Multiple hamartoma syndrome (Cowden's disease) associated with non-Hodgkin's lymphoma. *Arch Dermatol* 1986; 122: 572–575.
6. Starink TM. Cowden's disease: An analysis of fourteen new cases. *J Am Acad Dermatol* 1984; 11: 1127–1141.
7. Salem OS, Steck WD. Cowden's disease (multiple hamartoma syndrome). *J Am Acad Dermatol* 1983; 8: 686–695.
8. Mallory SB. Cowden syndrome (multiple hamartoma syndrome). *Dermatologic Clinics* 1995; 13: 27–31.
9. Weary PE, Gorlin RJ, Gentry WC, Comer JE, Greer KE. Multiple hamartoma syndrome (Cowden's disease). *Arch Dermatol* 1972; 106: 682–690.
10. Starink TM, Meijer CJLM, Brownstein MH. The cutaneous pathology of Cowden's disease: New findings. *J Cutan Pathol* 1985; 12: 83–93.
11. Johnson BL, Kramer EM, Lavker RM. The keratotic tumors of Cowden's disease: An electron microscopic study. *J Cutan Pathol* 1987; 14: 291–298.
12. Pujol RM, de Castro F, Schroeter AL, Su WPD. Solitary sclerotic fibroma of the skin: A sclerotic dermatofibroma? *Am J Dermatopathol* 1996; 18: 620–624.
13. McCalmont TH. Sclerotic fibroma: A fossil no longer. *J Cutan Pathol* 1994; 21: 82–85.
14. Requena L, Gutierrez J, Sanchez Yus E. Multiple sclerotic fibromas of the skin: A cutaneous marker of Cowden's disease. *J Cutan Pathol* 1991; 19: 346–351.

16
Gyrate Erythemas: Erythema Gyratum Repens and Erythema Chronicum Migrans

■ Synonyms:	EGR—None ECM—Erythema migrans
■ Etiology:	EGR—Unknown, hypersensitivity? ECM—Infection with *Borrelia burgdorferi*
■ Associations:	EGR—Internal malignancy, tuberculosis ECM—Outdoor activities in endemic areas for *Ixodes* ticks
■ Clinical:	EGR—Truncal arcuate erythematous bands with trailing scale ECM—Expanding erythematous solid or annular patch
■ Histology:	EGR—Mild spongiosis with superficial perivascular lymphocytic infiltrate ECM—Nonspecific superficial and deep lymphocytic perivascular infiltrate
■ IHC repertoire:	None
■ Staging:	EGR—None ECM—Early, early disseminated, chronic/late
■ Prognosis:	EGR—Poor with internal malignancy ECM—Good with appropriate antibiotic therapy, <5% with serious complications including encephalopathy, heart block, fetal death
■ Adverse variables:	EGR—Most cases associated with advanced visceral adenocarcinoma ECM—Neuroborreliosis, heart block, gestational disease
■ Treatment:	EGR—Supportive measures for disseminated carcinoma ECM—Uncomplicated: doxycycline 100 mg b.i.d. or amoxicillin 500 mg t.i.d. 14 days
■ Complicated:	as above, 30-day regimen or I.V. ceftriaxone

The gyrate erythemas are a heterogeneous group of dermatoses clinically defined by the presence of circinate, annular, and/or polycyclic lesions that are often associated with serious underlying systemic diseases (1). The gyrate erythemas consist of the entities erythema annulare centrifugum (EAC), erythema marginatum rheumaticum (EMR), erythema gyratum repens (EGR), and erythema chronicum migrans (ECM). The latter two entities, namely EGR and ECM, are associated with potentially deadly underlying disorders and thus will be discussed in greater detail.

Erythema Gyratum Repens

This distinctive dermatoses is the rarest of the gyrate erythemas with only 55 cases reported to date (2). Initially reported by Gammel in 1953 as a distinctive rash with a "wood-grain" appearance that appeared to move or "creep" (hence the Latin designation of *repens*), he correctly surmised its development in conjunction with underlying breast carcinoma and subsequent resolution with removal of the tumor.

Of the patients reported to date, there is a 2:1 male-to-female gender ratio with an average age at presentation of 66 years with most patients being greater than 40 years of age at diagnosis (3). All patients reported thus far have been Caucasian. Approximately 90% of patients possess an underlying malignancy, most commonly involving the lung and representing carcinoma. Lymphoreticular malignancy or sarcoma is seldom seen. Carcinoma of the breast, cervix, bladder, prostate, and kidney, among others, may also be seen (4). The rash usually precedes the discovery of the malignancy but may present concomitant with, or rarely, following the diagnosis of internal malignancy. Approximately 10% of the cases fail to show an internal malignancy and rare single cases of its association with pulmonary tuberculosis and the CREST syndrome have also been reported (5).

The pathogenesis of this disorder is unknown. Among the possible mechanisms postulated are immune mediated models in which cross-reactivity between tumor and endogenous skin antigens occurs, the tumor antigens bind *in situ* to endogenous skin antigens, or tumor antigen immune complexes circulate and deposit within the skin. Alternatively, the cytokine-rich milieu of malignancy may incite an abnormal localized inflammatory cell response resulting in increased matrix elaboration responsible for the observed clinical patterns and migration of the rash.

The clinical features consist of a pruritic rash with broad erythematous bands of polycyclic and arcuate arranged patches with a trailing scale that commonly assumes the appearance of wood-grain or marble (Figure 16.1). The lesions typically migrate at a rate of approximately 1 cm per day. The rash is usually located on the trunk and rarely involves the face or extremities. The most important diagnoses to exclude are ECM and EAC. In contrast to EGR, EAC generally produces more slowly evolving, palpable plaques that characteristically clear within the center. Although EAC may be associated with underlying malignancy, most cases are either idiopathic or follow drug hypersensitivity.

Histology shows epidermal spongiosis with surmounted scale-crust and exocytosis of lymphocytes (6). The dermis discloses a predominantly superficial perivascular lymphocytic infiltrate with interspersed eosinophils (Figure 16.2). Involvement of the deeper vascular plexus and abnormal collections of Langerhans cells have also been reported. Direct immunofluorescence may show granular deposits of IgG and C3 along the basement membrane (7). Laboratory abnormalities frequently include hypereosinophilia. Some patients have been shown to have abnormal numbers of circulating T- and B-lymphocytes.

Although the rash is itself innocuous, it is associated with underlying malignancy in the vast majority of cases. Many of the patients have advanced-stage visceral cancers at diagnosis and thus succumb to their underlying disease. However, a minority of patients, particularly those individuals discovered to have early-stage disease or less aggressive forms of cancer such as cervical carcinoma, may expect a favorable outcome and resolution of the rash following removal of the tumor.

Treatment should be principally aimed at timely diagnosis and removal of the underlying malignancy. Patients should undergo chest X-ray and CT scanning of the abdomen and pelvis, and should also be considered for esophagogastroduodenoscopy and colonoscopy. The rash

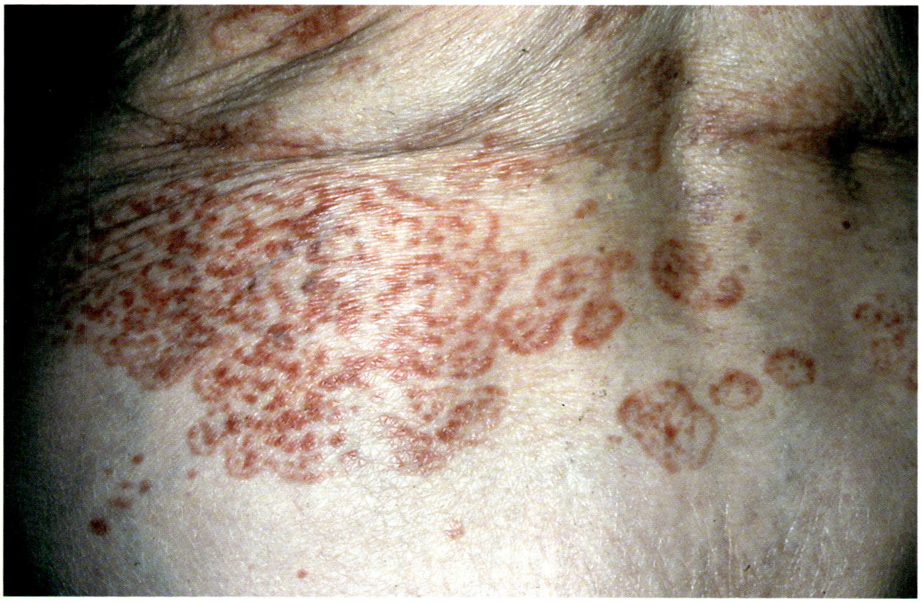

FIGURE 16.1. Multiple annular and serpiginous patches likened to the appearance of wood grain seen in erythema gyratum repens.

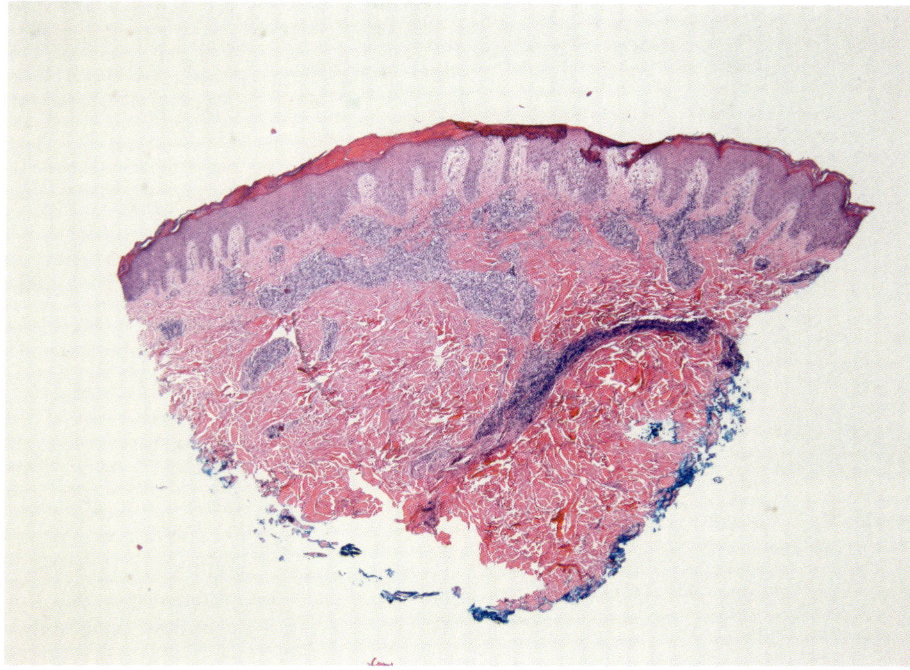

FIGURE 16.2. Low power photomicrograph depicting superficial and deep lymphocytic dermatitis and dermal edema seen in the gyrate erythemas including erythema gyratum repens.

itself does not respond to topical or intralesional corticosteroid therapy. Most cases resolve with removal of the underlying malignancy.

Erythema Chronicum Migrans

This dermatosis is one of the more common examples of gyrate erythema that derives its name from the distinctive manner of its clinical presentation. Coined by Afzelius as *erythema migrans* in 1909, it was later designated by Lipschutz as *erythema chronicum migrans* (8). Both investigators rightly surmised the relationship between the expanding erythematous rash and an antecedent tick bite. The association between tick bite and the constellation of neurologic and rheumatologic symptoms, however, would not come until 1977, with a landmark epidemiologic study conducted at the time around the communities neighboring Lyme, Connecticut. Shortly thereafter, the disease vector (*Ixodes* tick) and the etiologic agent (*Borrelia burgdorferi*) of Lyme disease, were determined.

ECM and Lyme disease afflicts persons of all ages and ethnic backgrounds, and with a nearly equal gender distribution. The disease has been reported across North America, Europe, and Asia and is the most common of the bacterial-borne arthropod diseases in North America. The common denominator for acquiring the disease is outdoor exposure or contact with the disease-carrying tick species *Ixodes*. Although most infections follow feeding with the hard tick *Ixodes*, infection following the bite of other tick genera and non-tick vectors has been reported. Human infection constitutes an exceptional event as the principal hosts of the infection are rodents, particularly the white-footed mouse, deer, and avian populations. The tick acquires infection with the spirochetal bacterial organism *Borrelia burgdorferi* following blood meal on an infected host and usually retains infectivity for life. Other cutaneous manifestations of Lyme borreliosis are *Borrelial lymphocytoma* and *acrodermatitis chronica atrophicans* (9).

The principal cutaneous manifestation of Lyme borreliosis is erythema chronicum migrans. The rash can initially be seen around the site of tick bite or may develop without the patient being aware of a previous tick bite (10). The rash typically follows an incubation period of 1 to 3 weeks but may occur as soon as 3 days following the bite or up to 3 months following exposure. The rash begins as a solid and slowly expanding erythematous patch that in time centrally fades, forming a distinctive annular appearance (Figure 16.3). Occasionally, the central site of the tick bite may persist as a small erythematous patch forming a bull's-eye-like or targetoid configuration. The erythematous band expands peripherally at a variable rate with the largest lesions generally occurring in individuals with the longest duration of symptoms. The band itself is generally between 1 and 2 cm wide and usually assumes a symmetrical annular pattern, although exceptional cases of eccentric or elliptical-shaped rings have been reported

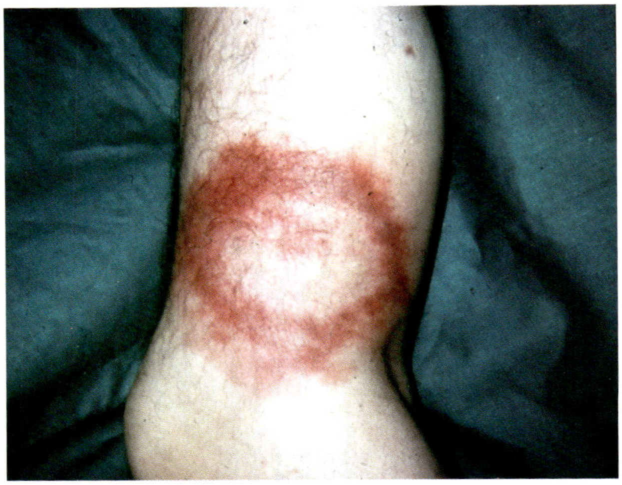

FIGURE 16.3. Annular erythematous patch with central clearing seen in erythema chronicum migrans.

(11). The rash has been rarely reported to form a scale or to vesiculate. The natural history of untreated cases is for gradual fading and complete resolution of the lesion within one year. The rash can develop anywhere on the skin surface with the lower extremities among the more common sites of involvement. Other signs commonly found in conjunction with the cutaneous manifestations include lymphadenopathy, and fever, additional complaints of headache, and malaise are common (12). Other less common cutaneous manifestations include the development of multiple erythema migrans lesions with secondary spirochetal dissemination, localized lymphocytoma usually involving the earlobe, and the sclerotic bands and nodules of the lower extremities seen in acrodermatitis chronica atrophicans. The latter entities are more commonly observed in Europe (13).

The histologic findings observed in Lyme disease are nonspecific and consist of a superficial or superficial and deep lymphocytic perivascular infiltrate with variable numbers of interstitial eosinophils and plasma cells (14,15). Spirochetes may be observed within the papillary dermis with the aid of the Warthin-Starry silver stain. Recent ancillary diagnostic methods incorporating the use of the PCR reaction and indirect immunofluorescence have also been reported. The diagnosis may be verified serologically by the demonstration of elevated IgM or IgG titers to *B. burgdorferi*. As outdoor enthusiasts often harbor antibody titers to the organism from previous exposure, borderline elevations in IgG antibody titers should be regarded with suspicion. Further compounding the limitations of serologic diagnosis are a lack of serologic standardization, low yield of the test in early infection, and false positive results in patients with relapsing fever and syphilis (16). Finally, *Borrelia* species may be cultivated using specialized media such as the modified Kelly media, although the procedure is laborious, requires a delay in diagnosis, and has a relatively low sensitivity (17).

Lyme disease can be staged or classified based upon the scope of disease activity. *Early* Lyme disease consists of the erythema migrans rash with or without lymphadenopathy and has an excellent prognosis with appropriate antibiotic therapy. *Early disseminated* disease consists of disseminated erythema migrans lesions with early manifestations of neurologic, cardiac, or rheumatologic involvement. The prognosis is excellent with longer-term administration of antibiotics. *Chronic or late* Lyme disease is associated with persistent or remitting neurologic, rheumatologic, or cardiac manifestations. The neurologic manifestations can include chronic depression, dementia, fatigue, and encephalopathy producing hemiparesis and ataxia. These symptoms develop in approximately 5% of untreated patients and may prove refractory to antibiotic therapy. Rheumatologic symptoms include intermittent episodes of asymmetric mono- or polyarthralgia and migrating musculoskeletal pain. Joint swelling may also be seen. The cardiac manifestations include atrioventricular conduction disturbances, myocarditis, pericarditis, and heart failure. Each of these complications may eventuate in death.

The treatment of uncomplicated Lyme disease involves the oral administration of either amoxicillin 500 mg t.i.d. or doxycycline 100 mg b.i.d. for 14 to 21 days. Complicated, disseminated, or chronic cases may be treated with the same regimen for 30 to 60 days or with intravenous ceftriaxone for 14 to 30 days.

References

1. Hurley H, Hurley J. The gyrate erythemas. *Semin Dermatol* 1984; 3: 327.
2. Gammel J. Erythema gyratum repens. *Arch Derm Syph* 1953; 66: 494.
3. Boyd A, Neldner K, Menter A. Erythema gyratum repens: A paraneoplastic eruption. *J Dermatol* 1992; 26: 757.
4. Appell M, Ward W, Tyring S. Erythema gyratum repens: A cutaneous marker of malignancy. *Cancer* 1988; 62: 548.
5. Langlois J, Shaw J, Odland G. Erythema gyratum repens unassociated with internal malignancy. *J Am Acad Dermatol* 1985; 12: 911.
6. Wakeel R, Ormerod A, Sewell H, et al. Subcorneal accumulation of Langerhans cells in erythema gyratum repens. *Br J Dermatol* 1992; 126: 189.
7. Albers S, Fenske N, Glass F. Erythema gyratum repens: Direct immunofluorescence microscopic findings. *J Am Acad Dermatol* 1993; 29: 493.
8. Trevisan G, Cinco M. Lyme disease: A general survey. *Int J Dermatol* 1990; 29: 1.

9. Asbrink E, Hovmark A. Cutaneous manifestations in *Ixodes*-borne *Borrelia* spirochetosis. *Int J Dermatol* 1987; 26: 215.
10. Berger B. Erythema chronicum migrans of Lyme disease. *Arch Dermatol* 1984; 120: 1017.
11. Krafchick B. Lyme disease. *Int J Dermatol* 1989; 28: 71.
12. Abele D, Anders K. The many faces and phases of borreliosis I. Lyme disease. *J Am Acad Dermatol* 1990; 23: 167.
13. Wu Y, Zhang W, Feng F, et al. Atypical cutaneous lesions of Lyme disease. *Clin Exp Dermatol* 1993; 18: 434.
14. Berg D, Abson K, Prose N. The laboratory diagnosis of Lyme disease. *Arch Dermatol* 1991; 127: 866.
15. Berger B, Clemmensen O, Ackerman A. Lyme diseases a spirochetosis. *Am J Dermatopathol* 1983; 5: 111.
16. Wienecke , Neubert U, Volkenandt M. Molecular detection of *Borrelia burgdorferi* in formalin-fixed, paraffin-embedded lesions of Lyme disease. *J Cutan Pathol* 1993; 20: 385.
17. Barbour A. Isolation and cultivation of Lyme disease spirochetes. *Yale J Bio Med* 1984; 57: 521.

17
Gardner Syndrome

- Synonyms: Familial adenomatous polyposis (FAP), adenomatous polyposis coli (APC)
- Etiology: Mutation in adenomatous polyposis coli (APC) gene, chromosome 5q21
- Associations: Colonic tubular adenomas and carcinoma, cutaneous epidermoid cysts, fibromas, desmoids, osteomas
- Histology: Epithelial cysts with pilomatrical differentiation, fibrous nodules
- Evaluation: Ophthalmologic examination, panoramic dental radiographs, lower GI tract evaluation, possible APC gene mutation evaluation
- Treatment: Prophylactic colectomy, periodic monitoring of upper GI tract and other organ systems for malignancy
- Prognosis: Good, with early detection and intervention

Gardner syndrome is a variant of familial adenomatous polyposis, an autosomal dominant disease characterized by multiple adenomatous polyps of the colon that inevitably transform into adenocarcinoma, usually by the fifth decade. Some cases are the result of spontaneous mutations. In 1951, Gardner described a familial adenomatous polyposis kindred with extracolonic manifestations, including bone tumors, and soft "cyst-like" surface tumors (1). Interestingly, the cutaneous lesions were not characterized in that report because one family member had expired shortly after having a cutaneous lesion removed, and others in the family were afraid they would meet the same fate if their lesions were removed.

Gardner syndrome (GS) was initially viewed as a distinct variant of familial adenomatous polyposis (FAP). However, it became clear that within a given kindred, there is highly variable expression of extracolonic manifestations. Some patients express prominent extracolonic manifestations, and others express only gastrointestinal tract disease. The notion that GS and FAP are a single disease is supported by genetic studies that have localized germline mutations in FAP families to chromosome 5q21, within the adenomatous polyposis coli (APC) gene (2–4). In a given kindred, the identical mutation may be associated with pure colonic disease or colonic disease with prominent extracolonic manifestations, implicating other genetic or environmental factors in disease expression (4). In one large kindred, there was a strong correlation of slow acetylators with extracolonic manifestations, but this has not been studied in other families (5). Somatic mutations in this same gene have been implicated as the cause of some cases of sporadic colon cancer (4).

The APC gene encodes a protein complex that functions as a tumor suppressor by its interactions with β-catenin. β-catenin is a protein that is a component of the adherens junctions at the plasma membrane. β-catenin also has an unbound soluble form that can act as a transcription factor with T-cell factor in the nucleus. This complex induces the expression of genes such as *c*-MYC, *cyclin* D1, and matrix metalloproteinase 7, which are involved in cell proliferation, migration, and metastasis. APC protein inhibits this process by phosphorylating β-catenin in the cytoplasm, precipitating its degradation. In the nucleus, it blocks β-catenin-induced transcriptional activity and aids in its removal from the nucleus. Once in the cytoplasm, β-catenin may be broken down or utilized at the adherens junctions (6). Thus, the effect of APC gene mutations is the cellular accumulation of β-catenin, with its resultant proliferative and tumorigenic effects. β-catenin stabilizing mutations have been implicated in some cases of colon cancer and cutaneous tumors with pilomatrical differentiation (7). β-catenin's resistance to breakdown in these cases results in the same cellular accumulation of the protein as occurs in APC mutations.

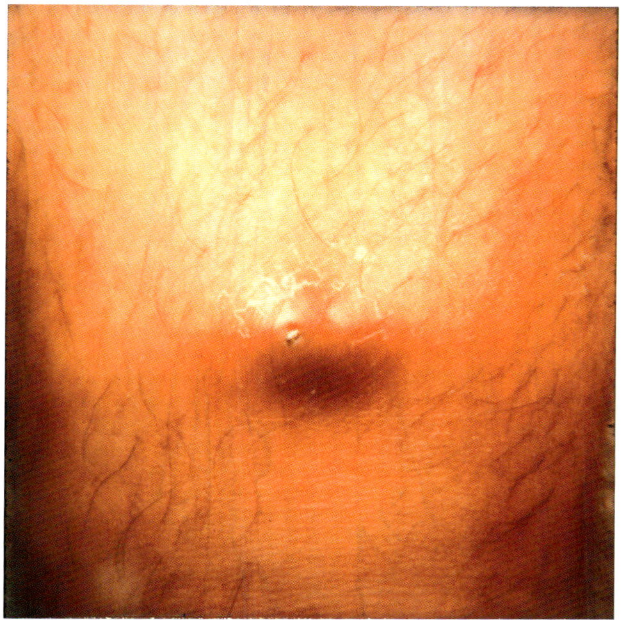

FIGURE 17.1. Epidermoid cyst with pilomatrical differentiation pretibial erythematous and violaceous cystic nodule.

FAP patients will usually develop tubular adenomas of the colon in the second and third decade, and most will develop carcinomas by the fifth decade if not treated by prophylactic colectomy. FAP accounts for fewer than 1% of cases of colon cancer, but implications of diagnosis and early treatment in affected kindreds are profound (8). Expression of extracolonic manifestations may allow for early diagnosis of FAP, potentially resulting in life-saving intervention. Given the highly variable expression of the disease within individuals, it is important to have an awareness of the spectrum of its features.

Ocular manifestations are present in a high percentage of FAP patients. They consist of round or oval pigmented patches of the retina, referred to as *congenital hypertrophy of the retinal pigmented epithelium* (CHRPE). These are probably choristomas or hamartomas (9). CHRPE is found in up to 90% of FAP patients, and is bilateral in 78%. It should be noted that this finding is not specific. Similar unilateral lesions are found in one-third of control patients, and bilateral lesions in 5% (10). Large or bilateral lesions are predictors of disease in the right clinical setting. Evaluation for CHRPE is particularly useful because such lesions are likely congenital, whereas other manifestations of the disease may not develop until adulthood.

Cutaneous manifestations of FAP help to define Gardner syndrome. These include epidermoid cysts and fibromas (Figure 17.1). Cutaneous cysts are usually multiple, and most occur on the scalp and face. Many begin to develop before puberty. While some cysts have no distinctive features, a study of cysts from a large kindred of Gardner syndrome patients revealed foci of pilomatrical differentiation in 63% of lesions (Figure 17.2A and 17.2B). Pilomatrical cells are those cells of the hair follicle that differentiate into the keratinizing cells that form the hair shaft. While the finding is of unknown specificity, such differentiation was not found in any of 100 randomly selected cysts (11). Multiple pilomatricomas may also be a cutaneous marker of Gardner syndrome (12). Nuchal-type fibroma is a deep-seated fibrous tumor, usually of the posterior neck, which may be associated with Gardner syndrome or, more commonly, diabetes mellitus. Tumors are composed of thick bundles of hypocellular collagen, which may entrap adipose tissue, and display traumatic

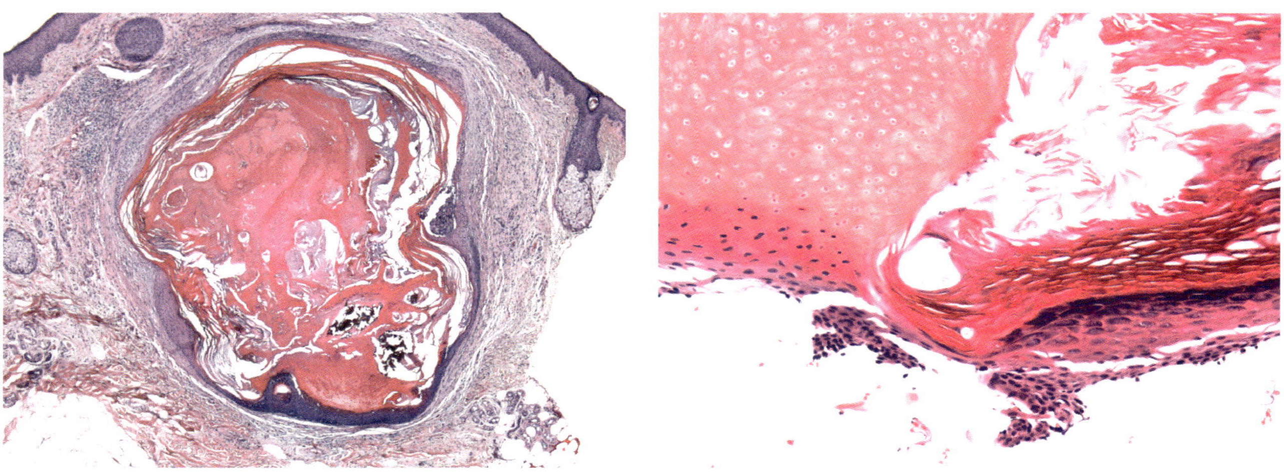

A B

FIGURE 17.2. (A and B) Dermal cyst with follicular infundibular (right on high power panel) and matrical (left on high power panel) differentiation.

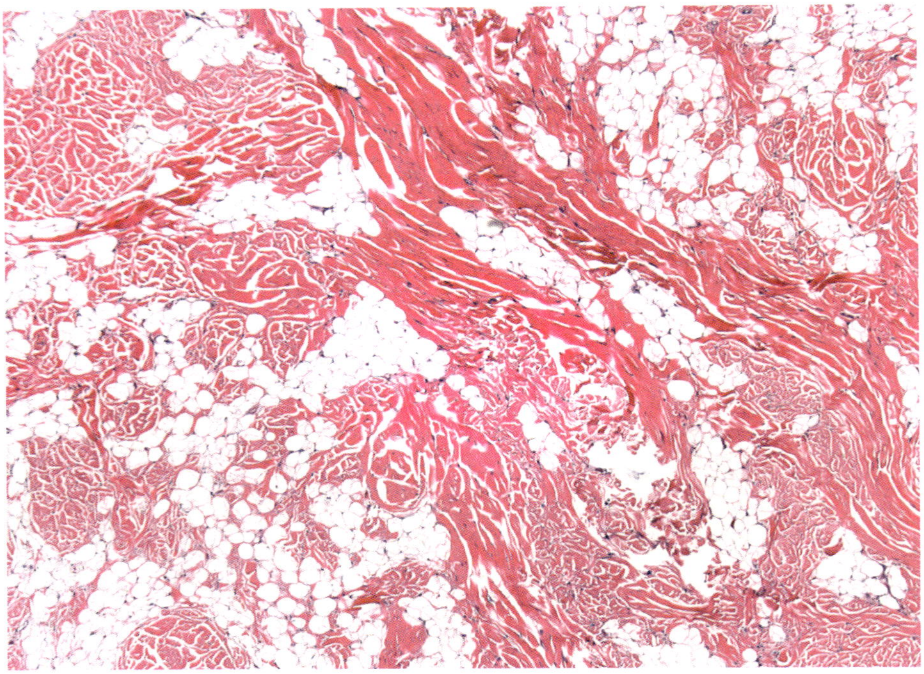

FIGURE 17.3. Nuchal-type fibroma: dense collagen bundles admixed with adipose tissue.

neuroma-like areas (Figure 17.3). A sparse population of CD34+ spindled cells is present (13,14). Similar lesions have been described at other anatomic sites in children with GS, as early as three months of age. In some, it represented the initial presentation of the disease. Nuchal-type fibromas may recur as desmoid fibromatosis, a myofibroblastic proliferation also known to occur in GS patients (14). Some patients with Gardner syndrome have oral and cutaneous fibromas that do not display the typical features of nuchal-type fibroma. This observation suggests that Gardner's fibroma and nuchal-type fibroma are not synonymous, and that GS should be regarded as being associated with a spectrum of benign fibrous lesions (15).

Desmoid fibromatosis, a benign-appearing myofibroblastic proliferation that may display a locally invasive growth pattern, occurs in approximately 10% of individuals with FAP (9). Abdominal cavity involvement, referred to as intra-abdominal fibromatosis, and abdominal wall involvement, are the most common sites of involvement. Desmoids may be induced by pregnancy, oral contraceptives, or surgical procedures. Microscopically, lesions have dense collagen with keloidal and myxoid change, vascular ectasia, and muscular hyperplasia of small arteries. Intra-abdominal fibromatosis occurs in the mesentery and in other peritoneal sites (Figure 17.4). Approximately 15% of those with intra-abdominal fibromatosis have Gardner syndrome, and most of that group have their disease induced by prior abdominal surgery, most commonly colectomy. Some have coexistent abdominal wall involvement (16).

Other extracolonic manifestations of FAP are numerous. The association of brain tumors with FAP was originally described as Turcot syndrome, but like Gardner syndrome, mutations within the APC gene will result in this phenotype. The noncutaneous extracolonic manifestations of FAP are summarized in Table 17.1. Of these, osteomatous jaw change is worthy of special mention, because it may have early onset and be fairly prevalent among those with APC mutations. This makes panoramic dental radiographs a worthwhile screening tool (17).

Cutaneous presentations of the Gardner syndrome variant of FAP usually consist of multiple cysts, or perhaps fibromas, nuchal-type or other, in childhood or early adulthood. Histopathologic evaluation of cysts is important because a finding of pilomatrical differentiation in such lesions should prompt a thorough evaluation for FAP. Family history may reveal FAP, but the lack of a history does not exclude the disease, since 25% of cases may represent spontaneous mutations. Evaluation in childhood should begin with ophthalmologic evaluation for pigmented retinal lesions, and panoramic dental radiographs or computed tomography for osteomatous change or other dental abnormalities. Genetic testing for APC mutations may be undertaken, but the false negative rate is approximately 20% (14). Direct visualization of colorectal mucosa should be a consideration in post-pubertal individuals depending upon the clinical setting.

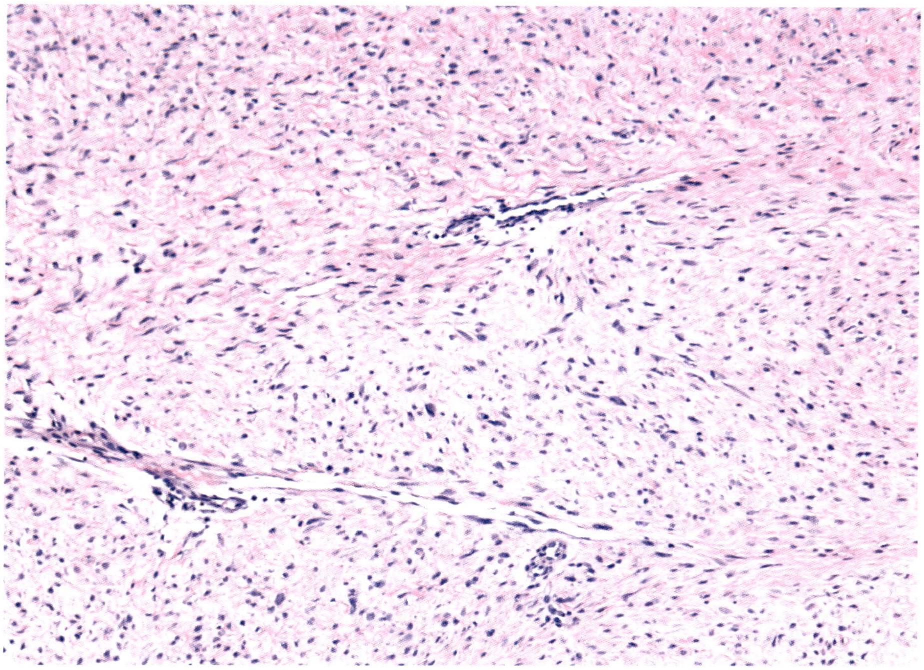

FIGURE 17.4. Desmoid fibromatosis: myofibroblastic spindle cell proliferation admixed with collagen and blood vessels.

Treatment of FAP consists of prophylactic colectomy since the incidence of carcinoma otherwise approaches 100% in the fifth decade. Polyps have been shown to regress with sulindac therapy, but they recur upon cessation of treatment (18). Since treatment is unlikely to prevent carcinoma, this therapy probably does not have a place in the management of FAP patients. Even with total colectomy, periodic evaluation of the upper gastrointestinal tract is indicated because of a 10%–12% estimated lifetime risk of developing duodenal or ampullary carcinomas (8). Thyroid screening has been advocated due to the occurrence of papillary carcinoma in some FAP patients (19). Onset of abdominal pain or gastrointestinal tract bleeding should prompt consideration of upper gastrointestinal tract tumors, obstructive pancreatitis due to periampullary tumors, or abdominal fibromatosis.

The Gardner syndrome variant of familial adenomatous polyposis is characterized by the presence of extracolonic manifestations, particularly cutaneous cysts and fibromas. The development of these markers early in life may herald the development of colonic polyposis and subsequent carcinoma, allowing for early diagnosis and potentially life-saving intervention for the patient and other affected family members.

TABLE 17.1. Noncutaneous Extracolonic Manifestations of FAP

1. **Dento-maxillary**—osteomas, diffuse osteomatous change, odontomas, dentigerous cysts, impacted teeth, hypercementomas, supernumerary teeth, fused or long roots
2. **Ocular**—congenital hypertrophy of the retinal pigment epithelium (CHRPE)
3. **Central nervous system tumors** (Turcot syndrome)—cerebellar medulloblastoma (most common), glioblastoma, craniopharyngioma
4. **Gastrointestinal tract**—duodenal and gastric polyps, periampullary adenoma and carcinoma (may cause obstructive pancreatitis), intra-abdominal fibromatosis
5. **Bone**—osteomas (facial or long bones)
6. **Other malignancy**—thyroid papillary carcinoma, hepatoblastoma, liposarcoma, osteosarcoma, testicular, renal

References

1. Gardner EJ. A genetic and clinical study of intestinal polyposis, a predisposing factor for carcinoma of the colon and rectum. *Am J Hum Genet* 1951; 3: 167–176.
2. Bodmer WF, Bailey CJ, Bodmer J, et al. Localisation of the gene for familial adenomatous polyposis on chromosome 5. *Nature* 1987; 328: 614–616.
3. Leppert, M, Dobbs M, Scambler P, et al. The gene for familial polyposis coli maps to the long arm of chromosome 5. *Science* 1987; 238: 1411–1413.
4. Nishisho I, Nakamura Y, Miyoshi Y, et al. Mutations of chromosome 5q21 genes in FAP and colorectal cancer patients. *Science* 1991; 253: 665–669.
5. Scott RJ, Taeschner W, Heinimann K, et al. Association of extracolonic manifestations of familial adenomatous polyposis with acetylation phenotype in a large FAP kindred. *Eur J Hum Genet* 1997; 5: 43–49.

6. Hildesheim J, Salvador JM, Hollander MC, Fornace AJ, Jr. CK2- and PKA-regulated APC and β-catenin cellular localization is dependent on p38 MAPK. *J Biol Chem* 2005; 280: 17221–17226.
7. Chan EF, Gat U, McNiff JM, Fuchs E. A common human skin tumour is caused by activating mutations in beta-catenin. *Nat Genet* 1999; 21: 410–413.
8. Burt RW, Bishop DT, Cannon-Albright L, et al. Population genetics of colon cancer. *Cancer* 1991; 70: 1719–1722.
9. Foulkes WD. A tale of four syndromes: Familial adenomatous polyposis, Gardner syndrome, attenuated APC and Turcot syndrome. *Q J Med* 1995; 88: 853–863.
10. Traboulsi EI, Krush AJ, Gardner EF, et al. Prevalence and importance of pigmented ocular fundus lesions in Gardner's syndrome. *N Engl J Med* 1987; 316: 661–667.
11. Cooper PH, Fechner RE. Pilomatricoma-like changes in epidermal cysts of Gardner's syndrome. *J Am Acad Dermatol* 1983; 8: 639–644.
12. Pujol RM, Casanova JM, Egido R, Pujol J, de Moragas JM. Multiple familial pilomatricomas: A cutaneous marker for Gardner syndrome? *Pediatr Dermatol* 1995; 12: 331–335.
13. Michal M, Fetsch JF, Hes O, Miettinen M. Nuchal-type fibroma: A clinicopathologic study of 52 cases. *Cancer* 1999; 85: 156–163.
14. Wehrli BM, Weiss SW, Yandow S, Coffin CM. Gardner-associated fibromas (GAF) in young patients. *Am J Surg Pathol* 2001; 25: 645–651.
15. Michal M, Boudova L, Mukensnabi P. Gardner's syndrome associated fibromas. *Pathol Int* 2004; 54: 523–526.
16. Burke AP, Sobin LH, Shekitka KM, Federspiel BH, Helwig EB. Intra-abdominal fibromatosis: A pathologic analysis of 130 tumors with comparison of clinical subgroups. *Am J Surg Pathol* 1990; 14: 335–341.
17. Utsunomiya J, Nakamura T. The occult osteomatous changes in the mandible in patients with familial polyposis coli. *Br J Surg* 1975; 62: 45–51.
18. Rigau J, Pique JM, Rubio E, Planas R, Tarrech JM, Bordas JM. Effects of long-term sulindac therapy on colonic polyposis. *Ann Intern Med* 1991; 115: 952–954.
19. Bell B, Mazzaferri EL. Familial adenomatous polyposis (Gardner's syndrome) and thyroid carcinoma: A case report and review of the literature. *Dig Dis Sci* 1993; 38: 185–190.

18 Multicentric Reticulohistiocytosis

- Synonyms: None
- Etiology: Unknown
- Associations: Mutilating osteoarthritis, visceral malignancies
- Clinical: Yellow papules on extremities
- Histology: Aggregations of histiocytes with "ground glass" cytoplasm
- IHC repertoire: CD68+, CD11b+, HAM-56+
- Staging: N/A
- Prognosis: Debilitating arthritis stabilizes
- Adverse variables: Visceral malignancies
- Treatment: Careful screening

Multicentric reticulohistiocytosis is a rare syndrome of adulthood characterized by the rapid appearance of multiple papules and nodules arising in conjunction with a severe, mutilating arthritis. When occurring as part of the syndrome, the reticulohistiocytomas are found on mucosal surfaces in up to 50% of cases (1–2). Visceral reticulohistiocytomas involving lymph nodes, bone marrow, lungs, and endocardium have also been described in patients with the syndrome (3,4). Cardiac involvement may result in cardiac failure in extreme cases. Xanthomatous lesions may also be present. The destructive osteoarthritis tends to be symmetrical and involves primarily the joints in the hands. The knees and wrists are also involved in greater than 50% of cases. The arthritis may precede, occur concurrently with, or follow the appearance of the cutaneous lesions but is the presenting sign in most cases. After a period of rapid deterioration, the arthritis usually stabilizes, but does not improve. In approximately 30% of cases, the constellation of multiple reticulohistiocytomas and destructive osteoarthritis has been associated with visceral malignancies (3,5,6). The types of cancer that have been reported in patients with multicentric reticulohistiocytosis are shown in Table 18.1 (7–12). In rare cases, multicentric reticulohistiocytosis has been reported in children, also associated with development of malignancy (9). Resolution of the arthritis has been reported in cases with effective treatment of the underlying neoplasm (13). Systemic vasculitis has also been reported in these patients (5).

Reticulohistiocytoma presents as one or several yellow-brown dermal papules or nodules, occasionally with overlying erythema. In most cases, there are no surface epidermal changes and the growths are most prominent on the dorsal surfaces of the hand, overlying joints (Figure 18.1) (1). The individual lesions are asymptomatic and raise a large clinical differential diagnosis. These lesions occur in adults, with a mean age of 40 years, and there is a slight female predominance. The diagnosis is made ordinarily only following biopsy. These lesions are benign and may resolve spontaneously after an initial period of growth. Affected patients have normal serum lipid levels.

The histologic features of a solitary reticulohistiocytoma and multicentric reticulohistiocytosis are identical. In either case, the growths demonstrate a compression of the overlying epidermis with a nodular aggregation of large cells within the superficial dermis (Figure 18.2). The aggregate is well-circumscribed, but not encapsulated and is separated from the epidermis by a thin Grenz zone. The histiocytes are large, with abundant eosinophilic cytoplasm and vesicular nuclei. In many cases, the cytoplasm has a characteristic "ground glass" or finely granular appearance. The granules stain with PAS with and without diastase predigestion. Occasional multinucleated cells may be seen, but these are less prevalent than the lipidized Touton giant cells in the similar appearing xanthogranuloma (Figures 18.2–18.4).

The histiocytes are admixed with lymphocytes and abundant eosinophils in many cases. There is

TABLE 18.1. Tumors Associated with Multicentric Reticulohistiocytosis

Breast carcinoma
Pancreatic adenocarcinoma
Squamous cell carcinoma—lung
Melanoma
Non-Hodgkin's lymphomas
Gastric adenocarcinoma
Ovarian mucinous adenocarcinoma
Colonic adenocarcinoma
Pleural mesothelioma
Cervical squamous cell carcinoma

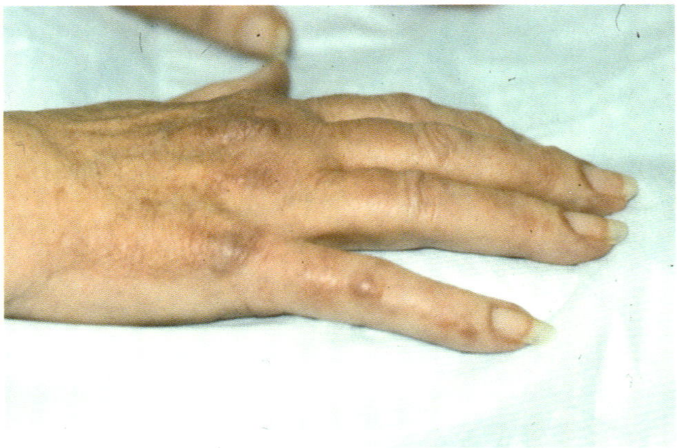

FIGURE 18.1. Multiple tan-red papules on digits with periungual accentuation seen in multicentric reticulohistiocytosis.

no tendency to form granulomas and caseation is not seen. Immunostains reveal the histiocytes to express CD68, CD3, CD45, CD11b, and HAM-56 (11). These cells do not express S100 protein, CD1a, or Mac387.

Multicentric reticulohistiocytosis appears, at least in some cases, to be a paraneoplastic phenomenon of unknown pathogenesis. Its recognition warrants a full systemic evaluation in order to screen for possible underlying malignancy and close clinical follow-up (11,12).

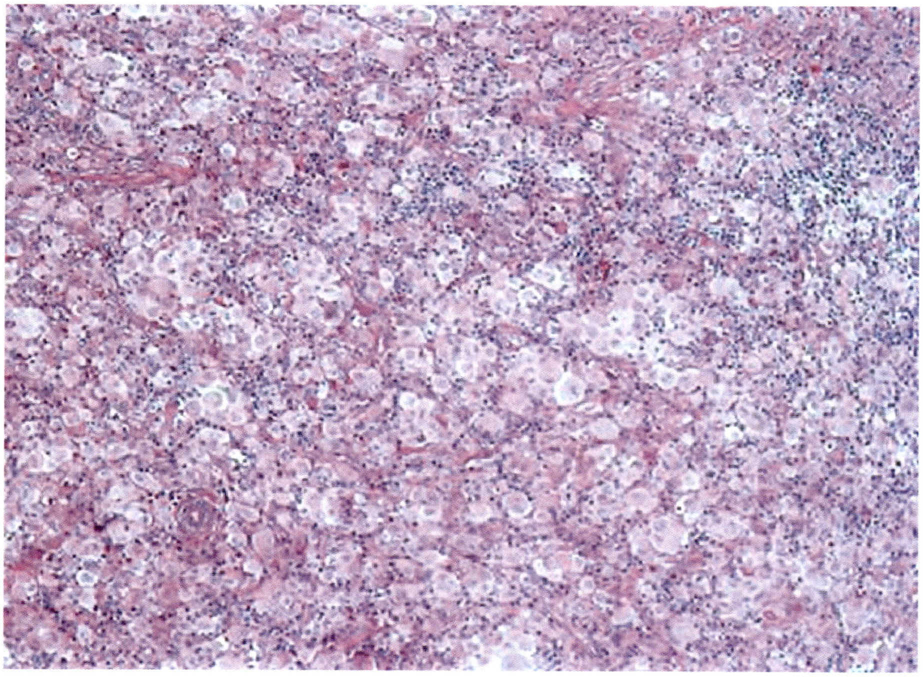

FIGURE 18.2. Low power photomicrograph depicting loose aggregates of giant cells with interspersed lymphocytes and neutrophils.

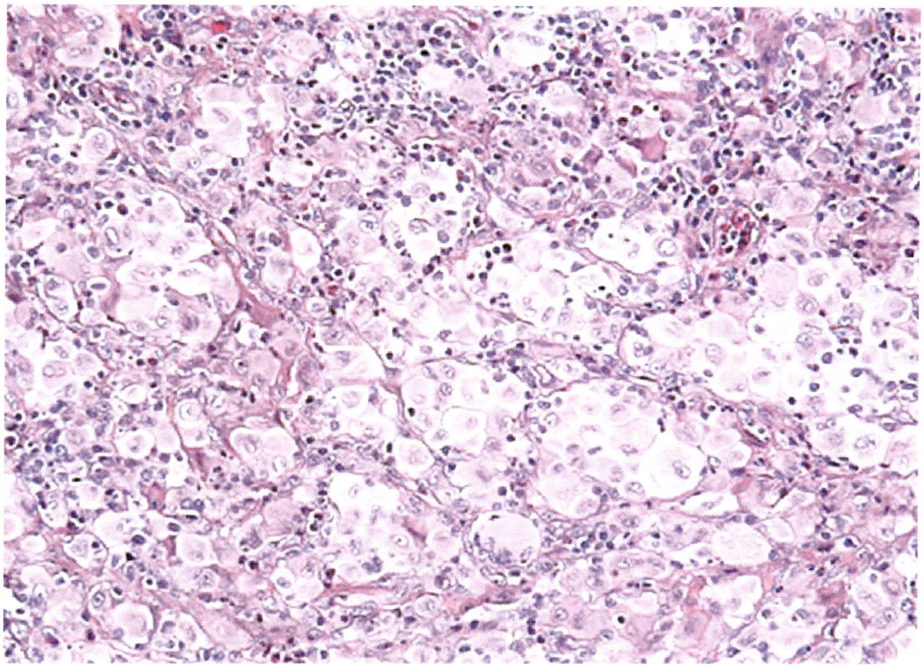

Figure 18.3. Medium power photomicrograph depicting giant cells with surrounding inflammatory cells.

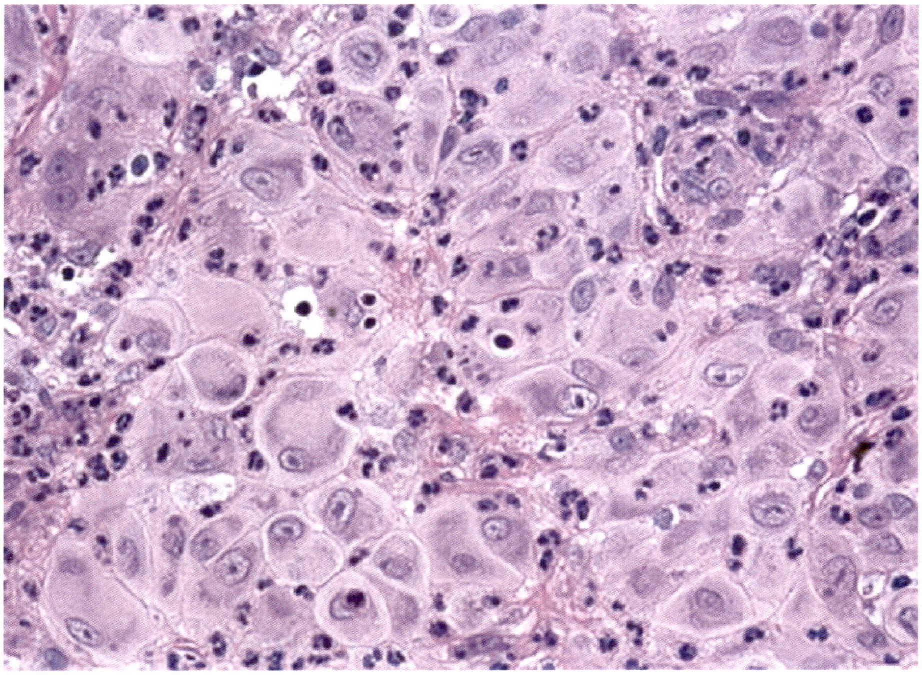

Figure 18.4. High power photomicrograph depicting two-toned cytoplasm (ground-glass) with darker periphery with central clearing characteristic of reticulohistiocytosis.

References

1. Caro MR, Senear FE. Reticulohistiocytoma of the skin. *Arch Dermatol Syphilol* 1950; 65: 701–713.
2. Barrow MV, Holubar K. Multicentric reticulohistiocytosis: A review of 33 patients. *Medicine* 1969; 48: 287–305.
3. Chevrant-Breton J. La reticulohistiocytose multicentrique: Revue de la literature recente (depuis 1969). *Ann Dermatol Venereol* 1977; 104: 745–753.
4. Moble MA, Taschen JA, Sairam S, McNearney T, Orsak G, Knox JM. Multicentric reticulohistiocytosis with pulmonary involvement. *J Am Acad Dermatol* 2003; 49: 1125–1127.
5. Olivier GF, Umbert IU, Winkelmann RK, Muller SA. Reticulohistiocytoma cutis: Review of 15 cases and an association with systemic vasculitis in two cases. *Clin Exp Dermatol* 1990; 15: 1–6.
6. Lotti T, Santucci M, Casigliani R, Fabbri P, Bondi R, Panconesi E. Multicentric reticulohistiocytosis: Report of three cases with the evaluation of tissue proteinase activity. *Am J Dermatopathol* 1988; 10: 497–504.
7. Ridgway HA, Rhodes EL. Multicentric reticulohistiocytosis with carcinoma-in-situ of the cervix. *Br J Dermatol* 1979; 101 supplement: 61–62.
8. Nunnick JC, Krusinski PA, Yates JW. Multicentric reticulohistiocytosis and cancer: A case report and review of the literature. *Med Pediatr Oncol* 1985; 13: 273–279.
9. Kuramoto Y, Iizawa O, Matsunaga J, Nakamura N, Tagami H. Development of Ki-1 lymphoma in a child suffering from multicentric reticulohistiocytosis. *Acta Derm Venereol* 1991; 71: 448–449.
10. Gibson G, Cassidy M, O'Connell P, Murphy GM. Multicentric reticulohistiocytosis associated with recurrence of malignant melanoma. *J Am Acad Dermatol* 1995; 32: 134–136.
11. Snow JL, Muller SA. Malignancy-associated multicentric reticulohistiocytosis: A clinical, histological and immunophenotypic study. *Br J Dermatol* 1995; 133: 71–76.
12. Valencia IC, Colsky A, Berman B. Multicentric reticulohistiocytosis associated with recurrent breast carcinoma. *J Am Acad Dermatol* 1988; 39: 864–866.
13. Lambert CM, Nuki G. Multicentric reticulohistiocytosis with arthritis and cardiac infiltration: Regression following treatment for underlying malignancy. *Ann Rheum Dis* 1992; 51: 815–817.

19 Multiple Cutaneous Leiomyomas

■ Synonyms:	Multiple cutaneous and uterine leiomyomatosis (MCUL) syndrome Hereditary leiomyomatosis renal cell cancer (HLRCC) syndrome
■ Etiology:	Mutation in fumarate hydratase gene, mapped to chromosome 1q42.3–q43
■ Associations:	Uterine leiomyomas and rarely leiomyosarcomas, renal carcinoma
■ Clinical:	Red-brown indurated papules, sometimes clustered or in linear array
■ Histology:	Reticular dermal fascicular tumor with cigar-shaped nuclei, amphophilic vacuolated cytoplasm, rare mitotic figures
■ IHC:	Smooth muscle actin+, desmin+
■ Evaluation:	Renal, uterine ultrasound, possible evaluation for fumarate hydratase function or mutation
■ Treatment:	Surgical management of underlying tumors, excision of painful cutaneous tumors, or nifedipine
■ Prognosis:	Excellent with early detection of underlying malignancy

Cutaneous leiomyomas are uncommon tumors that arise from arrector pili muscle (pilar leiomyoma), genital smooth muscle (genital leiomyoma), or vascular smooth muscle (angioleiomyoma). Angioleiomyomas are histologically distinct, and are not known to occur as multiple lesions. Most pilar leiomyomas occur singly, but can occur as multiple lesions. As multiple lesions, they may occur in association with uterine leiomyomas and, rarely, leiomyosarcomas, in the multiple cutaneous and uterine leiomyomatosis (MCUL) syndrome. More recently, cutaneous and uterine leiomyomas have been reported to occur in association with renal cell carcinoma in the hereditary leiomyomatosis renal cell cancer (HLRCC) syndrome (1). MCUL and HLRCC likely represent part of a spectrum of one disease. These syndromes are both familial and transmitted in an autosomal dominant pattern, with variable penetrance. The implicated gene encodes fumarate hydratase, an enzyme in the Krebs cycle that maps to chromosome 1q42.3–q43 (2). Fumarate hydratase (FH) is distributed predominantly within mitochondria, but also within the cytosol, of mammalian cells. In the cytosol, FH is involved in the purine nucleotide cycle. In mitochondria, it catalyzes the reversible hydration of fumarate into malate as part of the Krebs cycle. The previous step in the Krebs cycle is the conversion of succinate to fumarate by succinate dehydrogenase. Succinate dehydrogenase mutations are also associated with a cancer predisposition, specifically pheochromocytoma and paraganglionoma. The mechanism of tumorigenesis is unknown (3).

There is a spectrum of fumarate hydratase gene defects described in different clinical settings, but the type of defect does not appear to correlate with disparate clinical manifestations (4). Fumarate hydratase mutations cause multiple cutaneous and uterine leiomyomatosis (MCUL) syndrome, hereditary leiomyomatosis renal cell cancer (HLRCC) syndrome, and autosomal recessive FH deficiency, which manifests as severe developmental delay, and death in childhood. Autosomal recessive FH deficiency does not appear to be associated with development of malignancy. However, short life expectancy may not allow for its expression. Some parents of FH-deficient children develop leiomyomas as may be expected in the heterozygous state (2). In HLRCC and MCUL, the development of uterine and cutaneous leiomyomas and renal cell cancer occurs with one mutant allele and one wild type (normal) allele. Tumor development requires a "second hit," as suggested in Knudson's theory of tumorigenesis. Loss of expression of the wild type allele may occur by loss of heterozygosity, or second mutation in the previously normal allele. Loss of heterozygosity at the genetic locus for these syndromes is known to occur in the cutaneous and uterine leiomyomas and renal cell carcinomas in patients with the syndrome, supporting a role for FH in tumor suppression (5). Mutations of the FH gene are rare in sporadic leiomyomas, and not found in sporadic leiomyosarcomas. Therefore, the gene does not play a major role in the development of sporadic tumors (6).

Cutaneous leiomyomas usually present as red-brown dome-shaped papules, from several millimeters to approximately one centimeter in diameter (Figure 19.1). When they are multiple, they may be clustered or form a linear array. Solitary lesions usually occur on the extremities, and multiple lesions may occur on either the trunk or extremities. Pain is commonly reported, and may be precipitated by cold or pressure. The discomfort is described as sharp, burning, or throbbing (7). The differential diagnosis is wide for solitary lesions, and for multiple lesions may include such disparate entities as segmental neurofibromatosis, foreign body granuloma, dermatofibrosarcoma protuberans, and sarcoidosis.

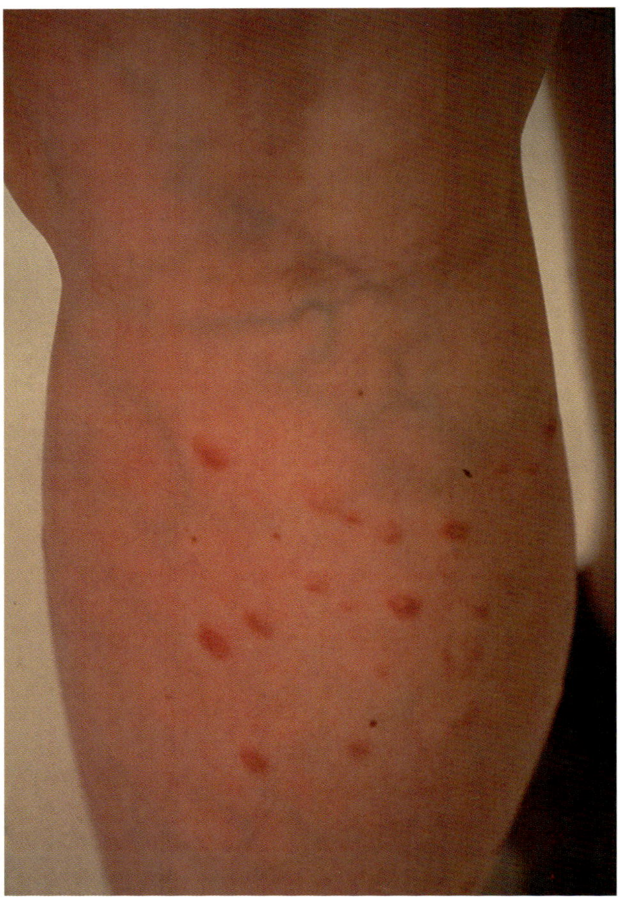

FIGURE 19.1. Clustered erythematous papules and small nodules of the calf. Photo courtesy of Cleveland Clinic Foundation, Department of Dermatology.

Histopathology reveals a reticular dermal tumor composed of fascicles of smooth muscle bundles, with cigar-shaped nuclei and eosinophilic to amphophilic vacuolated cytoplasm (Figure 19.2A and 19.2B). Tumor cells are highlighted by antibodies to smooth muscle actin and desmin. In one series, 55% of these tumors had epidermal hyperplasia, and 10% had focal infiltration of the fat. Twenty-eight percent had mitotic figures, but these were usually sparse. No recurrences were seen in the mitotically active lesions. A nodular, more circumscribed architecture appears to correlate with the presence of multiple lesions (7). Renal carcinomas occurring in association with FH deficiency are of the Type II papillary or collecting duct type (4).

Multiple leiomyomas are not exclusively a manifestation of fumarate hydratase deficiency. They have also been reported to occur in patients with chronic lymphocytic leukemia (8) and HIV infection (9). An association of leiomyosarcomas and leiomyomas with HIV infection and other forms of immunosuppression is well-established, and is known to be induced by Epstein-Barr virus (EBV) infection. In these tumors, EBV genomes are detectable within tumor cells by *in situ* hybridization (10).

Management of multiple leiomyomas is primarily surgical. Excision of symptomatic lesions may be warranted. Nifedipine has been used to alleviate the pain in the setting of multiple painful tumors (11). Affected individuals should undergo renal imaging studies, and in women, uterine imaging because of a risk of development of leiomyosarcoma. Evaluation of family members should also be undertaken. Genetic evaluation for fumarate hydratase mutations or functional assay should be considered.

Multiple cutaneous leiomyomas has recently been added to the list of cancer-susceptibility syndromes that may first present in the skin. These tumors may represent manifestations of multiple cutaneous and uterine leiomyomatosis (MCUL) syndrome or leiomyomatosis renal cell cancer (HLRCC) syndrome, which are closely related, if not the same entity. Recognition of the cutaneous leiomyomas may have life-saving implications for the patient and relatives.

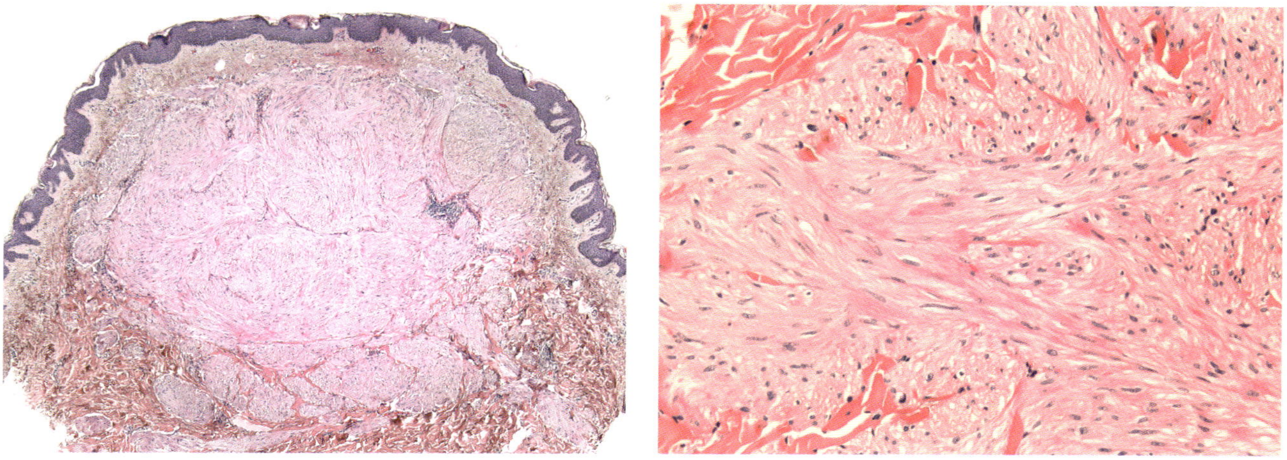

A B

FIGURE 19.2. (A and B) Dermal tumor composed of fascicles of smooth muscle cells with vacuolated cytoplasm and blunt-ended nuclei.

References

1. Launonen V, Vierimaa O, Kiuru M, et al. Inherited susceptibility to uterine leiomyomas and renal cell cancer. *Proc Natl Acad Sci* USA 2001; 98: 3387–3392.
2. Tomlinson IPM, Alam NA, Rowan AJ, et al. Germline mutations in *FH* predispose to dominantly inherited uterine fibroids, skin leiomyomata and papillary renal cancer. *Nat Genet* 2002; 30: 406–410.
3. Rustin P. Mitochondria, from cell death to proliferation. *Nat Genet* 2002; 30: 352–353.
4. Alam NA, Rowan AJ, Wortham NC, et al. Genetic and functional analyses of *FH* mutations in multiple cutaneous and uterine leiomyomatosis, hereditary leiomyomatosis and renal cancer, and fumarate hydratase deficiency. *Human Molec Genet* 2003; 12: 1241–1252.
5. Kiuru M, Launonen V, Hietala M, et al. Familial cutaneous leiomyomatosis is a two-hit condition associated with renal cell cancer of characteristic histopathology. *Am J Pathol* 2001; 159: 825–829.
6. Lehtonen R, Kiuru M, Vanharanta S, et al. Biallelic inactivation of *fumarate hydratase* (*FH*) occurs in nonsyndromic uterine leiomyomas but is rare in other tumors. *Am J Pathol* 2004; 164: 17–22.
7. Raj S, Calonje E, Kraus M, et al. Cutaneous pilar leiomyoma: Clinicopathologic analysis of 53 lesions in 45 patients. *Am J Dermatopathol* 1997; 19: 2–9.
8. Vergani R, Betti R, Uziel L, Tolomio E, Crosti C. Eruptive multiple sporadic cutaneous piloleiomyomas in a patient with chronic lymphocytic leukemia. *Br J Dermatol* 2000; 143: 907–909.
9. Kanitakis J, Carbonnel E, Chouvet B, Labeille B, Claudy A. Cutaneous leiomyomas (piloleiomyomas) in adult patients with human immunodeficiency virus infection. *Br J Dermatol* 2000; 143: 1338–1340.
10. McClain K, Leach C, Jenson H. Association of Epstein-Barr virus with leiomyosarcomas in children with AIDS. *N Engl J Med* 1995; 332: 12–18.
11. George S, Pulimood S, Jacob M, Chandi SM. Pain in multiple leiomyomas alleviated by nifedipine. *Pain* 1997; 73: 101–102.

20
Lethal Non-Langerhans Cell Histiocytoses: Necrobiotic Xanthogranuloma and Xanthoma Disseminatum

■ Synonyms:	NXG—Necrobiotic xanthogranuloma with paraproteinemia XD—Montgomery's syndrome
■ Etiology:	NXG—Unknown XD—Unknown
■ Associations:	NXG—Myeloma, Grave's disease, primary biliary cirrhosis, paraproteins XD—Myeloma, Waldenstrom's macroglobulinemia, paraproteins
■ Clinical:	NXG—Ulcerating red-orange plaques, particularly of the periorbital area XD—Disseminated red brown papules into plaques
■ Histology:	NXG—Palisading granulomatous dermatitis with bizarre giant cells XD—Diffuse epithelioid histiocytes, foam cells, and siderosis
■ IHC repertoire:	NXG—CD-68(+), S-100(–), CD-1(–) XD—CD-68(+), S-100(–),CD-1(–)
■ Staging:	NXG—None XD—None
■ Prognosis:	NXG—Overall 5% 5-year mortality XD—Overall 2% 5-year mortality
■ Adverse variables:	NXG—Cases associated with myeloma XD—Cases associated with myeloma and Waldenstrom's
■ Treatment:	NXG—Corticosteroids, alkylating agents XD—Corticosteroids

The histiocytic disorders encompass a broad range of malignant and nonmalignant entities capable of presenting in a variety of clinical and pathologic guises. The histiocytic disorders are generally classified by the cell of the origin, and specifically as bone marrow tissue-derived monocytes that migrate secondarily to the skin serving as either phagocytic macrophages or antigen-presenting dendritic or Langerhans cells. Langerhans cells typically reside closely to the epithelium and traffic to the lymph nodes. They are important in immunologic surveillance and are defined by the presence of Birbeck granules on ultrastructural examination, as well as S-100 and CD-1a immunopositivity. This discussion will focus upon the entities comprised of the phagocytic non-Langerhans cell macrophages and specifically the disorders within this category capable of producing or being associated with significant morbidity or mortality.

The two most important entities associated with serious systemic disorder including hematopoetic malignancy are necrobiotic xanthogranuloma (NXG) and xanthoma disseminatum (XD). Despite a marked difference in their clinical and histologic appearance, both share a common histogenesis, an association with abnormal amounts or types of circulating immunoglobulins (paraproteins) and hematopoetic malignancies including multiple myeloma.

Necrobiotic Xanthogranuloma

This rare non-Langerhans cell histiocytosis was first described in 1980 by Winkelman and Kossard, who correctly surmised its association with paraproteinemia and risk for development of multiple myeloma (1). Since its initial description, over 60 cases have been described with nearly all patients presenting as adults. There is no gender or ethnic predisposition (2). The etiology of the disorder is unknown but various theories regarding its development have been proposed, including abnormal immunoglobulin or lipid storage leading to the formation of xanthomatous histiocytic cells and faulty phagocytic mechanisms leading to the characteristic clinical and pathologic findings. Each of the theories, however, fails to wholly account for its rarity, associated laboratory findings, or peculiar anatomic predisposition.

NXG is associated with a variety of unrelated disorders including, most importantly, multiple myeloma (10% of patients), Hodgkin's disease, arthropathy, hypertension, neuropathy, primary biliary cirrhosis, and Grave's disease (3).

The clinical findings consist of firm red-orange to violaceous papules that typically enlarge into plaques, finally undergoing central atrophy and ulceration. The plaques may attain dimensions of greater than 25 cm and can be solitary or multiple. The lesions typically develop on the head and neck area, particularly the periorbital region (Figure 20.1). Lesions have been described on the trunk and extremities. Involvement in the oral mucosa has also been reported. The lesions themselves are typically asymptomatic although an antecedent pruritic and/or burning sensation has been documented. Other physical findings include hepatosplenomegaly, which has been documented in approximately 20% of patients. Although the skin is the principal organ involved, the eye, lungs, heart, and CNS may be afflicted.

The histopathologic features are distinctive and consist of a deep dermal and subcutaneous fat granulomatous inflammation with intervening zones of collagen degeneration, lymphoid follicles, and foam cells (Figure 20.2) (4). The granulomas take the form of palisading mono- and multinucleate giant cells with the latter often assuming irregular silhouettes and containing increased numbers of atypical nuclei as well as epithelioid granulomas, Touton-type wreath-like giant cells, and foreign body–type giant cells (Figures 20.3 and 20.4). The degenerated collagen foci often contain zones of cholesterol clefting (Figure 20.5). The histiocytes of NXG immunostain with CD-68, CD-15 and are negative with S-100 and CD-1a.

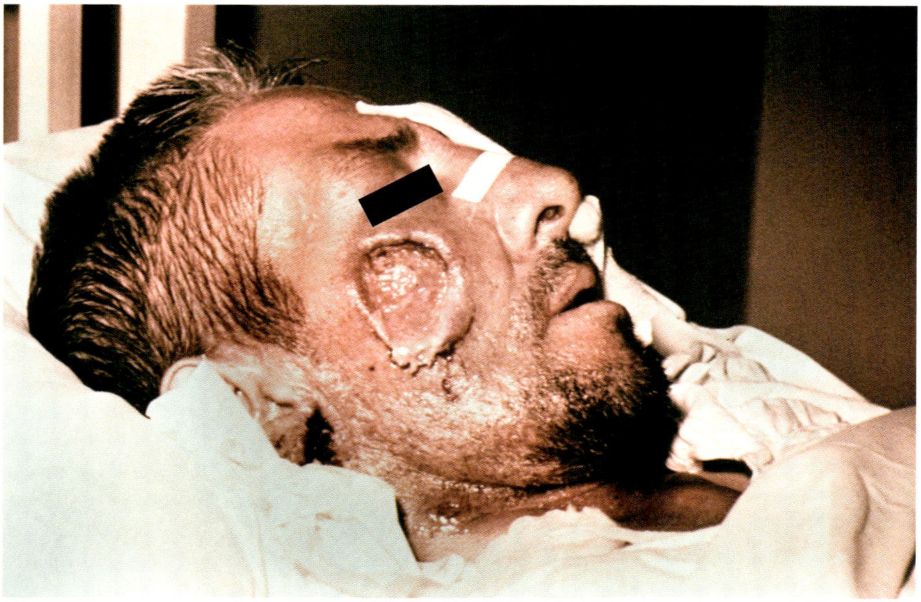

FIGURE 20.1. Infraorbital ulcer typical of necrobiotic xanthogranuloma.

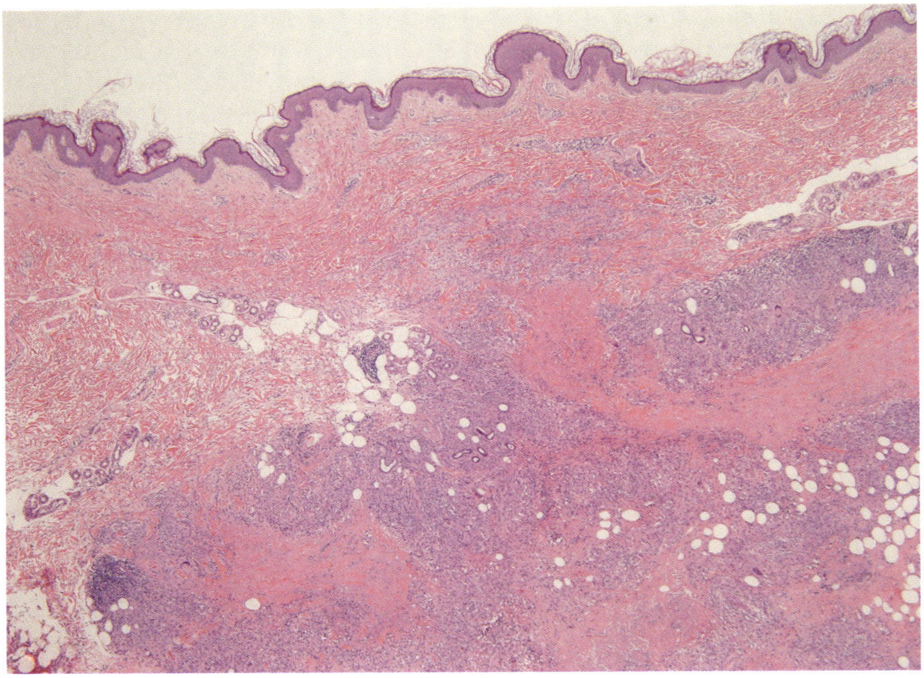

FIGURE 20.2. Low power photomicrograph depicting deep dermal palisading granuloma.

The most important diagnoses to consider in the histologic differential diagnosis are necrobiosis lipoidica, granuloma annulare, and rheumatoid nodule. Although each of the foregoing show palisading granulomatous foci, the collagen degeneration seen in NXG is more extensive, often extending deep into the panniculus, and is associated with cholesterol clefting.

Laboratory findings include paraproteinemia, found in approximately 90% of patients (usually IgG with mostly kappa or occasionally lambda light chains), cryoglobulins (~40% of cases), decreased complements, hyper/hypolipidemia, neutropenia, and elevated erythrocyte sedimentation rate. Bone marrow biopsy often yields increased numbers of atypical plasma cells.

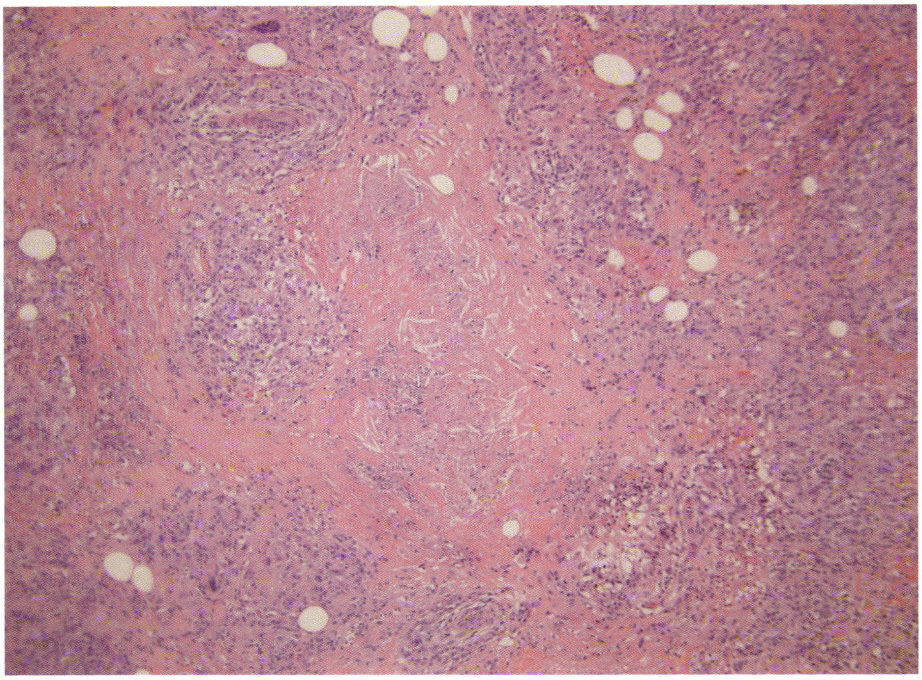

FIGURE 20.3. Medium power photomicrograph depicting central necrobiotic material replete with cholesterol clefts and peripheral palisade of granulomatous inflammation.

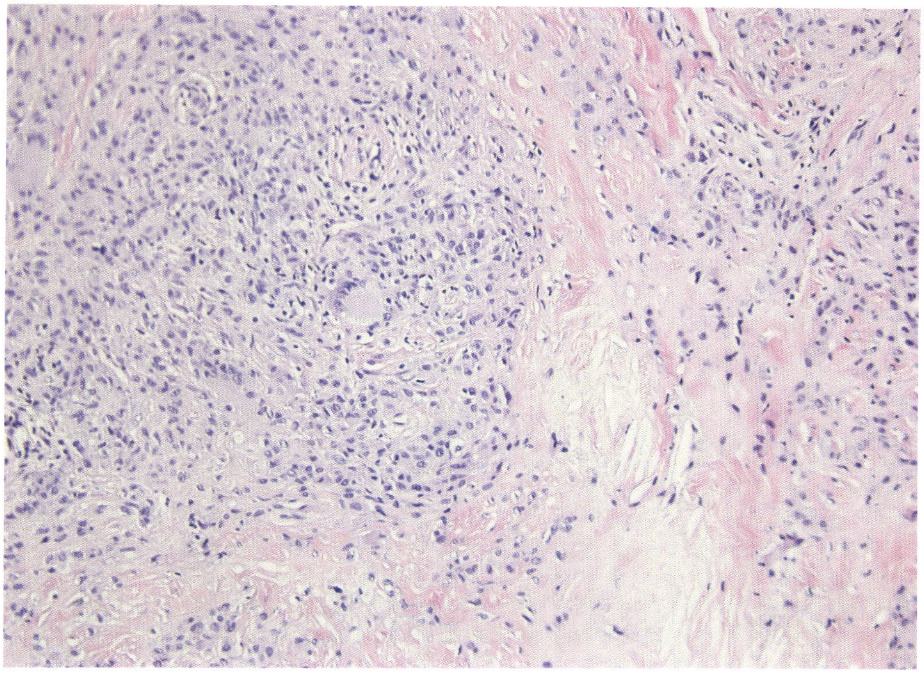

FIGURE 20.4. Medium power photomicrograph depicting nodular aggregates of lymphocytes with interspersed giant cells.

The course of NXG is usually chronic with episodic lesional development followed by healing and remission. Important complications involve its proximity to the eye and include conjunctivitis, keratitis, scleritis uveitis, cornel ulceration, and exceptionally, blindness. The development of multiple myeloma is particularly ominous and may present prior to, concomitant with, or following the diagnosis of NXG. The overall 5-year mortality of multiple myeloma is 40%.

The treatment consists of corticosteroids and low-dose alkylating agents such as chlorambucil and melphalan.

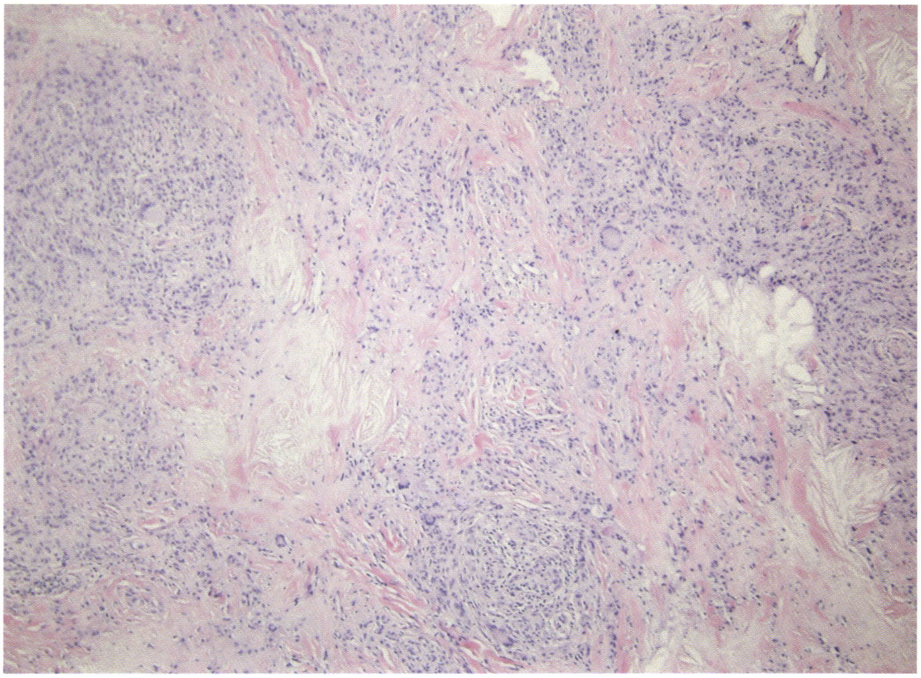

FIGURE 20.5. High power detail of lymphoid aggregates. Note central giant cell.

Temporary remission has also been reported with radiation therapy and plasmapheresis.

Xanthoma Disseminatum

This uncommon systemic non-Langerhans cell histiocytosis was first described by Montgomery and Osterberg in 1938. Since its initial description, over 100 cases have been described. The disorder is slightly more common among males and most patients described with this condition have been children (5). There is no ethnic predisposition. The etiology and pathogenesis of this disorder is unknown. Like NXG, it is associated with multiple myeloma, Waldenstrom's macroglobulinemia, and paraproteinemia (6,7). Notably, each of these disorders is typically exceptional among children.

The clinical findings consist of disseminated red-brown papules that have a tendency to become yellow and coalesce, forming plaques. Similar lesions are often found in approximately 50% of patients involving the mucous membranes of the mouth, pharynx, conjuctiva, and cornea. Lesions of the pharynx and larynx may produce symptoms of dysphagia, and an altered voice. Diabetes insipidus secondary to involvement of the hypothalamus and vasopressin deficiency is observed in approximately 50% of patients.

The histologic features of well-developed lesions are suggestive of the disorder and consist of diffuse dermal aggregates of foam cells with interspersed Touton-type wreath giant cells (8). Early lesions usually show an admixture of characteristically scalloped histiocytes with acute and chronic inflammatory cells. Extension into the subcutaneous fat or epidermal ulceration is exceptional. The lesional cells are CD-68 (+), S-100(−), CD-1a (−).

Laboratory findings usually show normal lipid levels. Serum vasopressin levels are typically depressed. The overall prognosis is favorable with the exception of those patients who develop hematopoetic malignancy. The dermatologic manifestations may pursue three clinical courses: spontaneous resolution; remain persistent; or rarely, progress. Important complications include diabetes insipidus and obstructive upper aerodigestive tract disease. Treatment consists of symptomatic removal of mucosal lesions and vasopressin administration in cases complicated by diabetes insipidus. The cutaneous lesions do not usually respond to topical or systemic medication.

References

NXG

1. Kossard S, Winkelman R. Necrobiotic xanthogranuloma with paraproteinemia. *J Am Acad Dermatol* 1980; 3: 257.
2. Finan M, Winkelman R. Necrobiotic xanthogranuloma with paraproteinemia: A review of 22 cases. *Medicine* 1986; 65: 376.
3. Macfarlane A, Verbov J. Necrobiotic xanthogranuloma with paraproteinemia. *Br J Dermatol* 1985; 113: 339.
4. Finan M, Winkelman R. Histopathology of necrobiotic xanthogranuloma with paraproteinemia. *J Cutan Pathol* 1987; 14: 92.

XD

5. Caputo R, Veraldi S, Grimalt R, et al. The various clinical patterns of xanthoma disseminatum. *Dermatology* 1995; 190: 19.
6. Maize J, Ahmed A, Provost T. Xanthoma disseminatum and multiple myeloma. *Arch Dermatol* 1974; 110: 758.
7. Goodenberger M, Piette W, Macfarlane D, et al. Xanthoma disseminatum and Waldenstroms macroglobulinemia. *J Am Acad Dermatol* 1990; 23: 1015.
8. Mishkel M, Cockshott W, Nazir D, et al. Xanthoma disseminatum: Clinical, metabolic, pathologic, and radiologic aspects. *Arch Dermatol* 1977; 113: 1094.

21 Pancreatic Panniculitis

■ Synonyms:	Pancreatic fat necrosis, nodular fat necrosis of pancreatic disease
■ Etiology:	In part, due to cutaneous enzymatic fat necrosis from circulating pancreatic enzymes
■ Associations:	Acute and chronic pancreatitis, acinar cell carcinoma
■ Clinical:	Erythematous subcutaneous nodules favoring lower extremities, may drain spontaneously; arthritis, serositis, abdominal pain, nausea, vomiting, lytic bone lesions
■ Histology:	Subcutaneous fat necrosis with loss of adipocyte nuclei, "ghost" cells, stippled basophilia of calcification, neutrophils early, mixed infiltrate late
■ Evaluation:	Serum amylase, lipase, CBC with differential (eosinophilia correlates with acinar cell carcinoma), pancreatic imaging studies
■ Treatment:	Correct underlying pancreatic disease
■ Prognosis:	Usually poor in carcinoma-associated disease because of advanced disease, and variable in pancreatitis-associated, depending upon severity of underlying disease

Pancreatic panniculitis is a form of subcutaneous fat necrosis that occurs as a rare manifestation of various pancreatic diseases, most commonly pancreatitis, or pancreatic carcinoma. Fat necrosis at remote sites occurs in only a small percentage of those with pancreatic disease. Its pathogenesis is uncertain. A review of 893 hospital admissions for various pancreatic diseases revealed only three cases of pancreatic panniculitis (1). Circulating pancreatic enzymes, lipase and amylase, are elevated in most but not all cases of pancreatic panniculitis (2). Human pancreatic lipase has been identified in lesions of pancreatic panniculitis, supporting its role in the pathogenesis of the disease (3). *In vitro* and clinical observations suggest that factors other than circulating amylase and lipase are necessary for the development of pancreatic panniculitis. *In vitro* incubation of human adipose tissue with pancreatic enzymes and serum from a patient with pancreatic panniculitis and elevated enzymes failed to induce fat necrosis, suggesting that there are other local factors or a labile circulating factor needed to induce the necrosis (4). Clinical observations indicate that pancreatic panniculitis occurs in only a small number of patients with pancreatic disease. It does not develop in many with striking elevation of pancreatic enzymes, and may arise in patients with normal circulating enzymes. Lesions of pancreatic panniculitis have been induced at sites of injury from a vascular procedure, suggesting that local trauma in a susceptible individual is capable of inducing disease (5). Localized lesions have also been induced by paracentesis in a patient with acute pancreatitis, most likely the direct effect of peritoneal pancreatic enzymes on subcutaneous fat reached via the needle tract from the procedure (6).

Most cases of pancreatic panniculitis occur in association with acute and chronic pancreatitis, and pancreatic adenocarcinoma. Most of the pancreatitis-associated cases are due to chronic alcoholism, but some are due to cholecystitis with biliary tract obstruction and trauma. Malignancy-induced pancreatic panniculitis is almost always due to acinar cell carcinoma. Although this tumor accounts for fewer than 5% of pancreatic malignant neoplasms, it produces large quantities of lipase and other digestive enzymes, likely accounting for the association (7). Other triggers of pancreatic panniculitis include pancreatic pseudocyst, post-traumatic pancreatitis (8), and structural anomalies such as pancreas divisum (9).

Patients who develop pancreatic panniculitis present with erythematous to brown, usually painful, subcutaneous nodules (Figure 21.1). The most common site of involvement is pretibial, but lesions may involve the upper extremities and trunk, and may spare the legs. Nodules are indurated, and many have some softening or fluctuation in the central portion, indicating liquefactive necrosis. In some patients, spontaneous ulceration occurs, with drainage of creamy or brown viscous fluid, representing degenerated adipose tissue. Spontaneous involution with lipoatrophy and dyspigmentation occurs in several weeks, and may or may not correlate with improvement of the underlying disease. Paradoxically, pancreatic panniculitis associated with alcoholic pancreatitis and markedly elevated pancreatic enzymes tends to have more localized cutaneous disease with less likelihood of spontaneous rupture, drainage, and ulceration than that associated with pancreatic carcinoma (8).

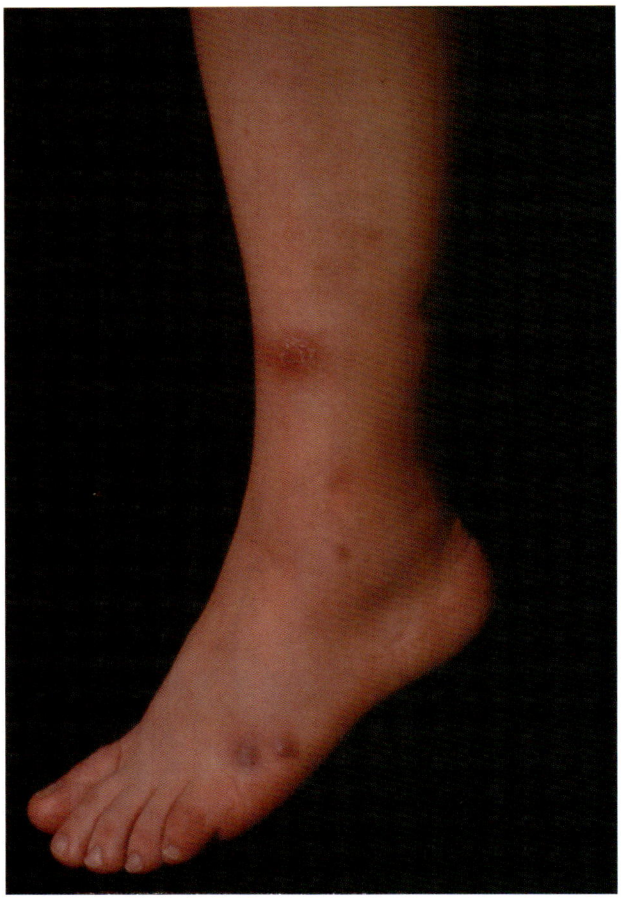

FIGURE 21.1. Pancreatic panniculitis: dusky acral subcutaneous nodules with some depressions from sites of prior spontaneous drainage. Photo courtesy of Cleveland Clinic Foundation, Department of Dermatology.

Many presentations of pancreatic panniculitis appear to represent localized disease, but others have numerous systemic manifestations, including those directly associated with pancreatitis such as abdominal pain, nausea, vomiting, chest pain, jaundice, and fever. Approximately 40% of pancreatitis-associated cases and 90% of malignancy-associated cases present without abdominal pain, nausea, or vomiting. Peripheral eosinophilia may occur, and is far more likely to be associated with underlying carcinoma than pancreatitis (10). Arthritis, described in approximately 60% of cases, usually represents periarticular fat necrosis. In some instances, the fat necrosis extends into the joint space resulting in a true arthritis. The most commonly affected joints are ankles, fingers, knees, and elbows (1). Ascites, pleural, and pericardial effusions may also occur (11). In one case with polyserositis, the presence of pleural deposition of IgG and C3 and reduced levels of hemolytic complement in blood, pleural, and pericardial fluid were detected, suggesting immune-mediated injury (11). Lytic bone lesions due to medullary fat necrosis have also been described. These may be mistaken for metastatic disease in malignancy-associated cases (12).

Pancreatic panniculitis may be the presenting sign of previously undiagnosed pancreatic disease. The clinical presentation of subcutaneous nodules with arthritis and serositis is not specific, but may suggest connective tissue disease accompanied by erythema nodosum. Pancreatic panniculitis is one of several disparate entities that may resemble erythema nodosum, but is readily distinguished from it based upon histologic features (Figure 21.2A and 21.2B). The epidermis and dermis are usually normal. The subcutaneous tissue has extensive fat necrosis with loss of adipocyte nuclei. Retained cell borders form "ghost-like" fat cells. There is stippled basophilia caused by calcification, and a mixed inflammatory cell infiltrate varying with the age of the lesion. Neutrophils predominate early (13). A septal pattern of inflammation has been described in an early lesion (14).

Most cases of pancreatic panniculitis wax and wane. The only effective treatment are to correct the underlying disease, tumor resection for localized malignancy, bowel rest and supportive measures for pancreatitis, or surgical correction of developmental anomalies or mechanical obstruction. This disease is important to recognize because it may closely mimic erythema nodosum, a common cause of panniculitis. A distinctive histologic pattern in pancreatic panniculitis is a valuable clue to the recognition of serious previously undiagnosed pancreatic disease.

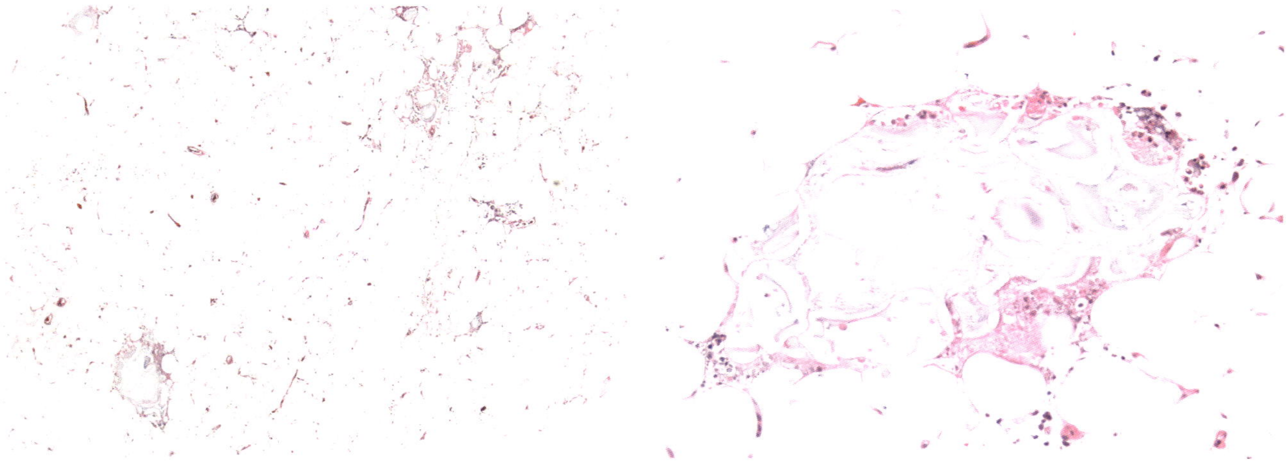

A B

FIGURE 21.2. (A and B) Multifocal fat necrosis with "ghost cell" formation, neutrophils, and stippled calcification.

References

1. Mullin GT, Ceperton EM, Crespin SR, et al. Arthritis and skin lesions resembling erythema nodosum in pancreatic disease. *Ann Intern Med* 1968; 68: 75–87.
2. Schrier RW, Melmon KL, Fenster LF. Subcutaneous nodular fat necrosis in pancreatitis. *Arch Intern Med* 1965; 116: 832–836.
3. Dhawan SS, Jiminez-Acosta F, Poppiti RJ, Barkin JS. Subcutaneous fat necrosis associated with pancreatitis: Histochemical and electron microscopic findings. *Am J Gastroent* 1990; 85: 1025–1028.
4. Berman B, Conteas C, Smith B, Leong S, Hornbeck L. Fatal pancreatitis presenting with subcutaneous fat necrosis: Evidence that lipase and amylase alone do not induce lipocyte necrosis. *J Am Acad Dermatol* 1987; 17: 359–364.
5. Cutlan RT, Wesche WA, Jenkins JJ, Chesney TM. A fatal case of pancreatic panniculitis presenting in a young patient with systemic lupus. *J Cutan Pathol* 2000; 27: 466–471.
6. Levine N, Lazarus G. Subcutaneous fat necrosis after paracentesis. *Arch Dermatol* 1976; 112: 993–994.
7. Thompson LDR, Heffess CS. Pancreas. In: Mills SE, Carter D, Greenson JK, Oberman HA, Reuter V, Stoler MH, eds. *Sternberg's Diagnostic Surgical Pathology*, 4th ed. Philadelphia: Lippincott Williams and Wilkins, 2004, 1623–1625.
8. Sibrack LA, Gouterman IH. Cutaneous manifestations of pancreatic diseases. *Cutis* 1978; 21: 763–768.
9. Haber RM, Assaad DM. Panniculitis associated with a pancreas divisum. *J Am Acad Dermatol* 1986; 14: 331–334.
10. Hughes PSH, Apisarnthanarax P, Mullins JF. Subcutaneous fat necrosis associated with pancreatic disease. *Arch Dermatol* 1975; 111: 506–510.
11. Potts DE, Mass MF, Iseman MD. Syndrome of pancreatic disease, subcutaneous fat necrosis and polyserositis. *Am J Med* 1975; 58: 417–423.
12. Good AE, Schnitzer B, Kawanishi H, Demetropoulos C, Rapp R. Acinar pancreatic tumor with metastatic fat necrosis: Report of a case and review of rheumatic manifestations. *Digestive Dis* 1976; 21: 978–987.
13. Szymanski FJ, Bluefarb SM. Nodular fat necrosis and pancreatic diseases. *Arch Dermatol* 1961; 83: 224–229.
14. Ball NJ, Adams SPA, Marx LH, Enta T. Possible origin of pancreatic fat necrosis as a septal panniculitis. *J Am Acad Dermatol* 1996; 34: 362–364.

22 Scleromyxedema

■ Synonyms:	Lichen myxedematosus, papular mucinosis, Arndt-Gottron syndrome
■ Etiology:	Unknown
■ Associations:	Paraproteinemia, multiple myeloma, hepatitis C, HIV disease, L-tryptophan syndrome
■ Clinical:	Coalescing indurated waxing papules
■ Histology:	Increased dermal mucin with increased fibroblasts
■ IHC repertoire:	N/A
■ Staging:	N/A
■ Prognosis:	Slowly progressive—increased mortality rate
■ Adverse variables:	Monoclonal gammopathy
■ Treatment:	Careful screening

Scleromyxedema is a cutaneous condition that is associated with paraproteinemia in more than 80% of cases (1). In the vast majority of cases, the paraprotein is an IgG heavy chain and a γ light chain. Rare cases of κ light chains have been reported, and polyclonal hypergammopathy is also seen in some cases. It has been reported that only 10% of patients with scleromyxedema and associated monoclonal gammopathy will progress to multiple myeloma (1). Overall, scleromyxedema is associated with an increased mortality rate, probably due to the manifold systemic associations.

Less commonly, scleromyxedema has been seen in association with Hodgkin's lymphoma, non-Hodgkin's lymphoma, leukemia, and Waldenstrom's macroglobulinemia (1,2). In about one quarter of patients, proximal muscle weakness may be encountered. Less commonly, peripheral neuropathies and central nervous system aberrations may be seen (3). Associated joint disease is characterized as a seronegative polyarthritis. Table 22.1 summarizes less common systemic associations.

Scleromyxedema is an unusual dermatosis that presents as the insidious onset of multiple firm, waxy, skin-colored papules that progress to confluence (Figure 22.1).

Middle-aged adults are most frequently affected (mean age 53) and there is no gender predilection (4,5). They are most common on the face, upper trunk, and extremities, and in the extreme form give rise to a leonine facies. The individual papules are only several millimeters in diameter and minimally elevated. Papules may be linearly aligned. When the glabella is involved, deep furrowing is apparent. When the eyelids are involved, ectropion may be a problem. In some cases, erythema and/or a brown discoloration may be present. The eruption tends to be relatively asymptomatic to minimally pruritic. When extensive, there may be diffuse thickening of the skin, resulting in decreased mobility of the fingers, joints, and mouth. Scleromyxedema is regarded by some authors as the generalized, lichenoid form of lichen myxedematosus (6).

The histologic features include a normal to somewhat flattened epidermis. The papillary dermis is characterized by increased neutral mucopolysaccharides and an increased number of fibroblasts (Figures 22.2 and 22.3).

There is minimal associated inflammatory response. In most cases, the increased dermal mucin is apparent with routine stains, though in some cases, it may be difficult to discriminate from dermal edema (Figure 22.4).

In these cases, colloidal iron or alcian blue stains done at a pH of 4.5 are helpful in identifying the increased amounts of mucin (Figure 22.5).

Table 22.1. Systemic Conditions Associated with Scleromyxedema (4)

Condition	Percent of Cases of Scleromyxedema with This Association
Paraproteinemia	83.2
Multiple myeloma	10
Proximal muscle weakness	27
Central or peripheral neuropathies	15
Joint involvement	10.5
Carpal tunnel syndrome	9.6
Raynaud's phenomenon	8.8
Dyspnea	16.7
Dysphagia	31.6
Renal disease/coronary artery disease	Reported
Ophthalmologic disorders (corneal opacities, ectropion, lagophthalmos)	18%
Hepatitis C	
AIDS	

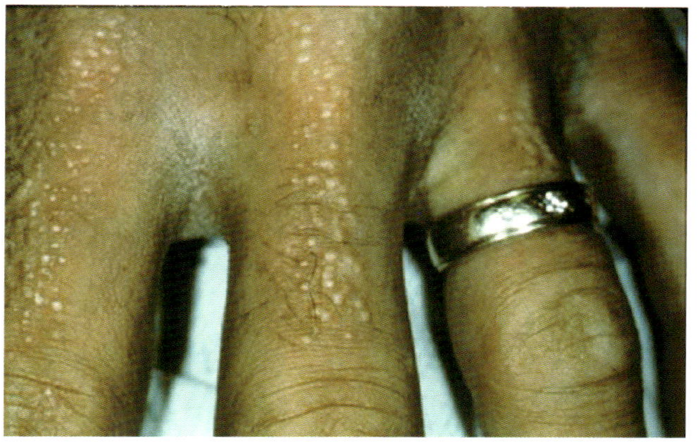

Figure 22.1. Multiple linearly arrayed waxy papules in scleromyxedema.

The increased cellularity and mucin deposition is centered in the upper portions of the dermis and rarely extends deeply into the reticular dermis. Collagen bundles have also been reported to be thickened in this condition (4).

The histologic differential diagnosis includes scleredema and pretibial myxedema. In scleredema, the increased ground substance is located primarily in the deeper reticular dermis and is not accompanied by a concomitant increase in cellularity. Pretibial myxedema demonstrates mucin within the papillary and superficial reticular dermis, similar to scleromyxedema, but rarely has a significant proliferation of fibroblasts.

There is a less common histologic variant in which pools of mucin are surrounded by fibroblasts and histiocytes. In these cases, the distinction from granuloma

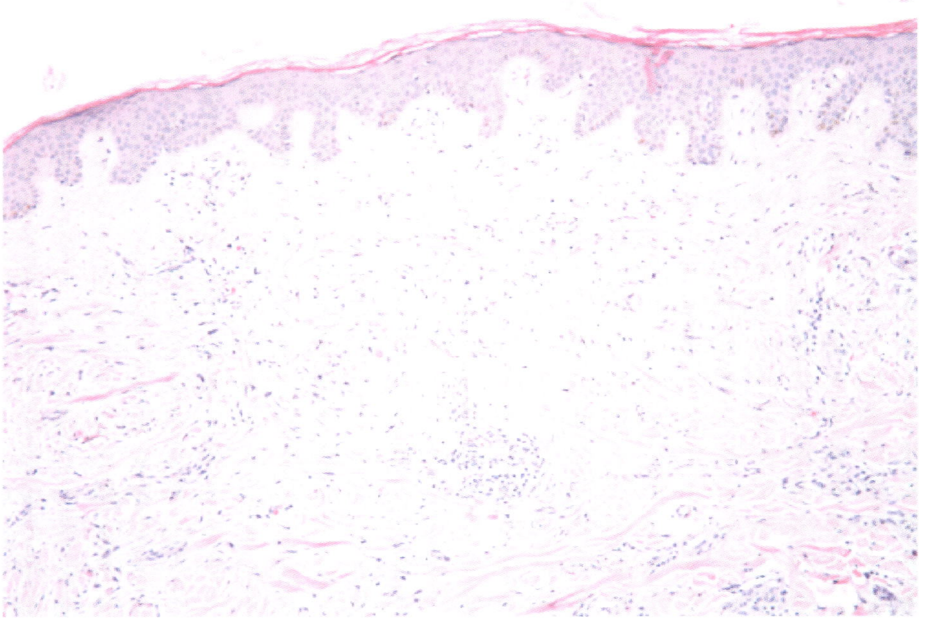

Figure 22.2. Low power photomicrograph depicting diffuse dermal fibroplasia.

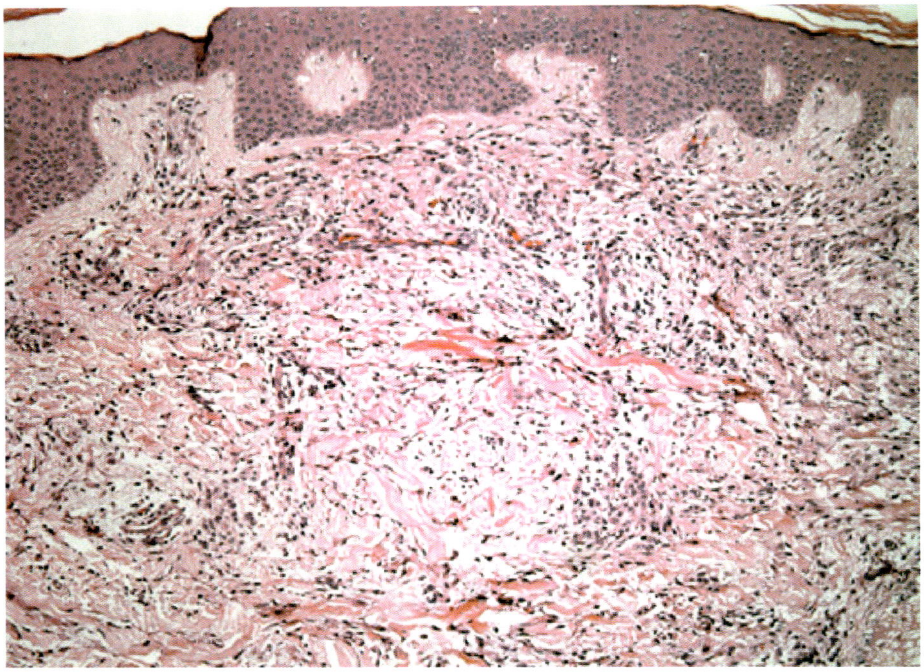

FIGURE 22.3. Medium power photomicrograph depicting increased number of spindled fibrocytes with interspersed lymphocytes.

annulare may be difficult and is most easily made based upon the clinical presentation.

The pathogenesis of scleromyxedema remains an enigma. Paraprotein levels do not correlate with extent or progression of disease (7).

Scleromyxedema is very difficult to treat effectively. A wide range of treatments including intralesional corticosteroids, PUVA, electron beam therapy, and plasmapheresis have demonstrated slight improvements. Low doses of melphalan and cyclophosphamide are effective, but may

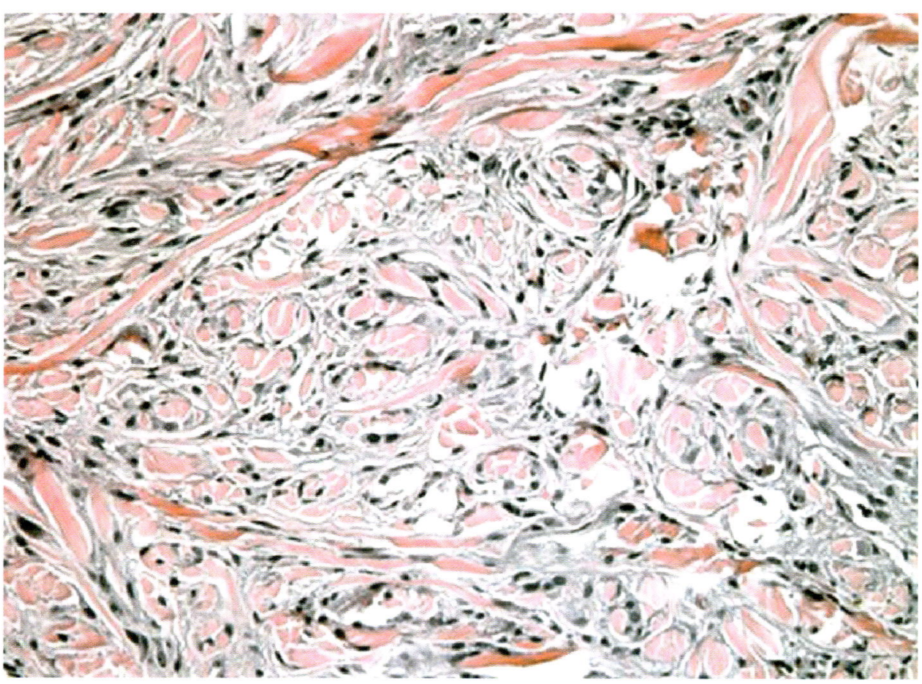

FIGURE 22.4. High power detail of spindled cells. Note stringy gray mucin deposits.

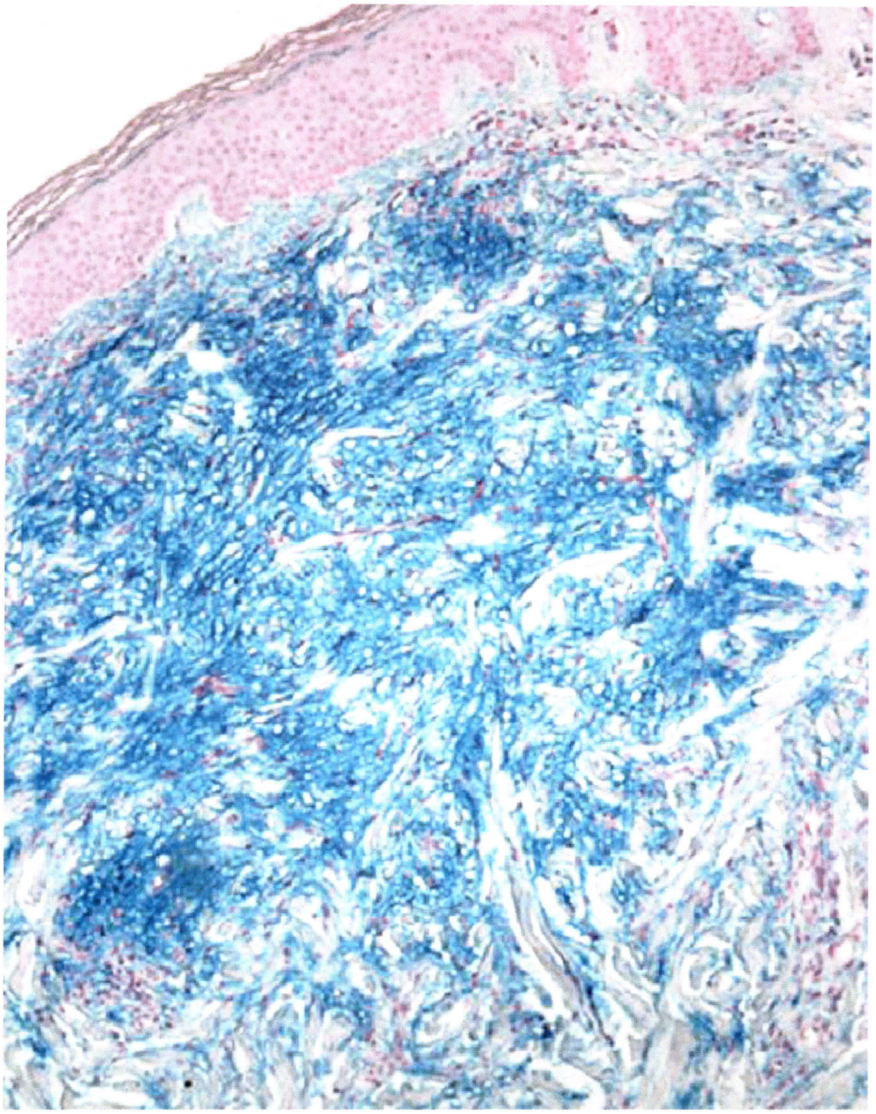

FIGURE 22.5. Colloidal iron diffuse dermal blue staining corresponding to the presence of increased dermal mucin (hyaluronic acid) deposits.

be related to subsequent development of hematologic malignancies.

References

1. Dineen AM, Dicken CH. Scleromyxedema. *J Am Acad Dermatol* 1995; 33: 37–43.
2. Alberts AS, Schulz EJ, Falkson G, Simson IW, Coccia-Portugal MA. Normalization of skin appearance in a patient with scleromyxedema after intensive chemotherapy for Hodgkin's disease. *Dermatologica* 1989; 178: 221–224.
3. Webster GF, Matsuoka LY, Burchmore D. The association of potentially lethal neurologic syndromes with scleromyxedema (popular mucinosis). *J Am Acad Dermatol* 1993; 28: 105–108.
4. Rongioletti F, Rebora A. Updated classification of popular mucinosis, lichen myxedematosus, and scleromyxedema. *J Am Acad Dermatol* 2001; 44: 273–281.
5. Gabriel SE, Perry HO, Oleson GB, Bowles CA. Scleromyxedema: A scleroderma-like disorder with systemic manifestations. *Medicine (Baltimore)* 1988: 67: 58–65.
6. Gottron HA. Skleromyxedema. *Arch Dermatol Syphilol* 1954; 199: 71–91.
7. Chanda JJ. Scleromyxedema. *Cutis* 1979; 24: 549–552.

23
Necrolytic Migratory Erythema

■ Synonyms:	Glucagonoma syndrome
■ Etiology:	Glucagon-secreting tumors, usually malignant and located principally in the pancreas
■ Associations:	MEN I syndrome, Zollinger-Ellison syndrome
■ Clinical:	Rash—erythematous, scaly patches intertriginous and acral area; angular chelitis, diabetes mellitus, diarrhea
■ Histology:	Mild epidermal acanthosis with confluent parakeratosis and vacuolar degeneration of the superficial epithelial layers
■ IHC repertoire:	N/A
■ Staging:	None
■ Prognosis:	Overall 5-year survival ~ 50%
■ Adverse variables:	Malignant pancreatic tumor, weight loss, metastases

Necrolytic migratory erythema (NME), referred to as the glucagonoma syndrome, is a rare paraneoplastic syndrome consisting of the classic triad of diarrhea, diabetes mellitus, and rash associated with serum hyperglucagonemia (1–3). The most common etiology involves the elaboration of glucagons from an islet cell tumor of the pancreas but may rarely follow the metabolic consequences of cirrhosis, pancreatic insufficiency, or celiac disease. There is no ethnic or gender predilection and age of onset is usually in the sixties. NME is associated with type 1 multiple endocrine neoplasia syndrome (MEN I) sequence and/or Zollinger-Ellison hypergastrinemia syndrome in a minority of the cases (4–6).

The cutaneous and systemic manifestations follow the metabolic consequences of glucagon elaboration. These consist of insulin antagonism with resulting hyperglycemia and hypoaminoacidemia. It is thought that the hypoaminoacidemia results in decreased available substrate for peptide synthesis that consequentially manifests in rapidly cycling tissues such as the skin, gut, and bone marrow. These profound metabolic disturbances underlie the clinical disorders of diabetes mellitus, rash, and diarrhea observed in this syndrome.

The rash consists of an expanding erythematous and scaly patch typically observed within the intertriginous areas including the inguinal creases, nasolabial sulcus, and popliteal fossae (Figure 23.1) (7). Other frequently involved areas include acral sites and the perineum. In time, the patches develop into blistering plaques with perilesional pustules. Lesional pain and intense pruritus are commonly observed. The rash typically waxes and wanes cyclically with concurrent lesions showing different levels of healing. Approximately 30% of patients develop angular chelitis and glossitis.

Other systemic manifestations that commonly accompany this syndrome include diabetes mellitus, weight loss, diarrhea, neuropsychiatric disorders, thromboembolic disease, and a host of laboratory abnormalities. Diabetes mellitus develops in approximately 85% of patients with NME. The hyperglycemia results from the antagonistic effect of glucagons upon insulin, by increasing gluconeogenesis in the liver and kidney, glycogenolysis in the liver and skeletal muscle and inhibiting glycogen synthesis in the liver (8). Glycemic management of patients with this syndrome can be difficult. Weight loss and tumor-associated cachexia is frequently observed and is particularly evident in the terminal stages of the disease. Diarrhea is observed in approximately one-third of patients and can be debilitating. Neuropsychiatric disturbances consist of depression, psychoses, as well as ataxia and visual disturbances. Thromboembolic complications are common and presumably due to tumor-associated hypercoaguability. Migratory thrombophlebitis (*Trosseau's syndrome*), deep venous thrombosis of the leg with

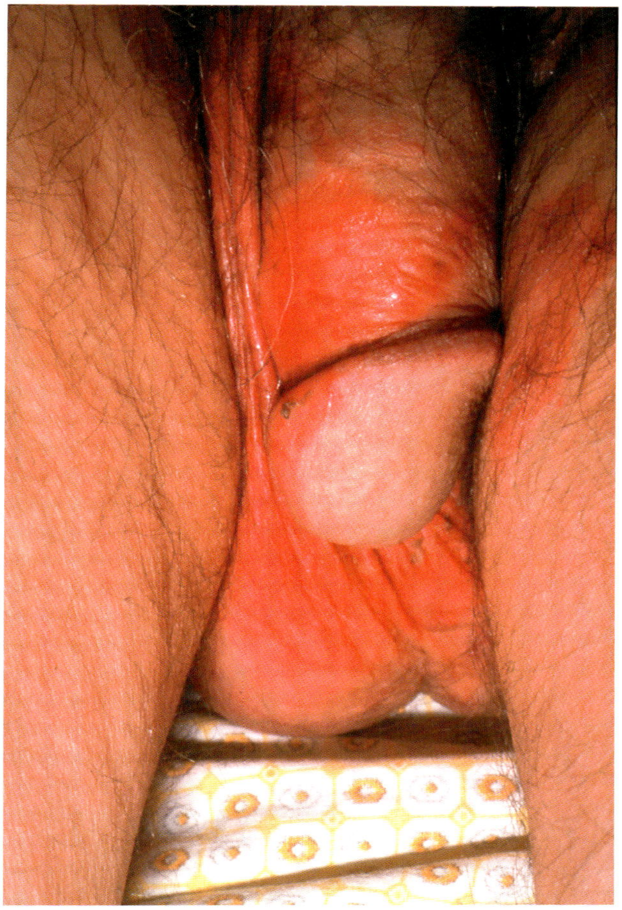

FIGURE 23.1. Erythematous and focally scaly eruption involving genitalia and inguinal regions seen in necrolytic migratory erythema. Photo courtesy of Cleveland Clinic Foundation, Department of Dermatology.

attendant risk of pulmonary embolism, and cerebral artery thrombosis are observed. Laboratory abnormalities include spectacular elevation of the serum glucagon level, elevated erythrocyte sedimentation rate, normochromic normocytic anemia, hypoalbuminemia, and hypoaminoacidemia.

The diagnosis can be established by histologic criteria in the appropriate clinical setting, or with laboratory testing (9). The histologic features are distinctive though not pathognomonic of the disorder. The histologic features are entirely limited to the epithelium and consist of alterations in all of its layers. Overall, the epithelium shows acanthosis, and confluent parakeratosis with loss of the granular layer (Figure 23.2). At high-power examination, the keratinocytes, particularly in the middle portion of the stratum spinosum, show ballooning and vacuolar degeneration. Intraepidermal bullae and neutrophilic exocytosis may also be observed (Figure 23.3). Although the differential includes disorders capable of showing exocytosis of neutrophils, such as psoriasis, as well as disorders that may induce keratinocyte degeneration, such as sunburn or viral infection, seldom do they constitute a diagnostic dilemma after clinical correlation. The most important disorders that are capable of producing histologic alterations that may mimic NME include the nutritional deficiency states of pellagra and acrodermatitis enteropathica. Pellagra or niacin deficiency has distinctive clinical attributes that usually permit its distinction from NME. *Pellagra* is primarily observed in two clinical settings including children with an inherited disorder involving tryptophan metabolism (*Hartnup disease*) and among nutritionally impoverished adults (10,11). The cutaneous manifestations include photodistributed erythematous and burning patches that in time develop into scaly and fissured hyperpigmented plaques. The cutaneous manifestations are often accompanied by diarrhea and dementia that, if not corrected in time, eventuate in death.

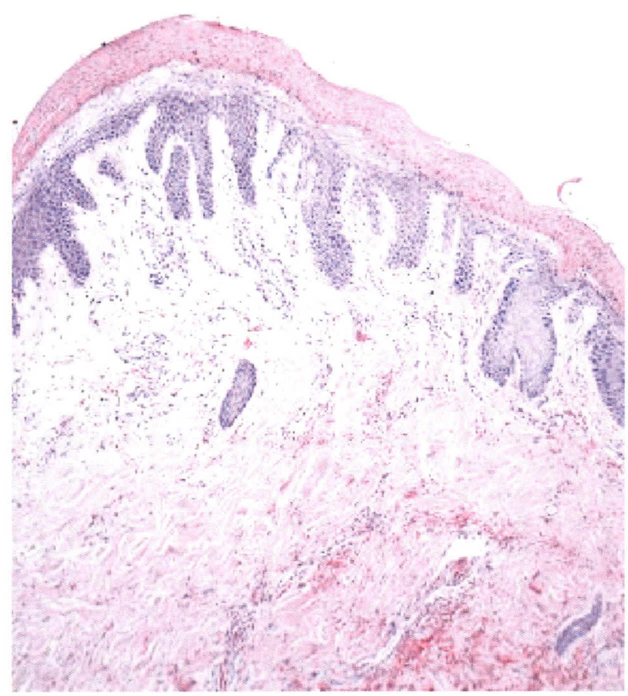

FIGURE 23.2. Low power photomicrograph depicting epidermal acanthosis with hyperkeratosis.

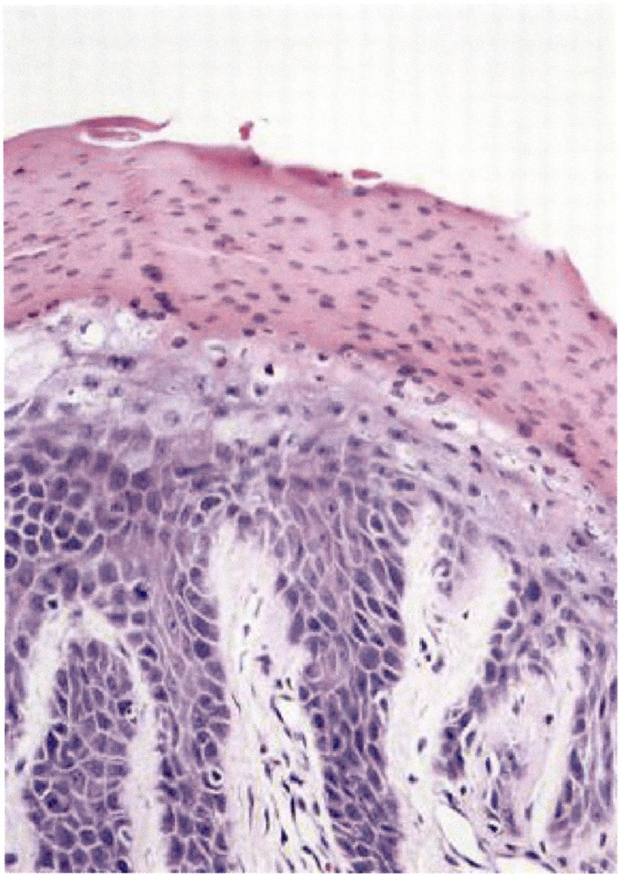

FIGURE 23.3. High power detail of stratum spinosum showing vacuolar alteration with loss of the granular layer and coarse parakeratosis typical of necrolytic erythema.

Additional settings in which niacin deficiency may be observed include the carcinoid syndrome in which the metabolic precursor of niacin, tryptophan, is usurped by the tumor. Niacin deficiency may follow impaired absorption or interaction with certain medications such as isoniazid, mecaptopurine, 5-fluoruracil, the sulfonamides, anticonvulsants, and antidepressants. *Acrodermatitis enteropathica* consists of a distinctive acral and periorifical rash observed in infants and less commonly adults, who are deficient in zinc or other micronutrients (Figure 23.4) (12–14). The metabolic defect in infants often involves a defect in the zinc transporter genes. Among adults, this condition may be observed in patients receiving total parenteral nutrition.

Laboratory confirmation can be achieved by measuring the serum level of glucagons. Levels are usually above 1000pg/ml (normal 100pg/ml). Although elevated serum glucagon levels are observed in 100% of cases, other causes of elevated serum glucagons include cirrhosis, renal failure, prolonged fasting, diabetic ketoacidosis, and with other islet cell tumors of the pancreas should be considered. Computerized tomography can be utilized to visualize the tumor that in the majority of cases resides within the pancreas. A minority of cases result from ectopic islet cell tumors located in the small intestine, stomach, or appendix. Selective celiac arteriography with serum sampling for glucagon also remains an important means of establishing the diagnosis.

In the largest study to date, approximately 50% of patients succumbed to their disease within 5 years of diagnosis (15). The majority of patients possess metastatic malignant islet cell tumors at the time of diagnosis. Early recognition of the disease is difficult as these tumors are rare and aggressive, and the clinical manifestations including the rash often develop following metastases. Adverse prognostic signs include the development of metastatic disease and weight loss. Treatment is aimed toward curative surgical extirpation of the tumor. Metastatic and unresectable disease may be palliated with various chemotherapeutic agents including streptzotocin and 5-fluoruracil. Clinical improvement of symptoms can in most instances be achieved with the administration of serotonin inhibitors such as octreotide.

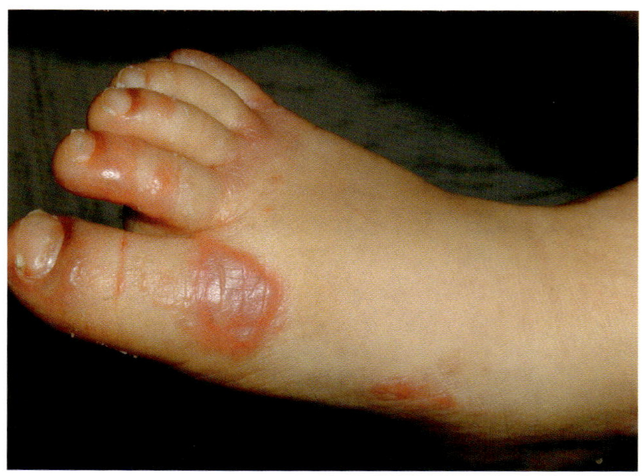

FIGURE 23.4. Acral distributed erythematous papules in child with acrodermatitis enteropathica because of zinc deficiency.

References

1. Leichter SB. Clinical and metabolic aspects of glucagonoma. *Medicine* 1980; 59: 100.
2. Hashizume T, Kiryu H, Noda K, et al. Glucagonoma syndrome. *J Am Acad Dermatol* 1988; 19: 377.
3. Frankton S, Boom SR. Glucagonomas. *Baillieres Clin Gastroenterol* 1996; 10: 697.
4. Chastain MA. The glucagonoma syndrome: A review of its features and discussion of new perspectives. *Am J Med Sci* 2001; 321: 326.
5. Boden G. Insulinoma and glucagonoma. *Semin Oncol* 1987; 14: 253.
6. Doll DC. Necrolytic migratory erythema. *Arch Dermatol* 1980; 116: 861.
7. Thorisdottir K, Camisa C, Tomecki K, et al. Necrolytic migratory erythema: A report of three cases. *J Am Acad Dermatol* 1994; 30: 324.
8. Goodenberger D, Lawley T, Strober W, et al. Necrolytic migratory erythema without glucagonoma: Report of two cases. *Arch Dermatol* 1979; 115: 1429.
9. Kheir SM, Omura EF, Grizzle W, et al. Histologic variation in the skin lesions of glucagonoma syndrome. *Am J Surg Pathol* 1986; 10: 445.
10. Hendricks W. Pellagra and pellagra-like dermatoses: Etiology, differential diagnosis, dermatopathology, and treatment. *Semin Dermatol* 1991; 10: 282.
11. Stratigos J, Katsambas A. Pellagra: A still existing disease. *Br J Dermatol* 1977; 96: 99.
12. Wong P, Pillai P. Clinical and biochemical observations in two cases of Hartnup disease. *Arch Dis Child* 1966; 41: 383.
13. Nedner K, Hambridge K, Walravens P. Acrodermatitis enteropathica. *Int J Dermatol* 1978; 17: 380.
14. Graves K, Kestenbaum T, Kalivas J. Hereditary acrodermatitis enteropathica in an adult. *Arch Dermatol* 1969; 99: 562.
15. Wermers R, Fatourechi V, Wyne A, et al. The glucagonoma syndrome: Clinical and pathologic features in 21 patients. *Medicine* 1996; 75: 53.

Part III
Infectious Diseases

24 Anthrax

■ Synonyms:	Woolsorter's disease (inhalational anthrax)
■ Etiology:	Inoculation or inhalation of spores of *Bacillus anthracis*, a gram-positive bacillus
■ Associations:	None
■ Clinical:	Cutaneous: papule, followed by vesicle, then ulcer with eschar at the site of inoculation; septicemia in approximately 20%
■ Histology:	Partial epidermal necrosis, dermal edema with fibrin, neutrophils, and abscess formation; positive gram stain expected
■ Evaluation:	Notifying local health department and laboratory of clinical suspicion, gram stain and culture of vesicle fluid or eschar base, skin biopsy with tissue culture
■ Treatment:	Ciprofloxacin or doxycycline
■ Prognosis:	99% survival for cutaneous disease if treated early, 20% survival for inhalational disease, and intermediate survival for gastrointestinal disease

Anthrax is an infection caused by the spore-forming bacterium, *Bacillus anthracis*. Infection occurs in mammals, particularly herbivores that ingest bacterial spores from soil. Human infection occurs from inhalation of spores, ingestion of animal meat contaminated with spores, or percutaneous inoculation of spores from exposure to infected animals or contaminated animal products. Anthrax has been an occupational disease of textile workers, farmers, butchers, veterinarians, and shepherds.

Anthrax is a historically important infection, thought to be the fifth and sixth plagues of ancient Egypt, brought by Moses. It was the cause of several disastrous animal plagues in Europe in the eighteenth and nineteenth centuries. In 1877, Robert Koch cultured *Bacillus anthracis*, the first proof of a microbial agent causing human disease (1). This discovery supported "germ theory" and gave birth to the science of modern microbiology. Subsequently, Pasteur and Greenfield successfully developed the first vaccine, composed of attenuated *B. anthracis* (2). Anthrax has been explored as an agent of biological warfare because of its exceptional virulence and capability to create an aerosol of odorless, invisible spores. Its spores could potentially be dispersed over densely populated areas, and generate disease in a multitude of people with high morbidity. This organism has gained notoriety more recently because of the anthrax attacks of 2001, in which anthrax spores were distributed by mail using the U.S. Postal Service, resulting in inhalational or cutaneous anthrax infection in 22 people.

Bacillus anthracis is a gram-positive, nonmotile, aerobic, spore-forming rod. The organism grows readily on standard culture media, especially sheep's blood agar, forming nonhemolytic irregular white-gray colonies, with tapered extensions (3). Gram stain of cultures reveals long chains of bacilli. Notifying the laboratory of clinical suspicion of *B. anthracis* is important because of the prevalence of the similar-appearing organism, *Bacillus cereus*, which is a frequent laboratory contaminant (4).

The infective unit of the organism is the endospore, which may reside in soil for decades. It is resistant to heat, ultraviolet and gamma irradiation, drying, and antimicrobial agents (5). Spores enter the body through broken skin, the lungs, or the gastrointestinal tract, and are engulfed by macrophages, and then transported to lymph nodes. Within the macrophage, they transform to the vegetative form and then multiply within the lymphatic system. They are eventually released in high concentrations into the bloodstream, resulting in sepsis. The organism achieves its virulence by the production of three polypeptides and an antiphagocytic capsule, encoded on two plasmids, pXO1 and pXO2. Both plasmids are needed for the organism to achieve complete virulence. pXO1 encodes the three polypeptides, protective antigen (PA), lethal factor (LF), and edema factor (EF), which combine as binary toxins. PA combines with LF to form lethal toxin, and combines with EF to form edema toxin. The PA component of the toxin facilitates access to the host cell by its binding to cellular receptors. The complex is cleaved by the serine protease furin, causing oligomerization and subsequent transport of toxins into the cell. The lethal toxin is a zinc metalloproteinase that activates oxidative burst pathways, forming reactive oxygen intermediates. It also induces the production of tumor necrosis factor-α and interleukin-1β, which are involved in inducing septic shock. Plasmid pXO2 encodes three genes involved in production of the polyglutamic acid capsule that inhibits phagocytosis of the vegetative state of *B. anthracis* (4,6,7).

The three forms of anthrax infection in humans are cutaneous, inhalational, and gastrointestinal. The disease is spread to humans via contact with infected animals or contaminated animal products. Naturally occurring anthrax has been almost eradicated in the United States and in Western Europe due to the presence of long-standing vaccination programs for at-risk livestock, but is still relatively common in Asia Minor.

Cutaneous anthrax is by far the most common form of the disease. Infection usually occurs from contact with infected animals or animal products such as hides, wool, hair, or bones. The primary lesion is a papule, sometimes pruritic, occurring three to five days after inoculation. The face, neck, and extremities are most commonly affected (4). Within two days, vesiculation occurs, with central necrosis, and formation of a 1–3 cm painless ulcer and subsequent eschar (Figure 24.1) (3). The eschar accounts for the derivation of the organism's name from the Greek word *anthrakos*, meaning coal (1). Lymphadenopathy and lymphangitis may develop, with satellite hemorrhagic vesicles and edema. Inoculation sites on the extremities usually result in "malignant pustule" formation. More central sites tend to have prominent edema, resulting in the "malignant edema" presentation (3). The latter form is more likely to be complicated by airway obstruction, requiring concomitant use of systemic steroids and antibiotics. Secondary bacterial infection of the site is common, so that treatment with extended-spectrum antibiotics may be needed. While many cases of cutaneous anthrax are self-limited, antibiotic treatment is recommended because of the approximately 20% of cases in which disseminated infection associated with high mortality occurs. Case fatality rate is less than 1% in treated cases (8). Cutaneous lesions are reported to heal without scarring in the large majority of cases (4). However, in a recent series, considerable scarring requiring reconstructive surgery in 23% of cases was noted (3).

Inhalational anthrax is exceptionally uncommon, but was more prevalent in occupational settings as "woolsorter's disease" before adequate hygienic standards were employed. In contrast to inoculation anthrax, disease caused by inhalation of anthrax spores is usually fatal because the disease causes nonspecific influenza-like symptoms followed by rapid onset of septic shock and death. Important information regarding inhalational anthrax was yielded by an accidental release of anthrax

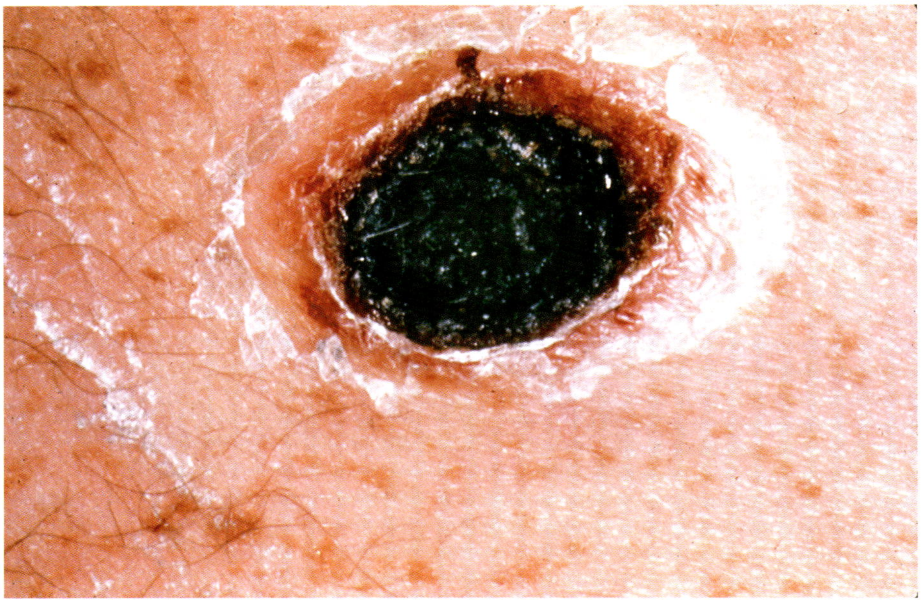

FIGURE 24.1. Cutaneous anthrax: ulcer, with central eschar, and surrounding erythema and edema.

spores from a biological weapons facility in Sverdlovsk in 1979, in which 66 deaths occurred. The incubation time ranged from 2 to 43 days, with an average of about 10 days. The mortality rate was approximately 80% (9). Despite its rarity, inhalational anthrax was the mode of infection in 50% of the anthrax cases in the 2001 attacks, and would be expected to be the prevalent form of the disease in a biological weapons attack (10). In the setting of an anthrax outbreak, clinical features favoring inhalational anthrax over an influenza-like illness include presence of dyspnea, hypoxemia, chest pain, lack of sore throat or rhinorrhea, and presence of mediastinal widening, pulmonary infiltrate, or pleural effusion on chest radiography. Laboratory evaluation may reveal neutrophilia with bandemia and elevated liver enzyme tests (11).

Gastrointestinal tract and oropharyngeal anthrax are also uncommon. These infections result from ingestion of contaminated meat from infected animals. The incubation period is two to five days. Infection probably occurs in a manner similar to that in the skin, with ulcer formation, and bacterial proliferation in lymphatic tissues. Inoculation may occur at any point along the gastrointestinal tract, including the oropharynx. Symptoms and signs vary depending on the site of inoculation, and may include fever, abdominal pain, nausea, vomiting, dysphagia, constipation, diarrhea, melena, and ascites. Mortality is considerable and may be the result of sepsis or intestinal perforation (4).

Cutaneous, inhalational, and gastrointestinal anthrax may all be complicated by anthrax meningitis, a complication occurring during bacteremia. Central nervous system involvement portends a grave prognosis despite therapy (4).

Diagnosis of anthrax may be made by blood culture in the setting of disseminated infection. Growth usually occurs in 6 to 24 hours (10). For cutaneous anthrax, vesicle fluid culture may grow the organism, and 64% of cases in one series had organisms identified by gram-stained smears of cutaneous lesion contents (3). The organism is unlikely to grow from skin or blood if the patient has received antibiotics prior to obtaining culture material (10). A new rapid diagnostic test for anthrax has recently been approved by the U.S. Food and Drug Administration that detects antibodies to anthrax-protective antigen in 45 minutes (12,13).

The differential diagnosis of cutaneous anthrax is considerable, and includes ecthyma, insect or arachnid bite reaction, tularemia, glanders, rickettsialpox, diphtheria, syphilitic chancre, ecthyma gangrenosum, and orf. In endemic or occupational settings, history of contact with animals or animal products is expected in cases of anthrax. Clinical features that may point to anthrax include relative lack of symptoms given impressive clinical findings, and prominent edema. Gram stain and culture of cutaneous vesicles or ulcers will yield the organism in the majority of cases. Skin biopsy specimens of *Bacillus anthracis* infection have prominent superficial dermal edema with variable epidermal necrosis, and an infiltrate of neutrophils throughout the dermis, with abscess formation. There is prominent dermal fibrin, with foci of vasculitis. Gram stain reveals gram-positive rods within the dermis (Figure 24.2A, 24.2B, and 24.2C) (14,15). Should there be

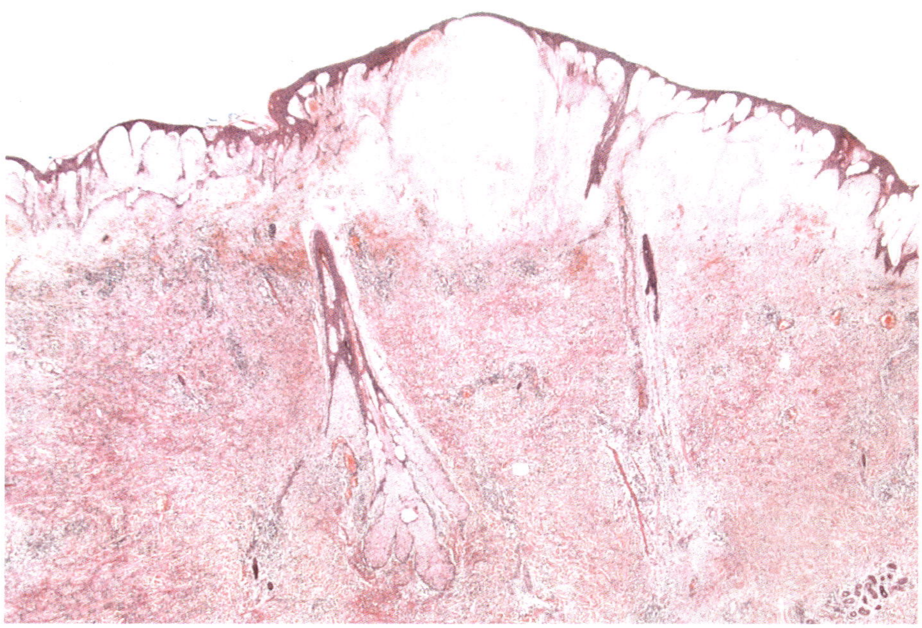

A

FIGURE 24.2. (A) Anthrax: mild epidermal hyperplasia and striking superficial dermal edema.

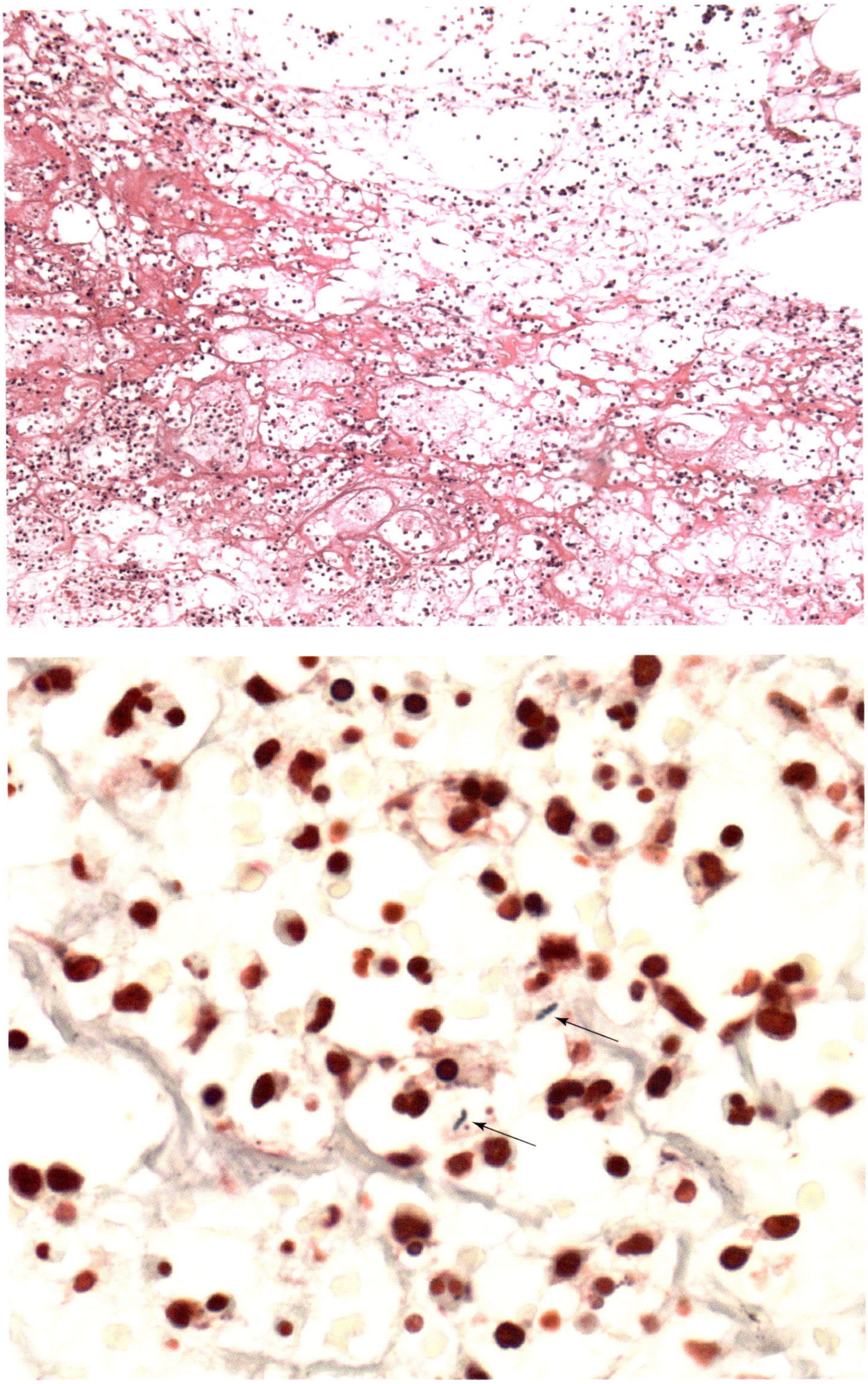

B

C

FIGURE 24.2. (B) Deep dermal and subcutaneous mixed inflammatory infiltrate of lymphocytes, neutrophils, and plasma cells, with edema and fibrin deposition. (C) Mixed inflammatory infiltrate with gram-positive bacilli (arrows). Courtesy of Eduardo Calonje, MD.

clinical suspicion of cutaneous anthrax, the following list of procedures should be employed:

Diagnostic Evaluation of Suspected Cutaneous Anthrax

1. Patient should be under contact precautions only, since the infective unit, the spore, is not shed.
2. Gram stain and culture of vesicle fluid, or unroofed eschar.
3. Two punch biopsy specimens, one for tissue culture, and one in formalin for routine processing.
4. Blood cultures if clinical suspicion of bacteremia is present.
5. Contact laboratory and local health department with clinical suspicion, bloodwork as recommended for serologic and diagnostic studies.

Diagnostic and management information on anthrax is available on the Internet from the U.S. Centers for Disease Control (16).

Cutaneous anthrax in endemic areas is treated successfully with penicillin, given intravenously in cases of "malignant edema" (3,17). However, treatment of cutaneous anthrax in the setting of a bioterrorism attack as recommended by the Working Group on Civilian Biodefense includes ciprofloxacin 500 mg p.o. twice daily for 60 days, or doxycycline 100 mg p.o. twice daily for 60 days. Complete treatment recommendations are delineated by the Working Group and U.S. Centers for Disease Control (10,16). The rationale for extended treatment is to cover the likelihood of concomitant inhalation of anthrax spores, which may incubate for close to 60 days before resulting in clinical infection. Penicillin was not recommended in this treatment protocol because isolates from the 2001 anthrax attacks showed an inducible β-lactamase that degrades the antibiotic. The clinical significance is uncertain, but suggests the potential for rapid onset of penicillin resistance (10). No resistance to fluoroquinolones has been identified, but *in vitro* high-level resistance can be induced by serial passage of *Bacillus anthracis* in media containing fluoroquinolones, suggesting that drug-resistant strains can be cultivated (18). No treatment other than antibiotics currently exists for anthrax. In a rodent anthrax model, infusion of antiprotective antigen antibodies with ciprofloxacin yielded greatly enhanced survival compared with ciprofloxacin alone, suggesting this as a potential therapeutic addition in humans (19).

Human anthrax vaccine is available as "anthrax vaccine adsorbed," a sterile filtrate of cultures of an attenuated unencapsulated, non-proteolytic strain of *B. anthracis*, containing predominantly protective antigen (2). Doses are given subcutaneously at 0, 2, and 4 weeks, with boosters given at 6, 12, and 18 months. Further boosters are recommended if continued exposure is a possibility. The vaccine has been widely used in military personnel and in some industries that have exposures to at-risk animals from endemic areas. Other immunizations are under investigation, including a transcutaneous system that has recombinant protective antigen of *Bacillus anthracis* and heat-labile toxin of *Escherichia coli* delivered by an adhesive patch. In a murine model, maximal immunity with protection against lethal doses of aerosolized anthrax spores was achieved with two doses, holding promise for future use in humans (20).

Naturally occurring cutaneous anthrax is a disease that has become almost nonexistent in the United States and Western Europe due to vaccination programs in at-risk animal reservoirs. However, the significance of this organism has been heightened recently because of its use in bioterrorism. The anthrax attacks of 2001 focus the potential for cutaneous presentations of this disease to be the first detectable manifestation of a terrorist biological weapons attack.

References

1. Turnbull PCB. Introduction: Anthrax history, disease and ecology. *Curr Top Microbiol Immunol* 2002; 271: 1–19.
2. Grabenstein JD. Anthrax vaccine: A review. *Immunol Allergy Clinics North Am* 2003; 23: 713–730.
3. Irmak H, Buzgan T, Karahocagil MK, et al. Cutaneous manifestations of anthrax in Eastern Anatolia: A review of 39 cases. *Acta Med Okayama* 2003; 57: 235–240.
4. Dixon TC, Meselson M, Guillemin J, Hanna PC. Anthrax. *New Engl J Med* 1999; 341: 815–826.
5. Watson A, Keir D. Information on which to base assessments of risk from environments contaminated with anthrax spores. *Epidemiol Infect* 1994; 113: 479–490.
6. Chensue SW. Exposing a killer: Pathologists angle for anthrax. *Am J Pathol* 2003; 163: 1699–1702.
7. Moayeri M, Leppla SH. The roles of anthrax toxin in pathogenesis. *Curr Opin Microbiol* 2004; 7: 19–24.
8. Brook I. The prophylaxis and treatment of anthrax. *Int J Antimicrob Agents* 2002; 20: 320–325.
9. Meselson M, Guillemin J, Hugh-Jones M, et al. The Sverdlovsk anthrax outbreak of 1979. *Science* 1994; 266: 1202–1208.
10. Inglesby TV, O'Toole T, Henderson DA, et al. Anthrax as a biological weapon, 2002: Updated recommendations for management. *JAMA* 2002; 287: 2236–2252.
11. Cinti SK, Saravolatz L, Nafziger D, Sunstrum J, Blackburn G. Differentiating inhalational anthrax from other influenzalike illnesses in the setting of a national or regional anthrax outbreak. *Arch Intern Med* 2004; 164: 674–676.
12. Stephenson J. Rapid anthrax test approved. *JAMA* 2004; 292: 30.
13. http://www.immunetics.com/anthrax.htm (accessed 1/23/05).

14. Lebowich RJ, McKillip BG, Conboy JR. Cutaneous anthrax: A pathologic study with clinical correlation. *Am J Clin Pathol* 1943; 13: 505–515.
15. Mallon E, McKee PH. Extraordinary case report: Cutaneous anthrax. *Am J Dermatopathol* 1997; 19: 79–82.
16. http://www.bt.cdc.gov/agent/anthrax/anthrax-hcp-factsheet.asp (accessed 1/23/05).
17. Kaya A, Tasyaran MA, Erol S, Ozkurt Z, Ozkan B. Anthrax in adults and children: A review of 132 cases in Turkey. *Eur J Clin Microbiol Infect Dis* 2002; 21: 258–261.
18. Karginov VA, Robinson TM, Riemenschneider J, et al. Treatment of anthrax infection with combination of ciprofloxacin and antibodies to protective antigen of Bacillus anthracis. *FEMS Immunol Med Microbiol* 2004; 40: 71–74.
19. Bast DJ, Athamna A, Duncan CL, et al. Type II topoisomerase mutations in Bacillus anthracis associated with high-level fluoroquinolone resistance. *J Antimicrob Chemother* 2004; 54: 90–94.
20. Kenney RT, Yu J, Guebre-Xabier M, et al. Induction of protective immunity against lethal anthrax challenge with a patch. *J Infect Dis* 2004; 190: 774–782.

25
Ecthyma Gangrenosum

▪ Synonyms:	None
▪ Etiology:	*Pseudomonas aeruginosa* and other gram-negative bacteria, similar lesions caused by opportunistic fungi
▪ Associations:	Immunosuppression, premature infants
▪ Clinical:	Indurated plaques with black eschar and rim of erythema, favors axillae, inguinal folds, and perineum
▪ Histology:	Mixed infiltrate of lymphocytes, neutrophils, plasma cells; special stains of affected skin usually demonstrate the organism
▪ Evaluation:	Blood cultures, skin biopsy with fresh tissue culture, special stains on touch preps of skin biopsy, consider frozen section
▪ Treatment:	Aimed at the specific infectious agent
▪ Prognosis:	High mortality rate; worse with extensive skin disease, prolonged immunosuppression, and delayed treatment

Ecthyma gangrenosum describes a cutaneous infection with *Pseudomonas aeruginosa* that is manifested by necrotic plaques with an eschar. The infection usually occurs in immunosuppressed patients. Three to six percent of *Pseudomonas* septicemia is complicated by ecthyma gangrenosum (1). The term *ecthyma gangrenosum* was given by Hitschmann and Kreibich in 1897 in Germany to describe necrotic cutaneous plaques due to cutaneous involvement in disseminated *Pseudomonas* infection. However, ecthyma gangrenosum is now known to be a morphologic pattern of cutaneous infection caused by a wide variety of organisms.

Ecthyma gangrenosum usually starts as an erythematous macule, which subsequently forms a vesicle. Multiple lesions may occur. Lesions rapidly become indurated and may develop pustules or bullae, which slough and leave an ulcer. An eschar forms, with a rim of erythema (Figure 25.1). The disease has a strong predilection for axillae, inguinal folds, and perineum, so-called "apocrine" areas. Extremities, trunk, and face are affected less frequently. Though once regarded as cutaneous seeding during *Pseudomonas* bacteremia, most cases represent aggressive primary infection, which may disseminate in immunosuppressed patients. Synchronous multiple lesions of the perineum, genitalia, and axillae are common. This pattern of infection supports the notion that ecthyma gangrenosum arises in the skin and then disseminates. In one series, folliculitis due to *Pseudomonas aeruginosa* O-11 from a hospital water supply rapidly developed into ecthyma gangrenosum in six hospitalized immunosuppressed patients (2). This represents a common scenario in which early lesions resemble a bacterial folliculitis, and then rapidly progress to typical ecthyma gangrenosum lesions. In the largest series of patients with ecthyma gangrenosum, over 75% were felt to originate in the skin, and two thirds primarily involved apocrine areas. Some patients developed septicemia (1).

The majority of patients who develop ecthyma gangrenosum are neutropenic, either secondary to chemotherapy or due to primary immunodeficiency. The disease has also been described in HIV-infected patients in the absence of neutropenia (3). A neonatal form of the disease termed *noma neonatorum* occurs in premature infants. In addition to anogenital involvement, this presentation has a distinct orofacial predilection (4). A necrotizing stomatitis, the mucosal equivalent of ecthyma gangrenosum, has also been described in immunocompromised patients (5).

Classical ecthyma gangrenosum is usually caused by *Pseudomonas aeruginosa*, but may be caused by several other gram-negative bacteria (Table 25.1). Similar lesions in immunosuppressed patients may be caused by a multitude of opportunistic fungi. These patients usually do not present with the typical apocrine folliculocentric lesions. However, the morphologic features of individual lesions

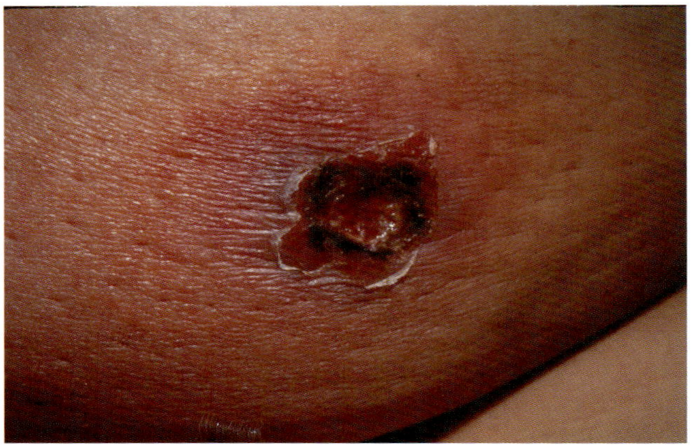

FIGURE 25.1. Indurated erythematous plaque with central ulceration and eschar.

may closely resemble ecthyma gangrenosum. As in bacterial ecthyma gangrenosum, cutaneous lesions due to opportunistic fungi may be a manifestation of hematogenous dissemination with secondary seeding of the skin. Alternatively, they may represent primary invasive infection, which may then disseminate. Gastrointestinal and respiratory tracts and skin are common portals of entry for disseminated infections. Invasive infections of the skin may occur in previously normal skin, but are more likely to occur in areas that have had a disrupted barrier, such as sites of vascular access, venipuncture, burns, or surgical procedures.

The clinical presentation of ecthyma gangrenosum in an immunosuppressed patient constitutes a medical emergency. Investigation into the etiologic agent must be pursued urgently, so that appropriate antibiotic therapy can be instituted. A list of organisms known to cause ecthyma gangrenosum or similar lesions in the immunosuppressed patient is given in Table 25.1.

The organisms listed in Table 25.1 cause ecthyma gangrenosum or lesions closely resembling it. However, numerous yeasts, and fungi causing hyalohyphomycosis and pheohyphomycosis, can cause invasive cutaneous infections in immunocompromised hosts. These cutaneous lesions may include subcutaneous and dermal nodules, or cellulitis. Since morphologic overlap with ecthyma gangrenosum could occur with a multitude of organisms, the list included in the table should not be viewed as comprehensive.

A clinical presentation of necrotizing papules and plaques in apocrine areas of an immunosuppressed patient strongly suggests ecthyma gangrenosum, but the differential diagnosis for a plaque or plaques with eschar is much wider, including true ecthyma caused by *Staphylococcus* or *Streptococcus* species, arachnid or arthropod bite reactions, anthrax, tularemia, diphtheria, syphilitic chancre, herpes simplex virus infection, and orf. Similar lesions may develop in patients with septicemic plaque (*Yersinia pestis*) (20). Also in the differential diagnosis is Fournier's gangrene, a polymicrobial acute necrotizing infection of the genitalia. Causes include *Streptococcus* and *Staphylococcus* species, usually in combination with various gram-negative and anaerobic bacteria. This infection differs from ecthyma gangrenosum in its frequent occurrence in diabetics, severe pain, and tissue crepitus.

Cultures of the blood will reveal the organism in most cases of septicemic ecthyma gangrenosum. Since bacterial and fungal causes are morphologically indistinguishable, both bacterial and fungal cultures should be performed. The laboratory should be notified of the suspicion of opportunistic infection to minimize the possibility that a true positive culture will be dismissed as a contaminant. Tissue evaluation may include skin biopsy with touch preps, microbial stains, and culture. Touch preps may be stained with gram stain for bacteria and calcofluor white for fungi. Frozen sections from affected tissue with and without special stains may aid in more rapid diagnosis.

Biopsy findings in ecthyma gangrenosum include dermal edema and an infiltrate composed of neutrophils, lymphocytes, histiocytes, and plasma cells within the dermis and subcutaneous tissue (Figure 25.2A and 25.2B). There is vascular proliferation, and variable epidermal necrosis. Organisms may be found with special stains in most cases. The organisms are usually located within the interstitium and adventitia of venules. The findings in ecthyma gangrenosum differ from those of bacterial septic

TABLE 25.1. Causes of Ecthyma Gangrenosum and Similar Lesions in Immunosuppressed Patients

Bacteria
Pseudomonas aeruginosa
Escherichia coli (6)
Morganella morganii (7)
Klebsiella pneumoniae (8)
Citrobacter freundii (9)
Xanthomonas maltophilia (10)
Aeromonas hydrophilia (11)
Fungi
Curvularia sp. (12)
Candida sp. (13)
Fusarium sp. (14)
Scytalidium dimidiatum (15)
Metarrhizium anisopliae (16)
Mucor sp. (17)
Exserohilum sp. (18)
Aspergillus niger (19)

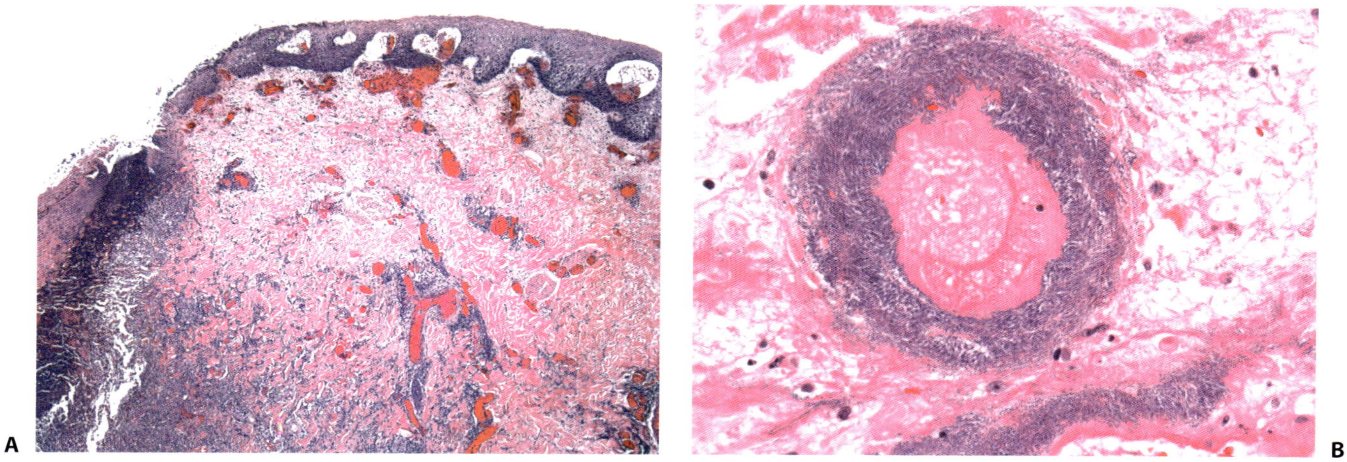

FIGURE 25.2. (A) Deep ulcer with vascular congestion and neutrophil-rich infiltrate. (B) Numerous intravascular, perivascular, and interstitial Pseudomonas bacilli.

vasculitis in which there is vascular damage associated with fibrin thrombi and intraluminal bacteria (21).

Treatment of ecthyma gangrenosum is directed by the etiologic agent. However, initially, broad spectrum antibiotic therapy must be undertaken urgently because of the high mortality associated with delayed treatment. Prognosis in ecthyma gangrenosum is dependent upon the infectious agent, but also the degree and duration of immunosuppression and the extent of cutaneous involvement (21).

References

1. El Baze P, Thyss A, Vinti H, Deville A, Dellamonica P, Ortonne JP. A study of nineteen immunocompromised patients with extensive skin lesions caused by *Pseudomonas aeruginosa* with and without bacteremia. *Acta Derm Venerol (Stockh)* 1991; 71: 411–415.
2. El Baze P, Thyss A, Caldani C, Juhlin L, Schneider M, Ortonne JP. *Pseudomonas aeruginosa* O-11 folliculitis: Development into ecthyma gangrenosum in immunocompromised patients. *Arch Dermatol* 1985; 121: 873–876.
3. Khan MO, Montecalvo MA, Davis I, Wormser GP. Ecthyma gangrenosum in patients with acquired immunodeficiency syndrome. *Cutis* 2000; 66: 121–123.
4. Freeman AF, Mancini AJ, Yogev R. Is noma neonatorum a presentation of ecthyma gangrenosum in the newborn? *Pediatr Infect Dis J* 2002; 21: 83–84.
5. Barasch A, Gordon S, Geist RY, Geist JR. Necrotizing stomatitis: Report of 3 *Pseudomonas aeruginosa*-positive patients. *Oral Surg Oral Med Oral Pathol Oral Radiol Endod* 2003; 96: 136–140.
6. Edelstein H, Cutting HO. *Escherichia coli* as cause of ecthyma gangrenosum. *Postgrad Med* 1986; 79: 44–45.
7. Del Pozo J, Garcia-Silva J, Almagro M, Martinez W, Nicolas R, Fonseca E. Ecthyma gangrenosum-like eruption associated with *Morganella morganii* infection. *Br J Dermatol* 1998; 139: 520–521.
8. Rodot S, Lacour JP, van Elslande L, Castanet J, Desruelles F, Ortonne JP. Ecthyma gangrenosum caused by *Klebsiella pneumoniae*. *Int J Dermatol* 1995; 34: 216–217.
9. Reich HL, Fadeyi DW, Naik NS, Honig PJ, Yan AC. Nonpseudomonal ecthyma gangrenosum. *J Am Acad Dermatol* 2004; 50: S114–117.
10. Vartivarian SE, Papadakis KA, Palacios JA, Manning JT, Anaissie EJ. Mucocutaneous and soft tissue infections caused by *Xanthomonas maltophilia*. *Ann Intern Med* 1994; 121: 969–973.
11. Shackleford P, Ratzan SA, Shearer T. Ecthyma gangrenosum produced by *Aeromonas hydrophilia*. *J Pediatr* 1973; 83: 100–101.
12. Bouduel M, Santos P, Turienzo CF, Chantada G, Paganini H. Atypical skin lesions caused by *Curvularia* sp. and *Pseudoallescheria boydii* in two patients after allogeneic bone marrow transplantation. *Bone Marrow Transplant* 2001; 27: 1311–1313.
13. File TM Jr, Marina OA, Flowers FP. Necrotic skin lesions associated with disseminated candidiasis. *Arch Dermatol* 1979; 115: 214–215.
14. Martino P, Gastaldi R, Raccah R, Girmenia C. Clinical patterns of *Fusarium* infections in immunocompromised patients. *J Infection* 1994; 28: SI, 7–15.
15. Benne CA, Neeleman C, Bruin M, de Hoog GS, Fleer A. Disseminating infection with *Scytalidium dimidiatum* in a granulocytopenic child. *Eur J Clin Microbiol Infect Dis* 1993; 12: 118–121.
16. Burgner D, Eagles G, Burgess M, et al. Disseminated invasive infection due to *Metarrhizium anisopliae* in an immunocompromised child. *J Clin Microbiol* 1998; 36: 1146–1150.

17. Kramer BS, Hernandez AD, Reddick RL, Levine AS. Cutaneous infarction. Manifestation of disseminated mucormycosis. *Arch Dermatol* 1977; 113: 1075–1076.
18. Levy I, Stein J, Ashkenazi S, Samra Z, Livni G, Yaniv I. Ecthyma gangrenosum caused by disseminated *Exserohilum* in a child with leukemia: A case report and review of the literature. *Pediatr Dermatol* 2003; 20: 495–497.
19. Panke TW, McManus AT, Spebar MJ. Infection of a burn wound by *Aspergillus niger*: Gross appearance simulating ecthyma gangrenosum. *Am J Clin Pathol* 1979; 72: 230–232.
20. Welty TK, Grabman J, Kompare E, et al. Nineteen cases of plague in Arizona: A spectrum including ecthyma gangrenosum due to plague and plague in pregnancy. *West J Med* 1985; 142: 641–646.
21. Greene SL, Su WPD, Muller SA. Ecthyma gangrenosum: Report of clinical, histopathologic, and bacteriologic aspects of eight cases. *J Am Acad Dermatol* 1984; 11: 781–787.

26
Rocky Mountain Spotted Fever and the Rickettsioses

■ Synonyms:	None
■ Etiology:	*Rickettsia rickettsii* following *Dermacentor* sp. tick bite
■ Associations:	Outdoor recreational activity
■ Clinical:	Fever/headache followed by macules and petechial eruption of wrists/ankles with subsequent generalization
■ Histology:	Lymphocytic vasculitis with vascular thrombosis, epidermal necrosis organisms with special stains seen in vascular wall
■ IHC repertoire:	Organisms identified by immunohistochemical and immunofluorescent antibodies
■ Staging:	Not applicable
■ Prognosis:	Fatality rate of 20%–30%, worse in the elderly or with coexisting G6PD deficiency
■ Adverse variables:	Renal failure, myocarditis, arrythmias, DIC and ARDS
■ Treatment:	Intravenous tetracycline, doxycycline, or chloramphenicol

The rickettsioses constitute a diverse group of arthropod-borne human diseases capable of producing significant morbidity and mortality. They share important pathologic and clinical attributes that permit their diagnosis in most instances (1). The rickettsioses are responsible for a great number of deaths seen particularly in times of war. It is estimated that over 3 million combatants and civilians in the First World War succumbed to epidemic typhus. Among the more deadly types of infection belonging to this group is Rocky Mountain Spotted Fever, the principal subject of this chapter.

The rickettsioses are endemic to most areas of the world where contact with arthropods, namely biting ticks, mites, fleas, and lice, can be found. They can be broadly categorized into tick-borne agents that principally include Rocky Mountain Spotted Fever (*R. rickettsii*) and Medditeranean fevers (*R. conorii*), mite-borne diseases including *rickettsialpox* (*R. akari*) and *scrub typhus* (*Orientia tsutsugamushi*, formerly *R. tsutsugamushi*), flea-borne *endemic typhus* (*R. typhi*), and louse-borne *epidemic thyphus* (*R. prowazekii*). *Q fever* is unique within the group as its etiologic agent *Coxiella burnetti* is acquired following aerosolization of infected tissues. They can also be subcategorized into the spotted fever group or the typhus group on the basis of shared immunologic or biologic properties (2). The infectious agents are among the smallest of bacteria at $0.3–10^{-6}\,\mu$m. They are considered to be gram-negative and exist as pleomorphic-appearing bodies either exclusive to the cytoplasm of infected cells (typhus group) or the nucleus and cytoplasm (spotted fever group). They require passage via blood-consuming arthropod vectors that use infected mammals and the arthropods themselves as a reservoir. Once introduced into the skin, the organisms attach to endothelial cell membranes until phagocytosed by inflammatory cells with subsequent hematogenous or lymphatic passage throughout the body.

Rocky Mountain spotted fever (RMSF) was first described in the late nineteenth century among settlers in the still-wild frontier of the American West, hence the term "Rocky Mountain" fever. RMSF is the most common rickettsial infection reported in North America and though found throughout the continent, is most common in the south Atlantic region of the United States (3). The most important vector for disease is the dog tick or *Dermacentor variabilis* and the Rocky Mountain wood tick *Dermacentor andersonii*. The etiologic agent *R. rickettsii* is transmitted with blood-meals of the infecting ticks, which usually requires at least a 6-hour interval of feeding (4).

Most infections occur during the summer and are most commonly seen in children or adult males engaged in outdoor recreational activity. Insect repellants, protective outer garments, periodic tick surveillance, and timely and efficacious extraction of feeding ticks are all important means of disease prevention (5).

The clinical manifestations are ushered in by high fever, chills, myalgia, and headache at an average of 7 days following exposure (range 2–14 days). The fever often exceeds 102 degrees and may be accompanied by gastrointestinal complaints (6). The cutaneous manifestation, namely rash, follows within 2 to 4 days after the initial complaints and consists of a macular followed by papular petechial rash (Figure 26.1). The rash initially begins on the wrists and or ankles and spreads to the trunk over the ensuing day. Palm and or sole involvement is fairly uncommon, yet can occur. The classic triad of fever, headache, and rash is present in about 60% of patients. A distinct minority (~10%) of patients may never develop rash, so-called *spotless fever*. This is most commonly seen in the elderly or among the dark-skinned races. The rash is most often accompanied by systemic manifestations including hypovolemia, tachycardia, and peripheral edema. Important complications include epidermal necrosis in conjunction with ischemic vascular thrombosis with digital or extremity loss, scarring, and visceral organ failure including hepatic or renal failure, cardiomyopathy with electrical instability, disseminated intravascular coagulation, the adult respiratory distress syndrome, and CNS involvement with delirium or seizure. Motor deficits, cranial nerve palsy, or coma may also be seen.

Important laboratory abnormalities routinely encountered in these patients include thrombocytopenia and normochromic normocytic anemia with increased prothrombin times and decreased fibrinogen, hyponatremia, hepatic transaminasemia with hyperbilirubinemia, and elevated BUN and creatinine levels.

Biopsies from the skin rash show perivascular lymphocytic infiltrates with variable degrees of vascular disruption including fibrin deposits and thrombosis (lymphocytic vasculitis), dermal purpura and edema (Figures 26.2–26.4) (7). The overlying epithelium may undergo necrosis in conjunction with ischemic vascular thrombosis. The organisms may be positively identified within the endothelia with the aid of immunohistochemical or immunofluorescent staining (8). Molecular-based methods including *in situ* PCR have also been utilized but are not widely available (9). Serologic methods remain the most important means of establishing a definitive diagnosis, although they suffer from a delay in diagnosis requiring comparison of acute and convalescent antibody titers. The Weil-Felix and complement-based serologic methods are antiquated due to poor sensitivity (10).

The differential diagnosis of RMSF is broad. Important viral entities to consider include measles, rubella, and infectious mononucleosis. Measles more often presents with upper (coryza) and lower respiratory (cough) complaints and less often produces a petechial rash. Rubella tends to be less symptomatic than RMSF and produces a less dramatic rash that typically begins on the face. Infectious mononucleosis (Epstein-Barr viral infection) less often produces a rash (~10% of patients) unless preceded

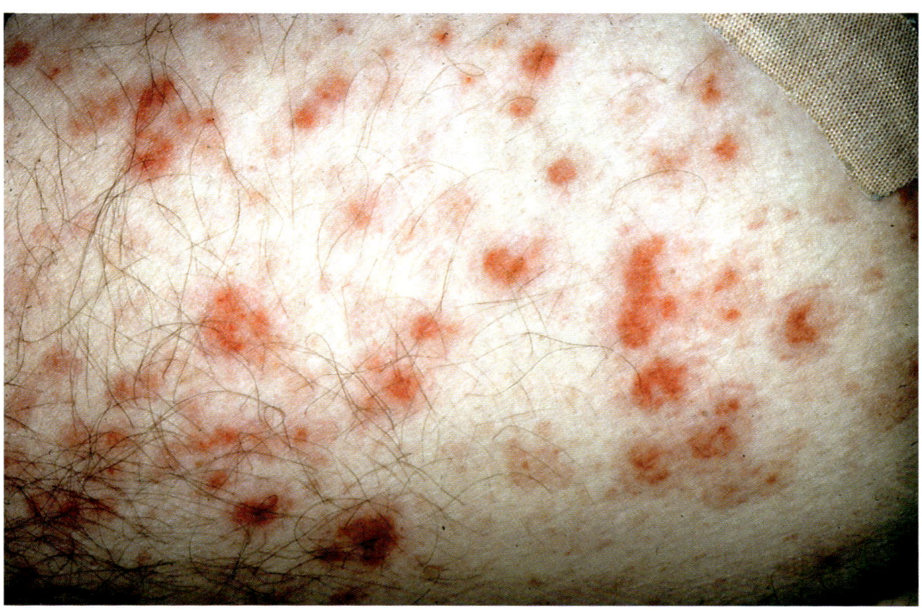

FIGURE 26.1. Maculopapular eruption with petechial hemorrhage in Rocky Mountain Spotted Fever.

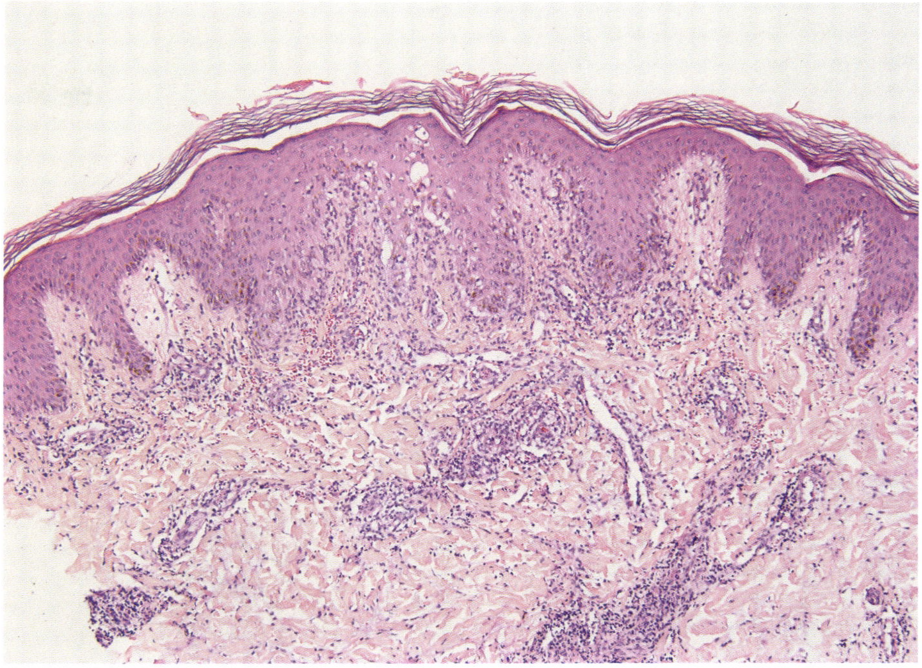

FIGURE 26.2. Low power photomicrograph depicting superficial and deep lymphocytic dermatitis with focal epithelial exocytosis. Note the prominent dermal hemorrhage.

by the administration of ampicillin. Important bacterial infections to exclude include in particular meningococcemia, tularemia, and leptospirosis. The rash of meningococcemia typically develops in conjunction with or shortly following the onset of symptoms and is often accompanied by leukocytosis. The rash of meningococcemia tends to produce larger and confluent stellate configured purpuric areas with an angulated border. Tularemia tends to produce solitary, often ulcerated or eschar-like cutaneous lesions with draining lymphadenopathy. Leptospirosis produces a rash that typically begins on the trunk, spreading later to the extremities. A clinical variant of leptospi-

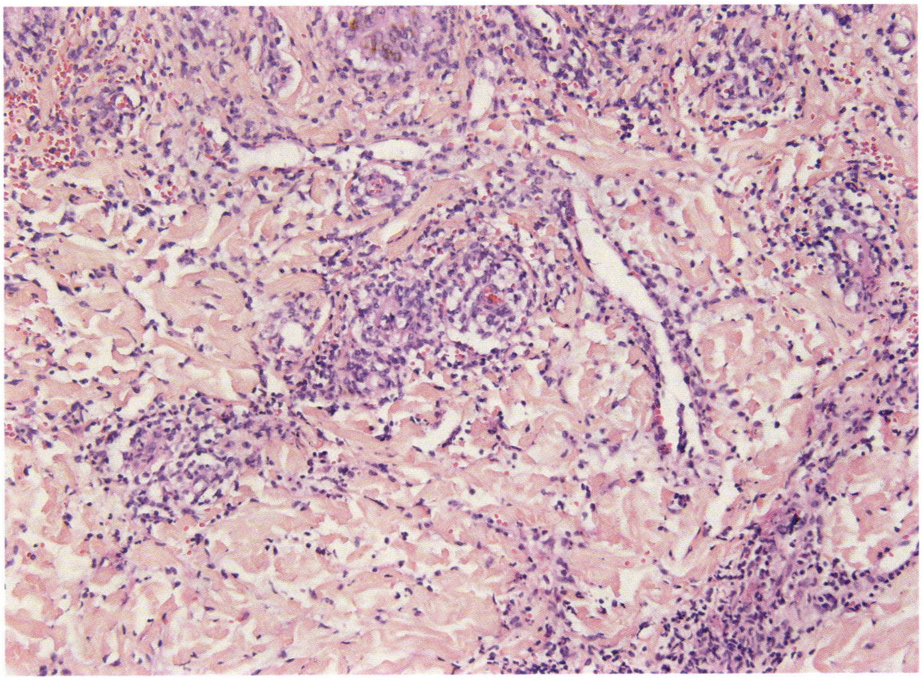

FIGURE 26.3. Medium power photomicrograph detailing perivascular lymphocytic infiltrate.

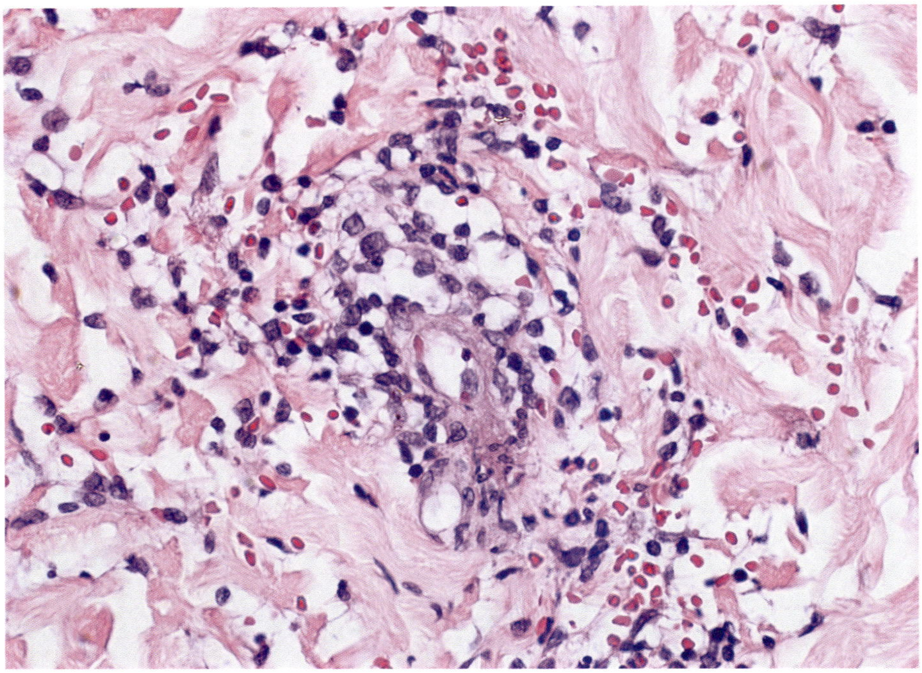

FIGURE 26.4. High power detail with perivascular lymphocytes and erythrocytes. Note fibrin deposits in proximity to the capillaries.

rosis termed Fort Bragg or pretibial fever produces a petechial rash confined to the pretibial surfaces.

Empiric intravenous antibiotics should be instituted prior to biopsy or serologic confirmation as the untreated mortality approaches 30% (6). Treatment recommendations are tetracycline 25–50 mg/kg q 6 hours or doxycycline 1 mg/lb q 12 hours or chloramphenicol 50–75 mg/kg q 6 hours for at least 7 days or until 2 days following resolution of symptoms. Aggressive fluid status and electrolyte balance management is essential. The overall mortality of RMSF is between 2% and 5% with appropriate antibiotic therapy. Most fatalities are observed between the eighth and fifteenth days of illness. Elderly patients and those individuals with coexisting glucose 6-phosphate dehydrogenase deficiency have been reported to have a worse prognosis.

References

1. Zaki M. Selected tickborne infections: A review of Lyme disease, Rocky Mountain Spotted Fever and babesiosis. *NY State J Med* 1989; 89: 320.
2. Boyd A, Neldner K. Typhus disease group. *Int J Dermatol* 1992; 31: 823.
3. Helmick C, Bernard K, d'Angelo L. Rocky Mountain Spotted Fever: Clinical, laboratory and epidemiological features of 262 cases. *J Infect Dis* 1984; 150: 480.
4. Woodward T. Rocky Mountain spotted fever: Epidemiological and early clinical signs are keys to treatment and reduced mortality. *J Infect Dis* 1984; 150: 465.
5. Cowan G. Rickettsial diseases: The typhus group of fevers—a review. *Postgrad Med J* 2000; 76: 269.
6. Weber D, Walker D. Rocky Mountain spotted fever. *Infect Dis Clin North Am* 1991; 5: 19.
7. Kao G, Evancho C, Ioffe O, et al. Cutaneous histopathology of Rocky Mountain spotted fever. *J Cutan Pathol* 1997; 24: 604.
8. Walker C, Cain B, Olmstead P. Laboratory diagnosis of Rocky Mountain spotted fever by immunofluorescent demonstration of *Rickettsia ricketsii* in cutaneous lesions. *Am J Clin Pathol* 1978; 69: 619.
9. Woodward T, Pederson C, Oster C, et al. Prompt confirmation of Rocky Mountain spotted fever: Identification of Rickettsiae in skin tissues. *J Infect Dis* 1976; 134: 297.
10. Kaplan J, Schonberger L. The sensitivity of various serologic tests in the diagnosis of Rocky Mountain spotted fever. *Am J Trop Med Hyg* 1986; 35: 840.

27 Smallpox

■ Synonyms:	Variola, alastrim, amaas
■ Etiology:	Infection with variola poxvirus
■ Associations:	Since eradication in 1979, confirmed presence should prompt consideration of biowarfare/terrorism
■ Clinical:	Influenza-like prodrome ~ 3 days prior to erythematous macular rash into vesiculating papules to umbilicated pustules and finally scars
■ Histology:	Intraepidermal and subepidermal vesiculation with neutrophils predominating, epithelium with eosinophilic (Guarnieri) inclusions
■ IHC repertoire:	N/A
■ Staging:	None
■ Prognosis:	Overall ~30% mortality
■ Adverse factors:	Confluent eruption, thrombocytopenia/DIC
■ Treatment:	Prevented with vaccination, cidofovir efficacious in animal studies

Smallpox, otherwise known as *variola*, was first described in ancient Chinese texts dating from the eleventh century B.C. The Chinese were the first to discover that purposeful inoculation of lesional material into the nose of the uninfected was preventative of disease in the sixth century B.C. (1). Although the disease was officially eradicated in 1979, known stocks of the material have been maintained in biolabs located in Russia and the United States, where they pose a potential source of public health concern if subverted as biowarfare agents (2–5). Smallpox belongs to the Poxvirus group of double-stranded DNA containing viruses that includes vaccinia, molluscum contagiosum, and cowpox. The poxviruses are among the largest of all human viruses, attaining a maximum diameter of 300 nm, and possess characteristic rectangular or cylindrical outer capsids and a central DNA core (6).

Natural infection follows contact with an infectious human most commonly via respiratory droplets but may also occur with skin inoculation or fomite spread. The virus is hearty and resistant to dessication. Scales and desquamated epithelium harbor viable virus for long periods. Following exposure, there is an asymptomatic 10- to 14-day period in which viral replication occurs within infected respiratory mucosa and associated draining lymphatic tissues. This phase of infection (primary viremia) coincides with generalized involvement of the reticuloendothelial organs including the liver, spleen, and lymph organs. Secondary viremia then follows in which systemic spread of the virus through the bloodstream occurs, heralding the onset of an influenza-like prodromal syndrome. Prodromal symptoms include high fever, severe headache, back pain, and vomiting. During this prodromal phase a characteristic and fleeting maculopapular rash involving the waist and proximal lower extremities may occur. The patient remains noninfectious during the prodromal phase, becoming infectious only when the exanthem appears. Laboratory testing during this period often yields abnormal coagulation parameters including thrombocytopenia and altered clotting times that may be associated with the development of the disseminated intravascular coagulation (DIC) syndrome. Abnormal bleeding is an ominous sign ascribed to the hemorrhagic form of the disease (*purpura variolosa*) with a generally fatal outcome. With secondary viremia, there is viral spread to the mucosa and skin epithelium, initiating the characteristic exanthematous rash of the disorder approximately 3 days after prodromal symptoms begin.

Although the morphology and course of individual rash lesions are similar, their number can vary (6). Mild forms of the disease (*alastrim*, *variola minor*) are charac-

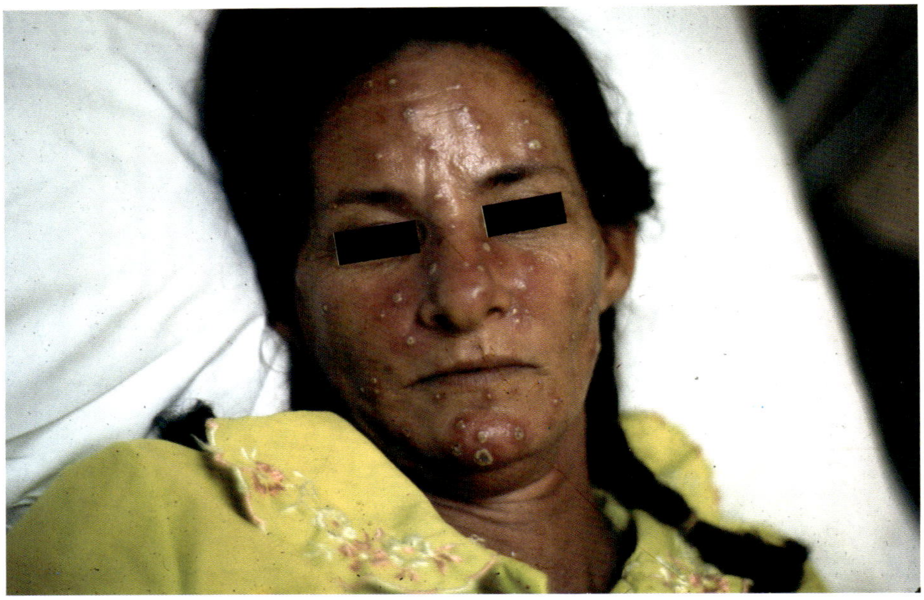

FIGURE 27.1. Multiple ulcerating pustules with erythematous bases seen in smallpox.

terized by a sparse number of lesions, whereas more severe forms may present with a confluent eruption. Lesions tend to be peripherally distributed with the greatest number located over the extremities and face (Figure 27.1). The earliest lesion consists of an erythematous macule that proceeds to a deep-seated papule with a cloudy appearing surmounted vesicle. The vesicle is multiloculated and resilient. The lesions mature generally within 7 days into pustules with characteristic central umbilication. Within 10 days, the surface forms a crusted scab, healing as a depressed scar. Occasionally, the lesions may present as crusted plaques or pass through the various stages without vesicle or pustule formation. Mucosal involvement often noted at the time of the exanthem includes ocular, genital, or oropharyngeal disease including upper airway obstruction with laryngeal and tracheal involvement. Visceral disease may take the form of pneumonitis, encephalitis, osteomyelitis, orchitis, or hepatitis. Pneumonia and encephalitis constitute serious complications that may eventuate in death.

The histologic features seen in variola are suggestive of the disorder (7). Early lesions show dermal edema with neutrophilic capillaritis. Developed lesions of smallpox show, in addition to the dermal edema, pronounced intrapidermal vesiculation with exocytosis of neutrophils (Figures 27.2 and 27.3). The blister cavity may contain or be surrounded by epithelial cells that possess characteristic eosinophilic granular inclusions known as *Guarnieri bodies* (Figure 27.4). Elementary or Paschen viral bodies may be demonstrated with Geimsa staining scrapped from or expressed from lesional material. Multinucleation, nuclear molding, and/or nucleus inclusions typical of the Herpesvirus infections are not identified.

Diagnosis of suspected cases of smallpox has obvious global implications and public health ramifications. Once presumptively diagnosed on the basis of the clinical presentation, the disease should now be confirmed by ancillary diagnostic techniques and in conjunction with public health agencies. Genomic-based technologies, including PCR techniques and fluorescent antibody testing of infectious material, provide fairly rapid and, presumptive results but the gold standard for identification involves tissue culturing and anti-serum neutralization. The diagnosis can also be achieved serologically through retrospective analysis of paired acute and convalescent sera.

The most important disorder to distinguish from smallpox is *chickenpox*. The latter typically produces little if any prodromal symptoms, and is associated with successive crops of lesions, thus showing lesions in various stages of development. There is a tendency of the lesions of smallpox to be peripherally distributed, larger, more often deep-seated, to possess central umbilication, and to become confluent compared to chickenpox.

There is no effective treatment for established cases. Ongoing trials with the antiviral agent cidofovir have been promising in animal models. Treatment with immune globulin, anti-vaccinia serum, and thiosemicarbazone has been attempted in the past with questionable efficacy. Supportive measures aimed at reducing secondary bacterial infection and monitoring fluid and electrolyte levels are important. Prevention remains the most important means of deterring smallpox. The Jennerian vaccination consists of the purposeful inoculation of vaccinia virus (a laboratory-altered form of smallpox) into the skin (8). Following inoculation, a crusted papule should develop at the site

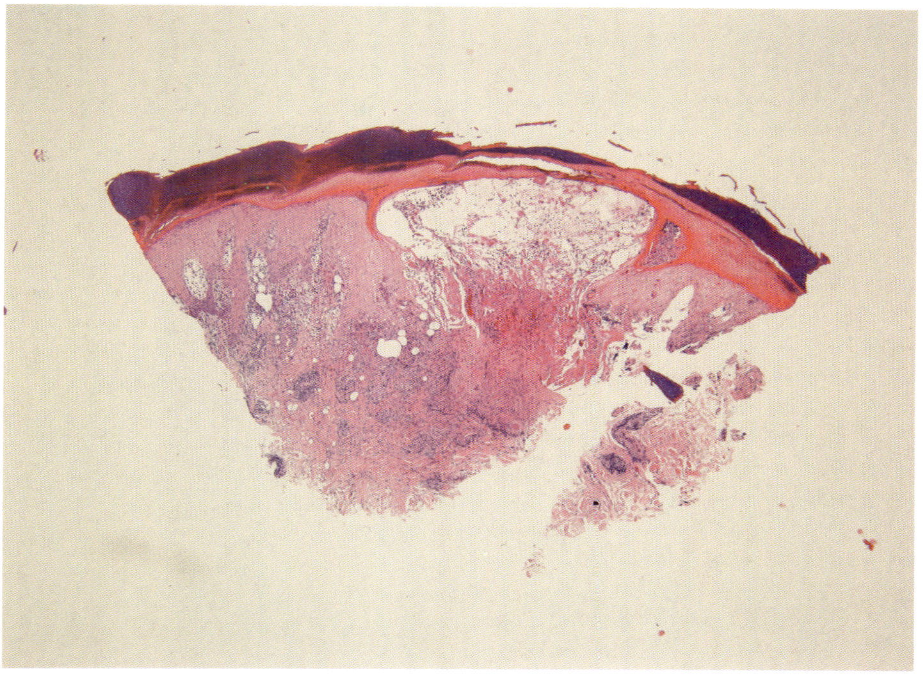

FIGURE 27.2. Low power photomicrograph showing epidermal blister with subepidermal necrosis.

within 10 days of administration. Failure to develop an inoculation site lesion is an indication of ineffective immunization or loss of vaccine potency and the immunization should be repeated. Vaccination is contraindicated in the immunosuppressed, infants, or individuals with atopy or other undisclosed dermatitis that may predispose them to dissemination of the virus. Vaccination against smallpox ended in 1972, leaving approximately 65% of the current U.S. population who have never received vaccination and, of those vaccinated, all have a questionable ability to mount an effective immune response. For these reasons, interest in vaccination, particularly among health care workers and those who might respond to its use as a bioterrorism agent, has emerged.

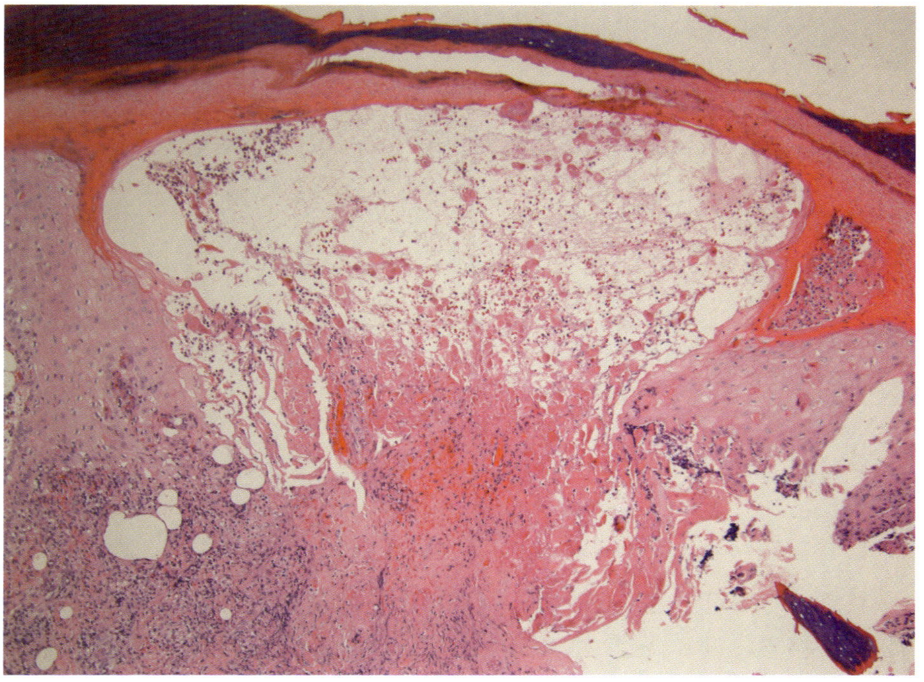

FIGURE 27.3. Medium power photomicrograph showing blister with reticular degeneration.

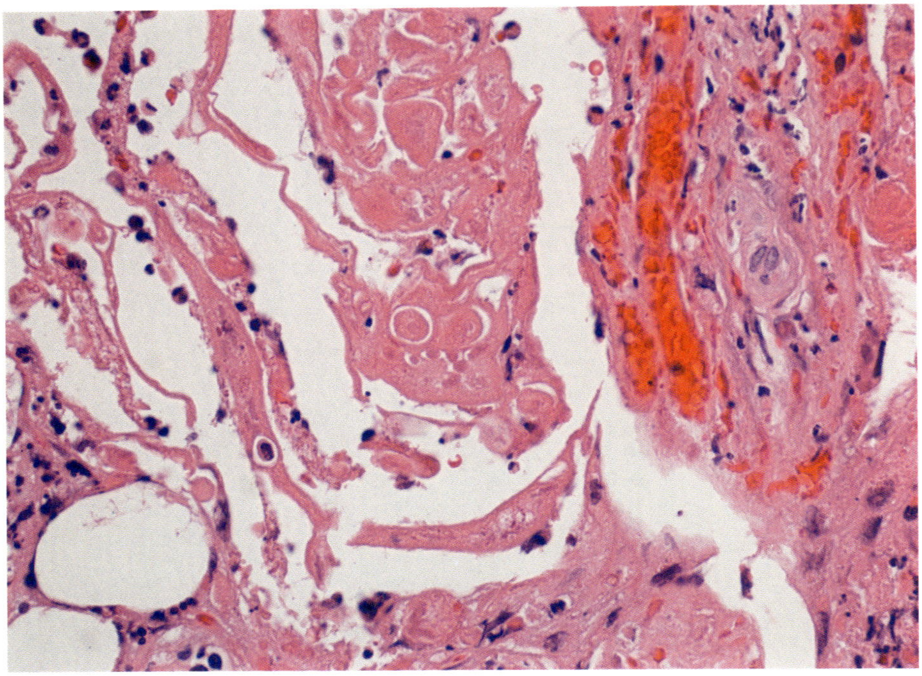

FIGURE 27.4. High power detail of blister cavity. Note central rounded eosinophilic bodies (Guarneri) associated with smallpox cytopathic effect.

Widespread immunization of the public engenders important practical and medical concerns. Vaccine production has only recently been reinstituted after a long hiatus and thus limited stocks are available. Important complications of the vaccine itself include hypersensitivity reaction, systemization or progressive cutaneous spread of the virus, encephalitis, and bacterial superinfection (8–10). An increased incidence of myocardial infarction among recipients of the vaccine has also been recently reported (11).

The overall mortality rate of smallpox is 30%. Individuals who develop disseminated or confluent lesions, DIC, encephalitis, or pneumonitis are at greater risk.

References

1. Breman J, Arita I. The confirmation and maintenance of smallpox eradication. *N Engl J Med* 1980; 303: 1263.
2. Breman J, Henderson D. Poxvirus dilemmas: Monkeypox, smallpox, and biologic terrorism. *N Engl J Med* 1998; 303: 556.
3. Albert M, Ostheimer K, Breman J. The last smallpox epidemic in Boston and the vaccination controversy, 1901–1903. *N Engl J Med* 2001; 344: 375.
4. Wehrle P. A reality in our time: Certification of the global eradication of smallpox. *J Infect Dis* 1980; 242: 636.
5. Fenner F. Global eradication of smallpox. *Rev Infect Dis* 1982; 4: 916.
6. Henderson D. Smallpox. Clinical and epidemiologic features. *Emerg Infect Dis* 1999; 5: 537.
7. Michelson H, Ikeda K. Microscopic changes in variola. *Arch Dermatol Syph* 1927; 15: 138.
8. Greenberg M. Complications of vaccination against smallpox. *Am J Dis Child* 1948; 76: 492.
9. Sarkany I, Caron G. Cutaneous complications of smallpox vaccination. *Trans St Johns Hosp Dermatol Soc* 1962; 48: 163.
10. Lane J, et al. Complications of smallpox vaccination, 1968: National surveillance in the United States. *N Engl J Med* 1968; 281: 1201.
11. CDC. Smallpox vaccine adverse events among civilians United States, March 2003. *MMWR* 2003; 52: 201.

28
Staphylococcal Toxin-Mediated Scalded Skin and Toxic Shock Syndromes

■ Synonyms:	SS—Ritter's disease, Ritter von Rittershain's disease TS—None
■ Etiology:	SS—Phage infected strains of *S. aureus* TS—Non-phage toxigenic strains of *S. aureus*
■ Associations:	SS—Children with head/neck Staph infections; adults with renal failure TS—90% menstruating women, 10% skin/soft tissue infection
■ Clinical:	SS—Red macular rash to generalized flaccid bullae TS—Fever, hypotension and macular erythroderma
■ Histology:	SS—Subcorneal (intragranular layer) cell-poor blister with acantholysis TS—Neutrophilic pustular dermatitis with necrosis
■ IHC repertoire:	SS—Not applicable TS—Not applicable
■ Staging:	SS—Not applicable TS—Not applicable
■ Prognosis:	SS—Children 2–3% mortality; adults ~40% TS—5%
■ Adverse signs:	SS—Bacteremia, renal failure TS—Shock, encephalopathy and renal failure
■ Treatment:	SS—Oral/intravenous antibiotics TS—Tampon removal, intravenous antibiotics/fluids

The toxin-mediated staphylococcal syndromes of *staphylococcal scalded skin syndrome* (SSSS) and *toxic shock syndrome* (TS) constitute important dermatologic entities capable of producing significant morbidity and mortality. Distinctive clinical and pathologic attributes usually permit their early recognition allowing for prompt institution of potentially life-saving therapy.

Credit for the first clinical description of SS belongs to Ritter von Rittershain, who in 1878 described 297 cases of a generalized exfoliative exanthem in neonates (1). An association with staphylococcus and subsequently the mechanism of phage-mediated toxin elaboration would be discovered in the 1940s and 1950s. Today, it is known that the epidermolytic toxins elaborated by viral phage-infected strains 71 and 55 of *Staphylococcal aureus* are responsible for the characteristic clinical and pathologic findings of this disorder. Interestingly, the target of the exfoliative toxin is pathogenically identical to superficial pemphigus (2,3). Both involve the disruption of the cadherin adhesion molecule desmoglein 1 antigen, hence the pathologic similarity between these two otherwise distinctive disorders. The toxin is renally excreted, thus the epidemiologic association between the relatively decreased renal clearance mechanisms characteristic of young children and among the renally impaired adult (4–6). Unlike children, adults with SS are more likely to have positive blood cultures. SS has been described in conjunction with HIV disease in the adult (7).

The historical experience with TS is much more brief. The association of a multiorgan systemic toxic syndrome with certain strains of staphylococcus and menstruating women using superabsorbent tampons would emerge in the early 1980s (8). Although most of the initial reports involved menstruating women, it was subsequently determined that the syndrome could occur in accordance with soft tissue and cutaneous infections by toxin-producing strains of *Staphylococcus aureus*. Important risk factors for non-menstrual TS include minor abrasions that serve as a portal for toxin entry, burns, trauma, and antecedent surgery (9,10). Since the removal of superabsorbent tampons from the market, non-menstrual TS is now the most common presentation of this illness. A common clinical antecedent of non-menstrual TS is streptococcal *necrotizing fasciitis*. Following entry into the bloodstream, the toxins themselves, termed TSST-1 and enterotoxin C1, are non-phage related and produce illness on the basis of *TNF*-like properties including hypotension, fever, and leukocyte activation (11).

The clinical presentations of these entities are distinctive. SS is broadly grouped into three different forms termed *generalized, localized,* and *abortive* disease (12). Generalized SS is the most important manifestation of the disease and is ascribed the greatest risk for complications. This form is associated with remote staphylococcal infection of the head and neck area including conjunctivitis or otitis media. The symptoms are heralded by the development of an orange-red, often tender macular rash. The rash may show periorificial or flexural accentuation. Within 24 to 48 hours, flaccid bullae typically develop. The blister roof is typically wrinkled and expands, forming large cavities, in particular involving flexural sites such as the groin or axillae. The blisters are typically Nikolsky's sign-positive and when removed, yield an erythematous glistening base. Despite widespread involvement of the bodily surfaces, the mucous membranes are characteristically spared. This stage is typically followed by desquamation and complete resolution within 5 to 7 days. Clinical improvement coincides with the presence of neutralizing serum antibodies to the toxin. The localized form of disease is synonymous with bullous impetigo and represents localized infection by toxigenic strains of *S. aureus*. As with the generalized form, this entity is typically encountered in children. The lesions are represented by superficial erosions with minimal gray exudates or by fragile vesicles or bullae filled with turbid fluid and surrounded by an erythematous rim. Lesions are typically encountered on the exposed surfaces of the skin and in particular, periorificial sites. Unlike the generalized form of the disease, wound cultures and Gram stains are positive for staphylococcus. The abortive form of the disease is less common and essentially consists of regionally limited bullae, the dermatologic manifestations of which may be confused with TS.

The clinical presentation of TS is ushered in by the precipitous development of high fever, hypotension, and macular rash (9). The rash is often localized to the site of infection and typically shows pronounced erythema with associated non-pitting edema (Figure 28.1). The conjunctivae are often injected and the oral mucosa may show petechiae and diffuse erythema. The rash is often followed by desquamation, in particular involving the palms and soles. Important systemic accompaniments to the rash to be cognizant of include painful skeletal muscles associated with rhabdomyolysis, decreased urine flow/hematuria associated with the azotemia and encephalopathy of renal failure, jaundice with hepatitis and hemorrhage associated with thrombocytopenia and disseminated intravascular coagulation. A related condition consisting of recurring erythematous rash and desquamation has been described in HIV patients, termed *recalcitrant erythematous desquamating disorder*, that produces a subacute illness of longer duration and high mortality (13).

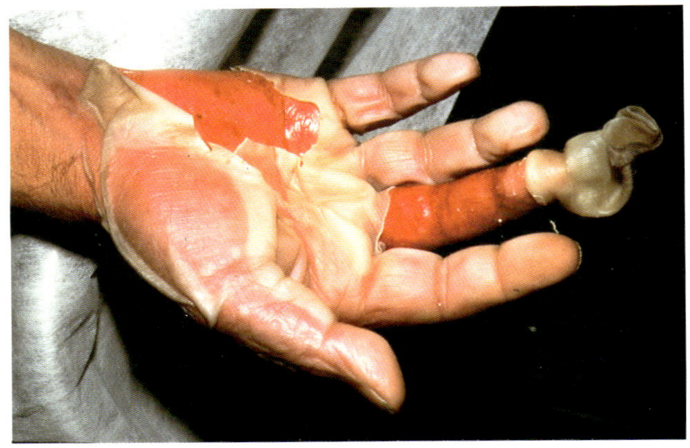

FIGURE 28.1. Epidermal loss with erythematous base seen in toxic shock syndrome.

Important considerations within the diagnostic differential of these entities include *Kawasaki's disease, drug eruption, scarlet fever,* and *toxic epidermal necrolysis* (TEN). Kawasaki's disease shows many of the features of TS, similarly sharing fever, conjunctivitis, and desquamative rash that can, however, usually be distinguished on the basis of the patient's age (Kawasaki's, 90% less than 5 years), lack of hypotension, and the presence of lymphadenopathy. Drug eruption and scarlet fever are seldom associated with hypotension. TEN is typically seen in adults and usually follows ingestion of an offending medication. Unlike TS, hypotension is not commonly seen in the early stages of TEN.

The histopathology of these entities is distinctive. SS shows blister formation situated within the epithelium just below the stratum corneum or within the granular layer (14) (Figures 28.2 and 28.3). The blister cavity typi-

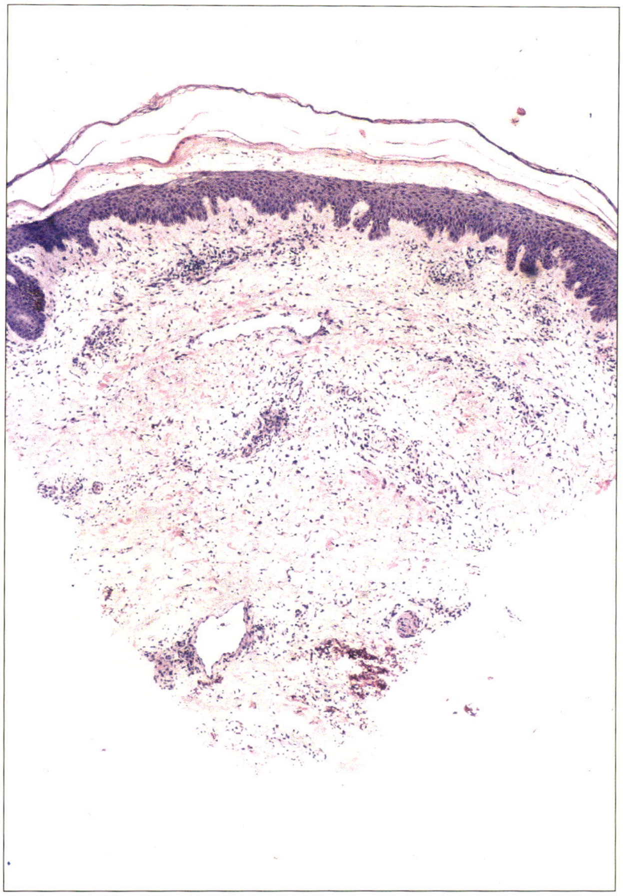

FIGURE 28.2. Low power photomicrograph of SSSS. Note subcorneal blister formation.

cally contains free-floating keratinocytes (acantholysis) and is devoid of inflammatory cells. Special (gram) stain for bacteria is negative. The dermis may show a sparse superficial perivascular lymphocytic or neutrophilic infiltrate. Localized forms of SS (bullous impetigo) show, in addition to the blister, copious numbers of neutrophils and pyogenic organisms. The histologic findings of TS show pustular collections of intraepithelial and subcorneal neutrophils with single and grouped dyskeratotic and necrotic keratinocytes. The dermis often shows edema with a perivascular and interstitial infiltrate of neutrophils and lymphocytes.

The therapy for SS should be directed toward treatment of the underlying infection. As most infections are produced by methicillin-resistant *Staphylococcus aureus*, appropriate intravenous penicillinase-resistant antibiotics are indicated. Attention to fluid and electrolyte balance and local wound care precautions are important. Complications include cellulitis, osteomyelitis, pneumonia, and, in the adult, sepsis. Measures that prevent the nosocomial transmission of the organism, including patient isolation, health provider handwashing, barrier functions, and oral antibiotic therapy for infected health care providers, should be considered.

The overall mortality rate of SS in children is about 3%, increasing to 40%–50% among immunosuppressed or renally impaired adults. The management of TS involves rapid intravenous resuscitation to ameliorate hypotension, removal of infected tampon or identification of the underlying infection, and appropriate intravenous antibiotics (15). Antimicrobial therapy generally consists of cell-wall active agents (i.e., penicillin) with adjunctive clindamycin. Intravenous gamma globulin and/or immunoglobulin containing fresh frozen plasma has also shown promise in therapy. The overall mortality of TS is approximately 5%.

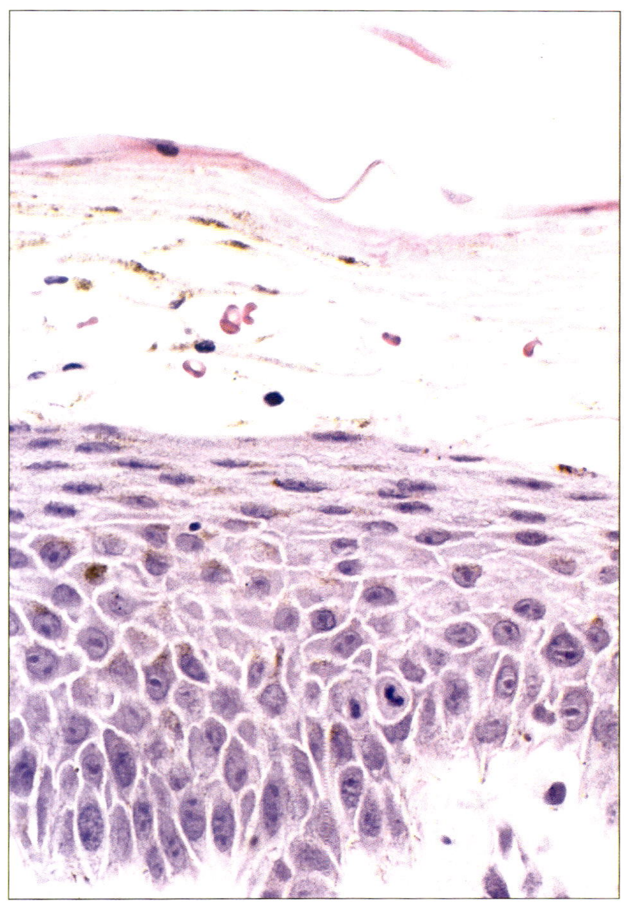

FIGURE 28.3. High power detail of subcorneal blister with scattered neutrophils. Note the absence of acantholysis.

References

SS

1. Ritter von Rittershain G. Die exfoliative Dermatitis jungerer Saugline. *Zentralzeitung fur Kinderheilkunde* 1878; 2: 3.
2. Melish M. Staphylococci, streptococci and the skin: Review of impetigo and the staphylococcal scalded skin syndrome. *Semin Dermatol* 1992; 1: 101.
3. Amagi M, Matsuyoshi N, Wang Z, et al. Toxin in bullous impetigo and staphylococcus scalded skin syndrome targets desmoglein 1. *Nat Med* 2000; 6: 1275.
4. Hardwick N, Richard M, Mathieu-Serra A. Staphylococcal scalded skin syndrome in a homosexual adult. *J Am Acad Dermatol* 1986; 15: 385.
5. Cribier B, Piemont Y, Grosshans E. Staphylococcal scalded skin syndrome in adults: A clinical review illustrated with a new case. *J Am Acad Dermatol* 1994; 30: 319.
6. Lyell A. The staphylococcal scalded skin syndrome in historical perspective: Emergence of dermopathic strains of *staphylococcus aureus* and discovery of the epidermolytic toxin. *J Am Acad Dermatol* 1983; 9: 285.
7. Richard M, Mathieu-Serra A. Staphylococcal scalded skin syndrome in a homosexual man. *J Am Acad Dermatol* 1986; 15: 385.
8. Institute of Medicine. National Academy of Science: Conference on the toxic shock syndrome. *Ann Intern Med* 1982; 96: 835.
9. Tofte R, Williams D. Toxic shock syndrome: Clinical and laboratory features in 15 patients. *Ann Intern Med* 1981; 94: 149.
10. Huntley A, Tanabe J. Toxic shock syndrome as a complication of dermatologic surgery. *J Am Acad Dermatol* 1987; 16: 227.
11. Manders S. Toxin-mediated streptococcal and staphylococcal disease. *J Am Acad Dermatol* 1998; 39: 383.
12. Elias P, Fritsch P, Epstein E. Staphylococcal scalded skin syndrome: Clinical features, pathogenesis, and recent microbiological and biochemical developments. *Arch Dermatol* 1977; 113: 207.
13. Cone L, Woodard D, Byrd R, Schulz K, Kopp S, Schlievert P. A recalcitrant, erythematous desquamating disorder associated with toxin-producing staphylococci in patients with HIV disease. *J Infect Dis* 1992; 165: 638.
14. Hurwitz R, Ackerman A. Cutaneous pathology of the toxic shock syndrome. *Am J Dermatopathol* 7: 563.
15. Schlievert P. Use of intravenous immunoglobulin in the treatment of staphylococcal and streptococcal toxic shock syndromes and related illnesses. *J Allergy Clin Immunol* 2001; 108: S107.

29
Meningococcemia and Purpura Fulminans

Meningococcemia

- Synonyms: Waterhouse-Friderichsen syndrome (with purpura fulminans and adrenal hemorrhage)
- Etiology: Invasive infection with *Neisseria meningitidis*
- Associations: Inherited or acquired deficiencies of complement or immunoglobulin in some cases
- Clinical: Upper respiratory tract symptoms, then fever, myalgias, arthralgias; cutaneous involvement—macules, papules, petechiae, palpable purpura; purpuric necrotic patches of purpura fulminans
- Histology: Skin biopsy with mixed lymphocyte and neutrophil infiltrate, ±vasculitis, organism may be found by Gram's stain
- Evaluation: Blood cultures, CBC with differential, platelets, PT/PTT, other coagulation parameters, Gram's stain of smears from purpuric lesions
- Treatment: Intravenous antibiotics—penicillin G or third generation cephalosporin, fluid and inotropic support; ±activated protein C infusion or bactericidal permeability increasing protein for severe sepsis
- Prognosis: Good if treated early, but guarded with signs of sepsis or purpura fulminans

Purpura Fulminans

- Synonyms: Symmetrical peripheral gangrene
- Etiology: Diffuse intravascular coagulation
- Associations: Inherited protein C or S deficiency, postinfectious, bacteremic sepsis
- Clinical: Widespread purpura with necrosis, skin and other organ systems
- Evaluation: PT/PTT, protein C and S, antithrombin III, CBC with differential, platelets, fibrinogen, fibrin degradation products
- Treatment: Reversal of underlying process
- Prognosis: High incidence of long-term deformity related to necrosis and amputations, high mortality in that associated with sepsis.

Meningococcemia is an invasive bacterial infection by the gram-negative diplococcus, *Neisseria meningitidis*, which is often rapidly fatal if not detected and treated early. *Neisseria meningitidis* infections occur both endemically and epidemically. Sporadic disease occurs more commonly during winter and early spring months, and affects predominantly children. The highest rate of infection is in infants six months to one year, with a steady decline in infection rate with age. This is likely explained by passive maternal immunity providing protection in the first six months, and gradual onset of acquired immunity with age. Approximately two-thirds of invasive meningococcal disease occurs in children (1). The human bacterial reservoir is the upper respiratory tract. In the general population, the carrier state is quite common, but in only rare cases do carriers develop invasive disease. There are many different serotypes of *Neisseria meningitidis*, but types A, B, C, W-135, and Y account for nearly all invasive disease. Worldwide, type A is responsible for most large epidemics, but in the United States, serotypes B and C account for approximately 90% of invasive infections. Most people exposed to an infected individual will become colonized in the upper respiratory tract. There is an approximately 5% chance of invasive infection developing in household contacts in the first 60 days after exposure. Most of these occur in the first week (2). Thus, treatment of close contacts of those with invasive infection is warranted.

The carrier state for *Neisseria meningitidis* is common, but invasive infection occurs in few individuals. The organism is able to survive in a carrier state by a number of different mechanisms. It may adhere to epithelial cells by pili and may produce IgA proteases—factors that inhibit ciliary activity. The bacterial polysaccharide capsule assists in adherence and inhibits phagocytosis (3). Invasive disease may be precipitated by antecedent viral infections, inhalation of dry, dusty air, or passive smoke inhalation, all factors that may disrupt the integrity of mucosal epithelium (3). Immunologic response to meningococcal disease utilizes all three components of the complement pathway, the classical pathway, the alternative pathway, and the mannose-binding lectin pathway. Patients with inherited defects of the terminal components of complement C6-C8 (4,5), properdin (6), and genetic variants of mannose-binding lectin (7) are susceptible to Neisserial infections, including fulminant or chronic meningococcemia. Acquired deficiencies of complement as may occur in chronic liver disease, systemic lupus erythematosus, and multiple myeloma also predispose to invasive meningococcal infection (4,8). In one series of patients presenting with a first episode of meningococcemia, 30% had either inherited or acquired deficiencies of complement (4). In addition to complement deficiencies, deficiencies of immunoglobulin IgG, IgG subclass 2, and IgA have been described in patients with meningococcal infections (9,10).

The clinical manifestations of meningococcal infection are varied. Tracheobronchitis, conjunctivitis, genital tract infection, pneumonia, and meningitis may all occur, with or without septicemia. Bacteremia may be occult. Acute meningococcemia usually begins with upper respiratory tract symptoms, progressing to fever, chills, myalgias, arthralgias, headache, and nausea and vomiting. Meningococcal meningitis usually presents without distinctive clinical features. It may closely resemble viral meningitis. Bacteremia is not necessarily present.

Cutaneous findings in meningococcemia are not consistently present. In one series of adult patients, 50% had no cutaneous findings or clinical evidence of meningitis (1). When present, skin findings are not specific. They may include a morbilliform eruption, urticarial papules and plaques, petechiae, or purpuric patches (Figure 29.1). Morbilliform eruptions, papules and urticarial plaques may occur early in the disease, and then purpura subsequently develops. Small purpuric necrotic papules and vesicles may occur in any anatomic site. These usually represent septic or immune complex vasculitis. Broad areas of purpura and necrosis are more likely to be manifestations of purpura fulminans, an ominous presentation

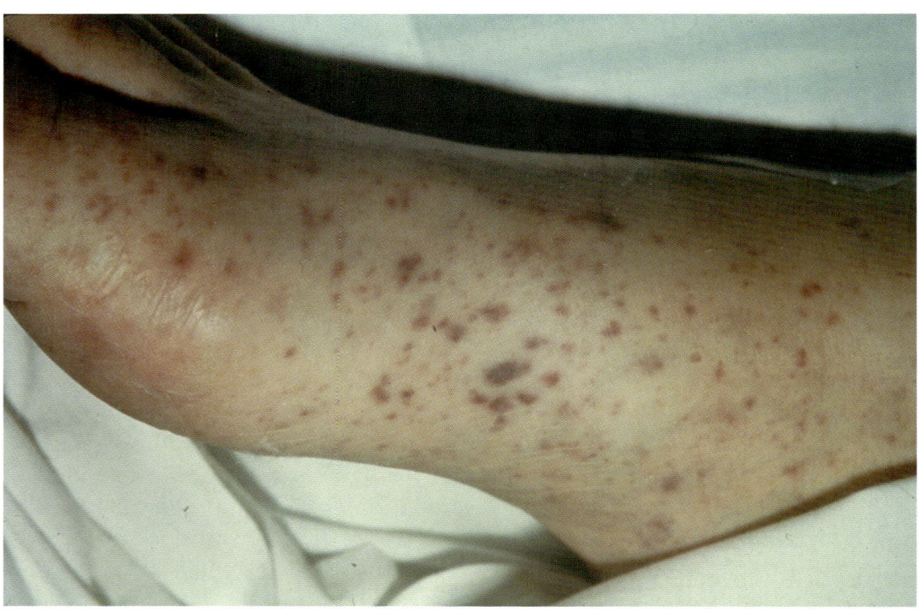

FIGURE 29.1. Meningococcemia: purpuric papules of the leg extremities.

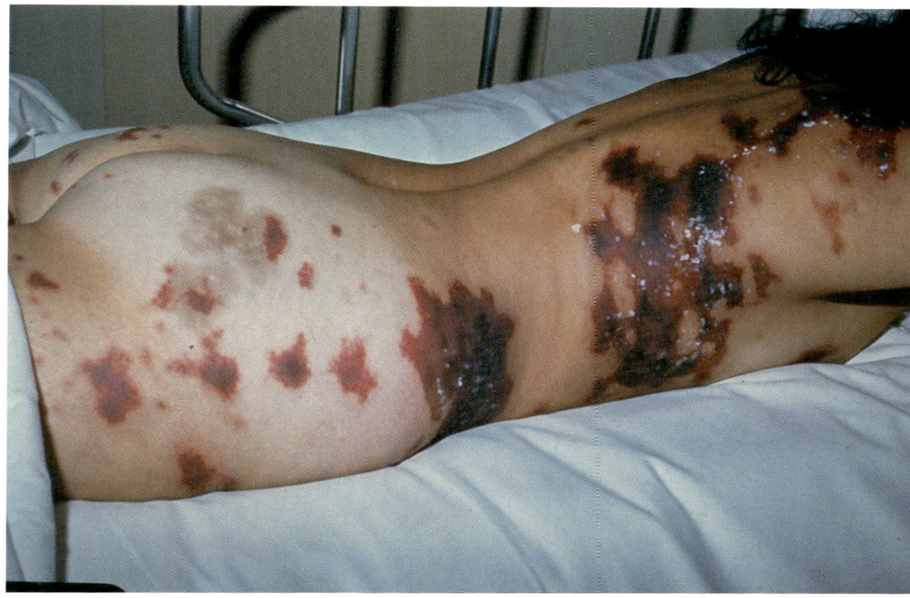

FIGURE 29.2. Purpura fulminans: extensive purpuric necrotic patches.

of sepsis-associated disseminated intravascular coagulation (Figure 29.2). Such cases may be rapidly fatal, and in the setting of adrenal hemorrhage are referred to as Waterhouse-Friderichsen syndrome. Early literature mistook manifestations of sepsis for adrenal insufficiency due to adrenal hemorrhage. Most patients with this syndrome have elevations in cortisol (2).

In the child presenting with fever and a purpuric eruption, one must be vigilant for the possibility of meningococcemia. However, in a series of such patients, bacterial sepsis comprises about 12% of the total, and of those, meningococcemia accounts for approximately two-thirds (2). Most children with fever and purpura have viral infections, particularly enterovirus. Enterovirus may cause aseptic meningitis, resulting in a clinical presentation similar to that of meningococcemia. The differential diagnosis also includes infection with parvovirus B19, Epstein-Barr virus, cytomegalovirus, as well as endocarditis, gonococcemia, typhus, drug eruption, and other forms of systemic vasculitis such as Henoch-Schönlein purpura.

A chronic form of meningococcemia also occurs, and generally presents with a less fulminant course and variable skin findings. These include macules, papules, erythema-nodosum-like lesions, or palpable purpura due to small vessel neutrophilic vasculitis. However, cutaneous involvement is not a constant feature of the disease, particularly in adults. Other manifestations include fever, malaise, myalgias, and arthralgias. Symptoms may persist for weeks prior to diagnosis. Chronic meningococcemia may occur in immunocompetent individuals or those with HIV infection or deficiencies of complement or immunoglobulin (11,12).

The diagnosis of meningococcal infection is made from isolation of the organism from usually sterile sites such as blood or cerebrospinal fluid. Surface cultures, especially those from oropharynx, are not useful because of high rates of carriage in the general population. Blood drawn from puncture wounds of purpuric lesions is reported to have a high yield for organisms by Gram's stain (13). The organism may be found in Gram's stains of biopsy specimens of skin lesions or even on the peripheral blood smear (14). Rapid serologic tests are available to detect *Neisseria meningitidis* capsular polysaccharide antigen. These may be particularly useful for CSF or if treatment has been instituted.

Fulminant sepsis may develop rapidly in meningococcemia. Endotoxin is a critical component of host immune activation, and its levels correlate with the severity of disease. Serotype C frequently has fulminant manifestations, probably because it has the highest production of endotoxin of any of the serotypes. In the circulation, CD14 on the surface of monocytes and endothelial cells is the principal receptor for endotoxin. The interaction causes production of pro-inflammatory cytokines such as TNF-α and IL-1β, which are important inflammatory mediators in sepsis (3). Neutrophils are activated via endotoxin and complement to produce proteases that result in tissue damage.

Complications of meningococcal sepsis may include septic arthritis, pericarditis, and endocarditis. One particularly deadly complication of meningococcemia is purpura fulminans, which occurs in 15%–25% of patients with meningococcemia (15). Patients develop a severe form of disseminated intravascular coagulation, clinically manifested by purpuric patches with extensive cutaneous necrosis, accompanied by high mortality rates. Purpura fulminans is not specific to meningococcemia, and occurs in several clinical settings.

Purpura Fulminans

Purpura fulminans (PF) occurs in three different clinical settings: neonatal homozygous protein C or S deficiency, after infection, and with bacterial sepsis. Homozygous protein C or S deficiency causes spontaneous intravascular coagulation in the neonatal period, clinically presenting as PF. Postinfectious PF usually occurs 7 to 10 days after an infectious trigger. Possible triggers include varicella, scarlet fever, viral exanthem, or even hypersensitivity reactions. This form is usually less severe than other forms, with disease more frequently limited to the skin. At least some cases seem to be mediated by autoantibodies induced against protein S (16). The third type of PF occurs in the setting of sepsis with endotoxin-producing bacteria. The majority of these cases are due to meningococcemia, but some occur in association with infection by *Streptococcus pneumoniae,* group A or B *Streptococcus,* and *Haemophilus influenzae,* among others. PF has also been induced by septicemia with *Capnocytophaga canimorsus* (DF-2), a complication of a dog bite (17). Hypercoagulable states such as Factor V Leiden mutation may predispose to some sepsis-induced PF (18).

Purpura fulminans likely represents a phenotype with multiple causes. A consumptive coagulopathy causes disseminated intravascular coagulation. In sepsis, circulating bacterial endotoxin and complement attack sequence disrupt endothelium, resulting in release of tissue factor. Tissue factor binds to coagulation factor VII, and the complex causes activation of factors V, X, VIII, and IX, with consequent formation of thrombin and other procoagulant proteins. Protein C is a vitamin K-dependent glycoprotein that circulates in plasma in an inactive form. In a prothrombotic state, thrombin forms a complex with endothelial membrane-bound thrombomodulin. Circulating inactive protein C binds to that complex and to membrane-bound endothelial protein C receptor, resulting in activated protein C. Once it is activated, it acts with its cofactor protein S to inactivate activated factors V and VIII, thus exerting an anticoagulant effect.

A dysfunctional protein C activation system likely contributes to PF in meningococcal sepsis. In meningococcal sepsis with PF, activated protein C in plasma is undetectable in most patients, and infusions of unactivated protein C concentrate do not increase activated protein C levels. Additionally, thrombomodulin and endothelial protein C receptor expression are reduced, theoretically leaving less available for use in protein C activation. The result of this imbalance in coagulation homeostasis is a thrombotic state (19).

The classical clinical presentation of purpura fulminans is acute onset of painful purpuric papules, plaques, and patches with a rim of erythema. Necrosis quickly ensues, sometimes with formation of vesicles and bullae, and subsequent eschar. Distal extremities are most commonly affected. Proximal involvement also occurs, but is more common in the postinfectious variant (15). Similar involvement of internal organ systems occurs. A consumptive coagulopathy develops in PF, which helps distinguish it from heparin and coumadin necrosis, thrombotic thrombocytopenic purpura, cryoglobulinemia, and thrombotic states associated with antiphospholipid antibody. Laboratory evaluation reveals reduced fibrinogen, platelets, factor V and VIII, protein C, S, and antithrombin III levels. There is a prolongation of PT and PTT, and an elevation in fibrin degradation products such as D-dimers. Histopathologic evaluation reveals thrombi of vessels, with fibrin, platelets, leukocytes, and, in the case of meningococcemia, sometimes gram-negative diplococci (Figures 29.3 and 29.4). In cases of PF associated with bacterial sepsis, a neutrophilic vasculitis may accompany the thrombi, distinguishing it from noninfectious causes (15).

The treatment of purpura fulminans is aimed at reversing the underlying cause, but may also include a variety of measures to counter the hypercoagulable state. Early surgical consultation is advised. Patients should be monitored for compartment syndrome, particularly if aggressive fluid resuscitation is implemented. "Compartments" are fascially delineated anatomic regions susceptible to ischemic necrosis in the setting of edema and low blood flow. Urgent fasciotomy may be necessary if compartment syndrome develops (20). Postinfectious PF may be induced by autoantibodies to protein S. These patients may benefit from plasmapheresis or intravenous immunoglobulin in addition to other therapies (16). Treatment for sepsis-induced purpura fulminans is discussed below.

Treatment in suspected cases of meningococcemia should be instituted immediately after cultures are obtained, because prognosis is dependent upon early intervention. Generally, intravenous treatment with a third-generation cephalosporin is given until cultures and susceptibilities allow narrowing the coverage. Fluid and inotropic support are given as needed. In patients who develop purpura fulminans, extensive cutaneous involve-

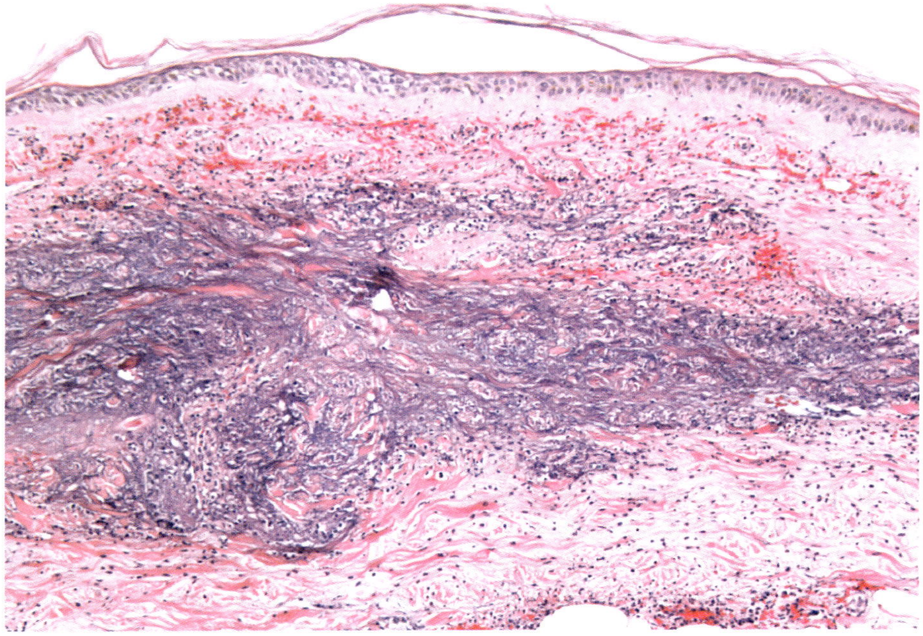

FIGURE 29.3. Meningococcemia: septic vasculitis with neutrophils, necrosis, and hemorrhage.

ment portends a poor prognosis. Beneficial effects in severe sepsis have been seen with infusions of activated protein C, and also bactericidal permeability increasing protein (which binds endotoxin, preventing the pro-inflammatory cascades), both in randomized controlled trials (21,22). In case reports, additional therapeutic measures reported to be of benefit include anti-endotoxin antibody, systemic steroids, anti-TNF-α antibody, anti-IL-1-β antibody, unactivated protein C infusion, fresh frozen plasma, antithrombin III, heparin, tissue plasminogen activator, plasmapheresis, and extracorporeal membrane oxygenation (3). Anticoagulation agents may be

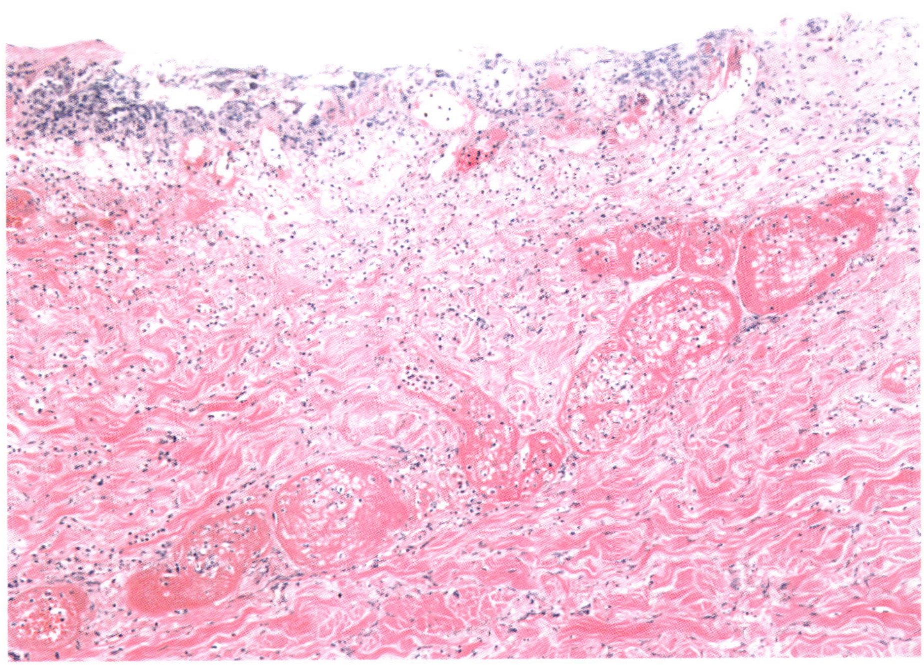

FIGURE 29.4. Purpura fulminans: prominent intravascular coagulation with occasional neutrophils and superficial necrosis.

associated with bleeding complications, so if used, it should be with great caution.

Poor prognostic features in meningococcemia include petechiae present for less than 12 hours prior to admission, hypotension (systolic blood pressure <70 mm Hg), absence of meningitis, peripheral WBC count <10,000, erythrocyte sedimentation rate <10 mm/hr, difference between rectal and skin temperature >3°C, and parental opinion that child's condition has deteriorated in the previous hour (23,24). The mortality rate is 8%–10% (2). Long-term complications usually result from ischemia during acute infection, and consist of amputations and abnormal bone growth. In those patients surviving the acute infection, evaluation for complement and immunoglobulin deficiency should be performed to determine if ongoing replacement therapy is needed.

Household and other close contacts should be treated prophylactically because of the potential for epidemic spread of invasive meningococcal disease. Meningococcal vaccine consists of tetravalent purified capsular polysaccharide with groups A, C, Y, and W-135. Group B is excluded because of its poor immunogenicity. Vaccine is routinely used in the military because of the potential for epidemics, and should be given to those with asplenia and complement deficiencies, both acquired and inherited.

References

1. Stephens DS, Hajjeh RA, Baughman WS, Harvey RC, Wenger JD, Farley MM. Sporadic meningococcal disease in adults: Results of a 5-year population-based study. *Ann Intern Med* 1995; 123: 937–940.
2. Salzman MB, Rubin LG. Meningococcemia. *Infect Dis Clin N Am* 1996; 10: 709–725.
3. Pathan N, Faust SN, Levin M. Pathophysiology of meningococcal meningitis and septicaemia. *Arch Dis Child* 2003; 88: 601–607.
4. Ellison RT, Kohler PF, Curd JG, Judson FN, Reller LB. Prevalence of congenital or acquired complement deficiency in patients with sporadic meningococcal disease. *N Engl J Med* 1983; 308: 913–916.
5. Adams EM, Hustead S, Rubin P, Wagner R, Gewurz A, Graziano FM. Absence of the seventh component of complement in a patient with chronic meningococcemia presenting as vasculitis. *Ann Intern Med* 1983; 99: 35–38.
6. Denson P, Weiler JM, Griffiss JM, Hoffmann LG. Familial properdin deficiency and fatal meningococcemia. *N Engl J Med* 1987; 316: 922–926.
7. Hibberd ML, Sumiya M, Summerfield JA, et al. Association of variants of the gene for mannose-binding lectin with susceptibility to meningococcal disease. Meningococcal Research Group. *Lancet* 1999; 353: 1049–1053.
8. Ellison RT, Mason SR, Kohler PF, Curd JG, Reller B. Meningococcemia and acquired complement deficiency: Association in patients with hepatic failure. *Arch Intern Med* 1986; 146: 1539–1540.
9. Bass J, Nuss R, Mehta KA, Morganelli P, Bennett L. Recurrent meningococcemia associated with IgG2-subclass deficiency. *N Engl J Med* 1983; 309: 430.
10. Castagliuolo PP, Nisini R, Quinti I, Fattorossi A, D'Amelio R. Immunoglobulin deficiencies and meningococcal disease. *Ann Allergy* 1986; 57: 68–70.
11. Ploysangam T, Sheth AP. Chronic meningococcemia in childhood: Case report and review of the literature. *Pediatr Dermatol* 1996; 13: 483–487.
12. Assier H, Chosidow O, Rekacewicz I, et al. Chronic meningococcemia in acquired immunodeficiency infection. *J Am Acad Dermatol* 1993; 29: 793–794.
13. McClean S, Caffey J. Endemic purpuric meningococcus bacteremia in early life: The diagnostic value of smears from the purpuric lesions. *Am J Dis Child* 1931; 42: 1053–1074.
14. Young EJ, Cardella TA. Meningococcemia diagnosed by peripheral blood smear. *JAMA* 1988; 260: 992.
15. Darmstadt GL. Acute infectious purpura fulminans: Pathogenesis and medical management. *Pediatr Dermatol* 1998; 15: 169–183.
16. Levin M, Eley BS, Louis J, Cohen H, Young L, Heyderman RS. Postinfectious purpura fulminans caused by an autoantibody directed against protein S. *J Pediatr* 1995; 127: 355–363.
17. Kullberg BJ, Westendorf RGJ, van't Wout JW, Meinders AE. Purpura fulminans and symmetrical gangrene caused by *Capnocytophaga canimorsus* (formerly DF-2) septicemia—a complication of dog bite. *Medicine* 1991; 70: 287–292.
18. Jackson RT, Luplow RE. Adult purpura fulminans and digital necrosis associated with sepsis and the Factor V mutation. *JAMA* 1998; 280: 1829.
19. Faust SN, Levin M, Harrison OB, et al. Dysfunction of endothelial protein C activation in severe meningococcal sepsis. *N Engl J Med* 2001; 345: 408–416.
20. Warner PM, Kagan RJ, Yakuboff KP, et al. Current management of purpura fulminans: A multicenter study. *J Burn Care Rehabil* 2003; 24: 119–126.
21. Levin M, Quint PA, Goldstein B, et al. Recombinant bactericidal/permeability-increasing protein (rBPi21) as adjunctive treatment for children with severe meningococcal sepsis: A randomised trial. rBPi21 Meningococcal Sepsis Study Group. *Lancet* 2000; 356: 961–967.
22. Bernard GR, Vincent JL, Laterre PF, et al. Efficacy and safety of recombinant human activated protein C for severe sepsis. *N Engl J Med* 2001; 344: 699–709.
23. Stiehm ER, Damrosch DS. Factors in the prognosis of meningococcal infection. *J Pediatr* 1966; 68: 457–467.
24. Sinclair JF, Skeoch CH, Hallworth D. Prognosis of meningococcal septicemia. *Lancet* 1987; 350: 38.

Part IV
Inborn Errors of Metabolism and Autoimmune Disease

30
Lethal Hereditary Vascular Disorders: Osler-Weber-Rendu, Ataxia-Telangiectasia, and Fabry's Disease

■ Synonyms:	OWR—Hereditary hemorrhagic telangiectasia AT—Louis-Bar syndrome FD—Anderson-Fabry disease, angiokeratoma corporis diffusum
■ Etiology:	OWR—AD, Chromosome 9 and 12-defect in endoglin or activin receptor-like kinase AT—AR, 11q22.3 phosphatidylinositol-3-kinase p53 checkpoint regulation FD—XL, Xq22.1, alpha-galactosidase A
■ Associations:	OWR—Arteriovenous malformations of the brain, lungs; hepatic fibrovascular tumors AT—B-cell non-Hodgkin's lymphoma, T-cell CLL, breast cancer, growth retardation FD—None
■ Clinical:	OWR—Mucocutaneous telangiectasias, epistaxis, hemoptysis, clubbing, cyanosis AT—Oculocutaneous telangiectasias, skin photoaging, cerebellar ataxia FD—Cutaneous nonblanching angiectases, neuropathic pain, cardiomyopathy, renal failure
■ Pathology:	OWR—Mucosal and dermal telangiectasias AT—Dermal elastosis, telangiectasias, pulmonary bronchiectasis, CNS demyelination FD—Mucosal and dermal telangiectasias and angiokeratomas, interstitial lipid deposits
■ Staging:	N/A
■ Prognosis:	OWR—Good in the absence of pulmonary or CNS malformation or abscess AT—Invariably fatal, usually early adulthood secondary to infection or lymphoma/leukemia FD—Poor without renal transplantation, better recent outcome with enzyme replacement
■ Complications:	OWR—Arteriovenous malformations and abscesses of CNS and lungs AT—Bronchiectasis, cerebellar ataxia, T-cell leukemia and B-cell lymphoma FD—Cardiomyopathy, cerebrovascular accident, renal failure
■ Treatment:	OWR—Supportive measures AT—Supportive measures FD—Alpha-galactosidase A gene therapy shows promise

Mucocutaneous vascular ectasia, otherwise referred to as telangiectasia, can be an important harbinger of serious systemic disease. Among a variety of acquired conditions, including hepatic cirrhosis that are responsible for their development, are a heterogeneous group of inherited conditions that entail the development of multiple cutaneous and mucous membrane vascular lesions associated with other life-threatening complications. This chapter deals with the clinical and pathologic features of three such conditions, namely Osler-Weber-Rendu syndrome, ataxia-telangiectasia, and Fabry's disease.

Osler-Weber-Rendu (OWR) syndrome synonymously referred to as hereditary hemorrhagic telangiectasia, was first described by Dr. William Osler in 1907 (1). He described many of the attributes of this distinctive disorder known today, including the characteristic triad of the superficial cutaneous vessels that undergo irreversible dilatation forming *telangiectasis*, bloody nasal discharge (*epistaxis*), and its familial tendency (2). The disorder affects all races, although it has been described with a higher incidence in the Dutch Antilles and parts of France. It is known to be an inherited or spontaneously acquired autosomal dominant trait. The overall incidence of the disorder is about 1 in 100,00 persons. The defect involves segments of chromosomes 9 and 12, which encodes for two important endothelial transmembrane receptors, termed endoglin and activin receptor-like kinase 1, respectively. The latter protein is the receptor for transforming growth factor beta, an important modulator of tissue repair and angiogenesis that when defective is thought to lead to defects in endothelial cell junctions and weakness of the supporting perivascular connective tissue resulting in telangiectasis and *arteriovenous malformation*. The disease typically manifests in early to mid-adulthood with the development of epistaxis. Other common presenting signs include mucosal and cutaneous telangiectasis, and other signs of bleeding diathesis including melena and hemoptysis. The telangiectasias consist of discrete red puncta, spider-like branching, and/or linear vascular lesions located in particular on the face, fingers, and oral and nasal mucous membranes (3) (Figure 30.1). Less common findings include headaches stemming from complications associated with cerebral arteriovenous malformation, cyanosis and/or clubbing associated with pulmonary arteriovenous malformation, signs and symptoms of high output cardiac failure produced from pulmonary vascular shunting, fatigue from blood loss and anemia, visual disturbances following intraocular hemorrhage, and fever associated with abscesses following bacterial seeding of the pulmonary or cerebral vascular anomalies (4). Important complications to consider include gastrointestinal and pulmonary bleeding, often necessitating transfusion, cerebrovascular accident, and infectious complications stemming from the vascular anomalies. The overall mortality is approximately 10% with patients generally succumbing to one of the aforementioned complications. Although estrogen has been reported in the past as producing some measure of therapeutic improvement, current recommendations include supportive measures including prompt recognition and cessation of bleeding (5).

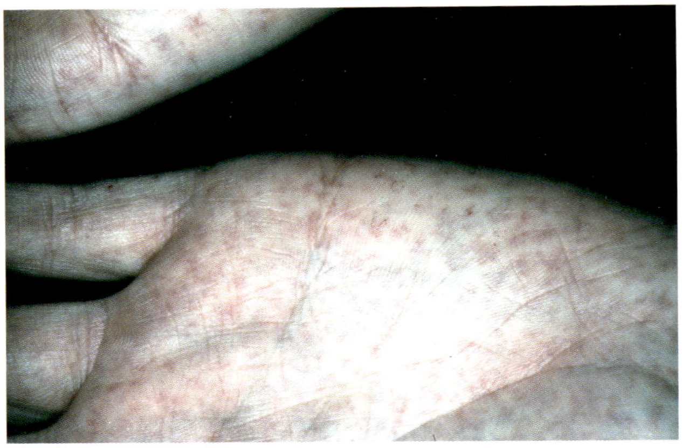

FIGURE 30.1. Diffuse palmar telangiectasis in Osler-Weber-Rendu syndrome.

Ataxia-telangiectasia (AT), or *Louis-Bar syndrome*, was first described by Syllaba and Henner in 1926 and later by the Belgian neuropathologist Dr. Denise Louis Bar in 1941, who detailed the progressive nature of the cerebellar ataxia and distinctive cutaneous telangiectasis of the disorder (6). Its final designation of ataxia-telangiectasia would come in 1957 with the discovery of its association with immunologic defects and the predisposition of afflicted patients to develop recurrent sinopulmonary infections. Today, we know this autosomal recessively inherited disease to involve the 11q22–23 gene that encodes for the ATM protein (7). This protein is an important regulatory phosphoprotein involved with p53-regulated cell cycling and DNA maintenance. Defective ATM function results in increased unregulated DNA synthesis and defective DNA strands predisposed to instability and a hypersensitivity to ionizing radiation. These defects are thus thought to predispose to neoplastic transformation and the increased risk these patients possess for solid organ and lymphoreticular malignancy as well as impact upon T-lymphocyte receptor function leading to immunologic dysfunction and a predisposition toward certain types of infection (8,9). The mechanisms that underlie the cerebellar ataxia, growth retardation, and mucocutaneous telangiectasis are not known but have been hypothesized to involve accelerated telomere loss. The disease affects all races and regions of the world and has an estimated incidence of 1 in 100,000 individuals (10). The disease is generally heralded by the development of ataxia in the first years of life. The ataxia commences with abnormal head movements and progresses to involve the gait and abnormal arm movements including tremor and myoclonus, later. Other neurologic findings include choreoathetosis, mask-like facies, and saccadic eye deviation with absent optokinetic nystagmus. The pathogenesis involves *spinocerebellar degeneration* with demyelination. The mucocutaneous telangiectasias develop by the age of 5 years and in particular involve the conjunctival angles and adjacent periocular skin (Figure 30.2). Accelerated aging (*progeric changes*) including graying of the hair, facial skin atrophy, seborrheic dermatitis, and mottled pigmentation are also common. Other cutaneous findings include café au lait macules, vitiligo, hypertrichosis, acanthosis nigricans, keratosis pilaris, actinic keratosis, and the presence of nonmelanoma skin cancer. The other major impairment associated with AT is immunologic dysfunction with increased sinopulmonary and ear infections associated with thymic hypoplasia, defective cell-mediated immunity, and reduced serum IgA and IgE immunoglobulin levels. Less prominent features of the disease include mental retardation, atherosclerotic heart disease, diabetes mellitus, and growth impairment. Pathology of the brain shows degeneration of the cerebellar Purkinje and granular cells and spinal column anterior horn and spinal tract degeneration and demyelination. The cutaneous findings include epidermal atrophy with solar elastosis and capillary telangiectasis. Less common findings include the presence of dermal non-caseating granulomas, pigmentary incontinence, and superimposed changes of seborrheic dermatitis or keratosis pilaris. The dermal granulomas consist of epithelioid granulomas that may masquerade as sarcoidosis. Cases of ulcerating or perforating granulomatous dermatitis and palisaded granulomatous dermatitis have been described as well (11). Actinic keratosis, basal cell and squamous cell carcinoma may be seen in young patients and as such may suggest the possibility of this disorder. Important complications primarily involve neoplastic and infectious diseases. AT patients have an estimated 100-fold increase in the incidence of malignancy, particularly Hodgkin's and non-Hodgkin's lymphoma, leukemia, and gastric and breast adenocarcinoma (9,10). An important complication of recurrent pulmonary infection is bronchiectasis. AT is invariably fatal with few afflicted individuals living beyond their third decade. The major causes of mortality include pulmonary infection and malignancy. Treatment consists of the aggressive management of infectious disease with antibiotics and prevention with prophylactic administration of immunoglobulins and vaccination. Sunscreens and sun avoidance are important with respect to the cutaneous complications. Increased awareness of oncologic disease with appropriate screening is recommended. Physical, speech, and occupational therapies should be instituted and genetic counseling for the patient and family is encouraged.

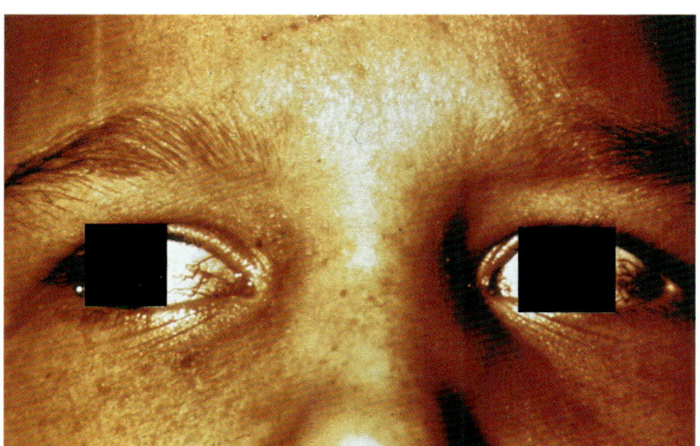

FIGURE 30.2. Conjunctival telangiectasis in ataxia-telangiectasia.

Fabry's disease, otherwise referred to as Anderson-Fabry disease or angiokeratoma corporis diffusum, was independently described by Drs. Anderson and Fabry in 1898 (12,13). The disease is inherited as an *X-linked trait* and involves a defect in glycosphingolipid metabolism caused by a deficiency of *alpha-galactosidase A*. Over 160 mostly missense-type mutations have been identified within encoding gene segments for alpha-galactosidase (14). Although males are predominantly afflicted, females may rarely present with milder forms of the disease. The disease is worldwide in distribution and although it afflicts all races, whites are overrepresented. The estimated incidence is 1 in 40,000 individuals. The etiology involves the accumulation of glycosphingolipid substrate following lack of enzymatic activity in the tissues of the principal organs involved with the disease (15). As the gene is located on Xq22, males are more severely afflicted, possessing very low to absent galactosidase levels. Carrier females and females with incomplete lyonization of the abnormal X-chromosome allele may develop milder disease stigmata. The disorder has been rarely reported in individuals with normal measured enzyme activity (16). The most important glycosphingolipids that accumulate due to the enzymatic defect are globotriaosylceramide and galabiosylceramide. These compounds accumulate primarily within the lysosomes and cytosol of endothelial, pericyte, and smooth muscle cells of the skin, renal, and neurovascular organs. The pathologic alterations stem from endothelial accumulation and disruption with consequent ischemic and degenerative changes. Symptoms are generally ushered in by the development of limb neuropathic pain and cutaneous vascular anomalies in late adolescence or early adulthood. The limb pain is usually exacerbated by exposure to cold and is typically described as burning in quality. The cutaneous changes consist of the development of myriad punctate red-to-blue nonblanching angiectasias particularly situated in the "bathing-suit" area of the lower abdomen and perineum (Figure 30.3) (15). The nonblanching quality of the lesions is an important contrast with telangiectasia, which typically blanches with external pressure or diascopy. Similar vascular lesions can be found on the oral mucosa. Other attendant cutaneous findings include lymphedema and hypohidrosis. Important additional systemic signs include various lens opacities that are pathognomonic for the disorder. Distinctive corneal opacities referred to as *cornea verticillata* are also commonly seen. The cutaneous and ocular findings are overshadowed by the serious systemic complications of visceral organ involvement. The kidneys are severely affected and renal failure is common by the fourth decade. Important signs of renal disease include increasing proteinuria and the demonstration of characteristic birefringent lipid globules with a "Maltese cross" pattern in the urinary sediment. The heart is particularly prone to complications stemming from the accumulation of lipids within the vessel walls and myocardium resulting in ischemic complications as well as left ventricular hypertrophy. Congestive heart failure and myocardial infarction are important causes of morbidity and mortality. Additional organs involved include the brain, where cerebrovascular accident is a common complication, and the gastrointestinal tract, where intestinal ischemia may be observed. The pathologic changes involve the progressive dilatation of capillaries and post-capillary venules within the dermis (Figure 30.4). Over time, the abutment adjacent to the epithelium produces epidermal hyperplasia

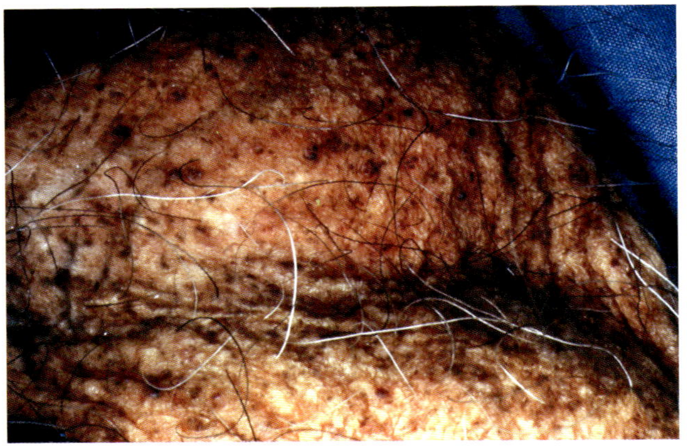

FIGURE 30.3. Diffusely scattered telangiectatic papules on scrotum of patient with angiokeratoma corporis diffusum.

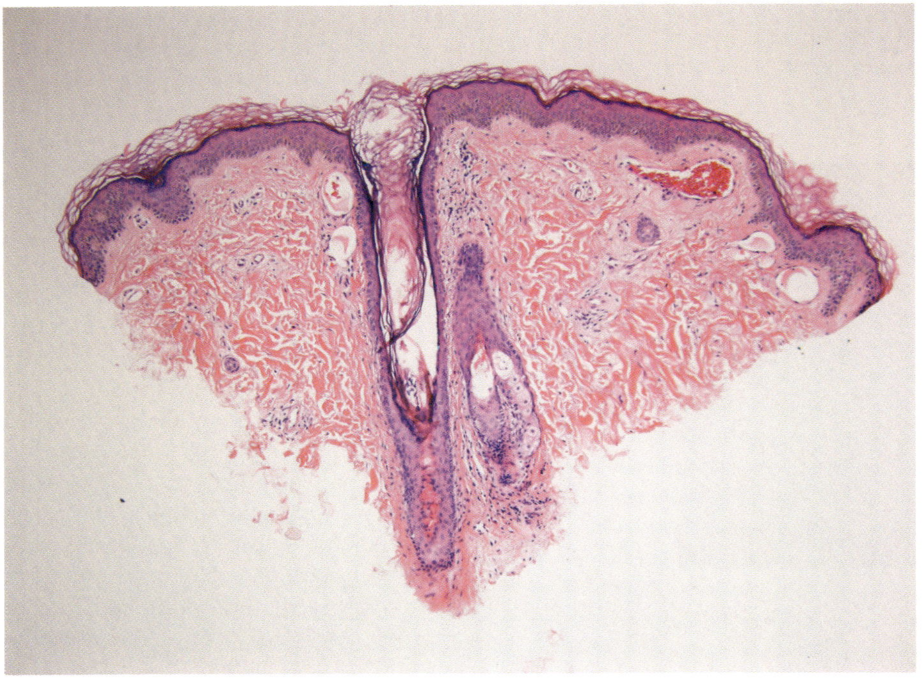

FIGURE 30.4. Low power photomicrograph depicting superficial dermal capillary telangiectasis in Osler-Weber-Rendu syndrome.

and angiokeratoma formation. Systemic pathologic changes additionally include vascular ectasia, accelerated atherosclerosis, and degenerative changes ascribed to ischemic alteration. The heart shows increased interstitial fibrous and lipid deposits. Glomerular and renal tubular deposits are seen in the kidney. Characteristic lysosomal organelle lamellar inclusions are observed ultrastructurally. The diagnosis can be confirmed by direct enzymatic assay of serum, leukocytes, or cultured fibroblasts, or by DNA analysis of the gene. A presumptive diagnosis can be rendered upon careful assessment of the ophthalmologic findings, the widespread nature of the angiokeratomas, and/or the urinary sediment findings. Important entities to consider in the differential diagnosis are other inherited enzyme deficiency syndromes with similar clinical stigmata. These disorders include L-fucosidase and neuraminidase deficiency, among other rarer entities (16–17). Important clues that suggest the latter entities include disseminated angiokeratomas in a female patient and psychomotor and cognitive impairment. The long-term prognosis of patients is determined by renal function status. Renal transplantation has dramatically improved the outcome of patients as transplanted kidneys generally possess normal enzyme activity. Important morbidities, including neuropathic pain and cerebrovascular and cardiovascular disease, are treated symptomatically with pain and anti-seizure medications, aggressive blood pressure control, and smoking cessation. Recent advances in recombinant gene therapy will likely revolutionize the treatment and long-term outlook of these patients. Recent clinical trials with the recombinant enzyme Fabrazyme (Genzyme Corporation Cambridge, MA) have shown great promise (14).

References

OWR

1. Osler W. On multiple hereditary telangiectasis with recurrent ring hemorrhages. *Q J Med* 1907; 1: 53.
2. Perry W. The clinical spectrum of hereditary hemorrhagic telangiectasias (Osler-Weber-Rendu). *Am J Med 1987*; 5: 989.
3. Chandler D. Pulmonary and cerebral arteriovenous fistula with Osler's disease. *Arch Intern Med* 1965; 116: 277.
4. Swanson D, Dahl M. Embolic abscesses in hereditary hemorrhagic telangiectasia. *J Am Acad Dermatol* 1991; 24: 580.
5. Vase P. Estrogen treatment of hereditary hemorrhagic telangiectasia: A double blind controlled clinical trial. *Acta Med Scand* 1981; 209: 393.

AT

6. Smith L, Conerly S. Ataxia-telangiectasia or Louis-Bar syndrome. *J Am Acad Dermatol* 1985; 12: 686.
7. Li A, Swift M. Mutations at the ataxia-telangiectasia locus and clinical phenotypes of A-T patients. *Am J Med Genet* 2000; 92: 170.
8. Khanna K. Cancer risk and the ATM gene: A continuing debate. *J Natl Cancer Inst* 2000; 92: 795.
9. Swift M, Morrell D, Massey R, et al. Incidence of cancer in 161 families affected by ataxia-telangiectasia. *N Engl J Med* 1991; 325: 1831.
10. Peterson R, Funkhouser J. Speculations on ataxia-telangiectasia: Defective regulation of the immunoglobulin gene superfamily. *Immunol Today* 1989; 10: 313.
11. Drolet B, Drolet B, Zvulunov A, et al. Cutaneous granulomas as a presenting sign in ataxia-telangiectasia. *Dermatology* 1997; 194: 273.

FD

12. Anderson W. A case of angiokeratoma. *Br J Dermatol* 1898; 10: 113.
13. Fabry J. Ein Beitrag Zur Kenntis der Purpura haemorrhagica nodularis. *Arch Dermatol Syphilol* 1898; 43: 187.
14. Eng C, Guffon N, Wilcox W, et al. Safety and efficacy of recombinant human alpha-galactosidase A replacement therapy in Fabry's disease. *N Engl J Med* 2001; 345: 9.
15. Wallace H. Anderson-Fabry disease. *Br J Dermatol* 1973; 88: 1.
16. Holmes R, Fenson A, McKee P, et al. Angiokeratoma corporis diffusum in a patient with normal enzyme activities. *J Am Acad Dermatol* 1984; 10: 384.
17. Epinette W, Norins A, Drew A, et al. Angiokeratoma corporis diffusum with a L-fucosidase deficiency. *Arch Dermatol* 1973; 107: 754.

31
Eruptive Xanthoma

■ Synonym:	Diabetic xanthoma, xanthoma diabetacorum
■ Etiology:	Serum hypertriglyceridemia and/or elevated VLDL
■ Associations:	Diabetes mellitus, oral estrogens, acute ethanol ingestion, lipoprotein lipase deficiency, Type IV/V hyperlipoproteinemia, pregnancy, nephrotic syndrome, hypothyroidism, intravenous miconazole, oral 13-*cis*-retinoic acid
■ Clinical:	Crops of red-yellow papules on buttocks and thighs
■ Histology:	Normal epithelium, early-perivascular lipid and neutrophils, later perivascular histiocytes and foam cells seen
■ IHC repertoire:	N/A
■ Staging:	None
■ Prognosis:	5% mortality
■ Adverse variables:	Acute pancreatitis, serum triglycerides >2000 mg/dL
■ Treatment:	Dietary modification, weight loss

Eruptive xanthoma (EX) is a serious systemic dyslipidemia with distinctive cutaneous features. Although the dermatologic manifestations are not in themselves serious, their presence may be the harbinger of serious visceral disease. EX is an uncommon disease with a near equal gender incidence, principally seen in two age groups with different predisposing factors. Among children and young adults genetic disturbances in lipid metabolism are largely responsible and include *lipoprotein lipase deficiency* and Type I and V hyperlipoproteinemia (1). In older adults, acute ethanol ingestion and endocrinologic disturbances including hypothyroidism and diabetes mellitus are often observed. Common to these clinical settings is the presence of serum hypertriglyceridemia and/or elevated very low-density lipoproteins (VLDL) (2). Triglycerides are transported in the serum as a composite, known as a chylomicron, consisting of lipid with the apolipoproteins B-48, C-II, C-III, E, A-I, and A-IV. The apolipoproteins are critical in the metabolism of the chylomicrons. Chylomicrons are synthesized in the intestine and circulate in the serum, passing off triglycerides to the peripheral tissue endothelial capillaries via the enzymatic action of lipoprotein lipase and the binding of apolipoprotein C-II. Chylomicron remnants return to the liver via apolipoprotein E receptors for metabolic breakdown. VLDL particles originate within the liver, contain relatively more cholesterol than triglyceride, yet perform a similar function, delivering triglycerides to the peripheral tissues and returning to the liver for breakdown. These lipids are usually markedly elevated in the serum as a directly inherited consequence of faulty lipid metabolism such as lipoprotein lipase or *apolipoprotein C-II deficiency* or as an indirect mechanism following heavy ethanol consumption (3). As the liver is critical to the metabolism of lipoproteins, ethanol and various medications including miconazole and retinoic acid that are similarly metabolized within or are affected by the status of the liver may result in lipid abnormalities (4,5). Similarly, serious endocrinologic disturbances, such as hypothyroidism or diabetes mellitus, or intrinsic liver disorders, such as the condition of fatty liver of pregnancy, may affect the metabolism of liver lipoprotein synthesis (6). Combined elevation of chylomicrons and VLDL constitutes Type 5 hyperlipoproteinemia, the most common hereditary-mediated cause of EX (7). This disorder is aggravated by secondary acquired factors such as obesity, which is known to be associated with elevated VLDL levels and insulin resistance. Insulin resistance and diabetes mellitus are also associated with defective lipolysis of chylomicrons and VLDL (8,9). The pathogenesis of the skin lesions and associated visceral findings relate to the presence of intravascular lipid as well as the escape of lipids from the circulation, evoked inflammation, and resulting foam cell formation. Marked elevation in intravascular lipids may induce platelet clumping and vascular plugging as observed in the retinal artery, and the complications of *lipemia retinalis,* capable of inducing blindness. Extravascular lipids may incite acute inflammation that, in conjunction with the lipid itself, produces free radical and oxidant-mediated cell membrane destruction. These mechanisms underlie the formation of the typical cutaneous lesions and the development of the most important systemic complication of *acute pancreatitis.* The risk for acute pancreatitis rises precipitously when triglyceride levels exceed 2000 mg/dL. In time, through a less-well understood mechanism, the extravascular lipid is scavenged by histiocytes forming foam cells.

EX presents as 1- to 4-mm reddish-yellow papules on the buttocks or extensor surfaces of the thighs and arms (Figure 31.1) (3). The lesions may be surrounded by an erythematous halo and usually occur in crops that may coalesce, forming plaques. Their presence is indicative of a triglyceride level that typically exceeds 2000 mg/dL. Other clinical stigmata of EX include ocular, abdominal, and pulmonary findings. The most important ophthalmic complication is lipemia retinalis. On fundoscopic examination, the retinal arteries and veins appear white and engorged. The risk of lipemia retinalis increases when serum triglyceride levels exceed 4000 mg/dL. Abdominal pain is a common accompaniment to EX. The source of the pain may be due to acute pancreatitis or hepatosplenomegaly. Chest pain or dyspnea may also occur due to decreased pulmonary oxygen diffusing capacity that may be aggravated by abnormal hemoglobin oxygen affinity. The natural history of the cutaneous lesions is gradual resolution with successful treatment within 6 to 8 weeks of instituting therapy.

The histologic changes of EX are often subtle, particularly in early lesions (10). The changes principally involve the dermal capillaries and perivascular tissue and consist of initial accumulations of neutrophils that in time are replaced by lymphocytes and histiocytes, including foam cells (Figures 31.2–31.4). Extravascular lipid or fibrin may be identified as a granular precipitate seen within the vicinity of the blood vessels.

The prognosis of EX is generally favorable with prompt recognition and institution of therapy (2,3). Delayed diagnosis, marked elevation of serum triglycerides, or acute pancreatitis is associated with a worse prognosis. In its initial setting, acute pancreatitis constitutes the most important cause of mortality with an overall rate of 5%. Important complications additionally include lipemia retinalis and hepatosplenomegaly.

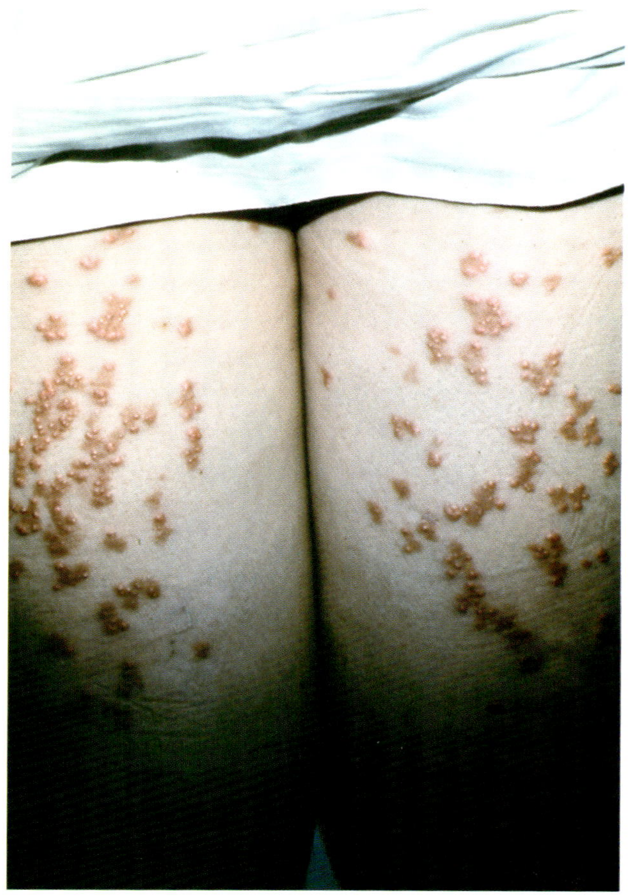

FIGURE 31.1. Orange-yellow grouped papules on buttocks of patient with eruptive xanthoma.

Therapy should be aimed at measures that reduce serum levels of triglyceride and/or VLDL and that palliate complications of EX or its disease associations such as diabetes mellitus, obesity, or ethanolism (2,3). Long-term dietary fat restriction, weight loss, and appropriate glucose-lowering measures aimed at maintaining serum triglyceride levels below 1500 mg/dL should be instituted.

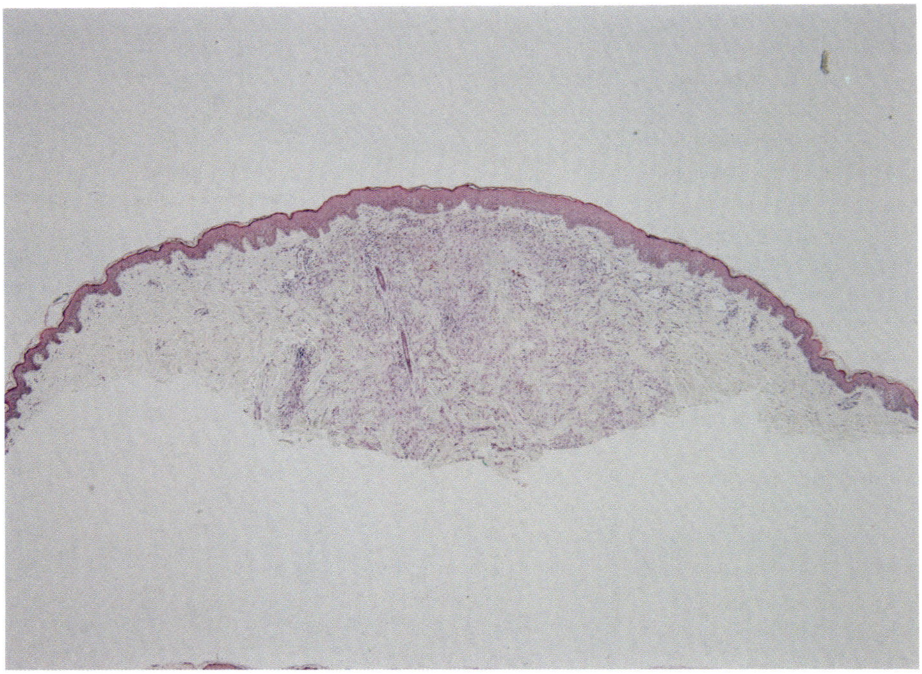

Figure 31.2. Dome-shaped papule with dermal inflammatory infiltrate.

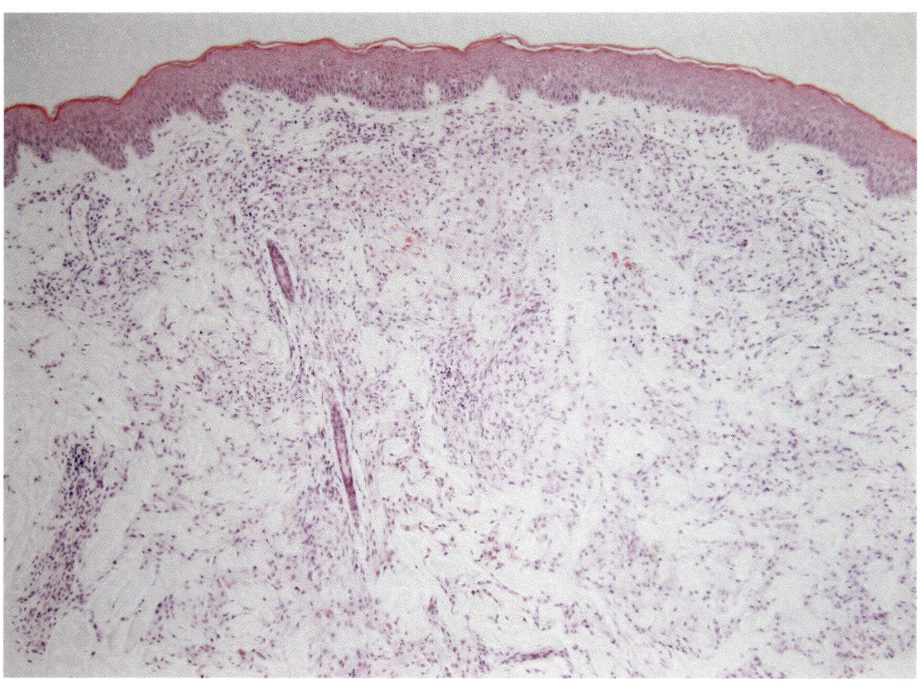

Figure 31.3. Medium power photomicrograph depicting perivascular and interstitial inflammatory infiltrate.

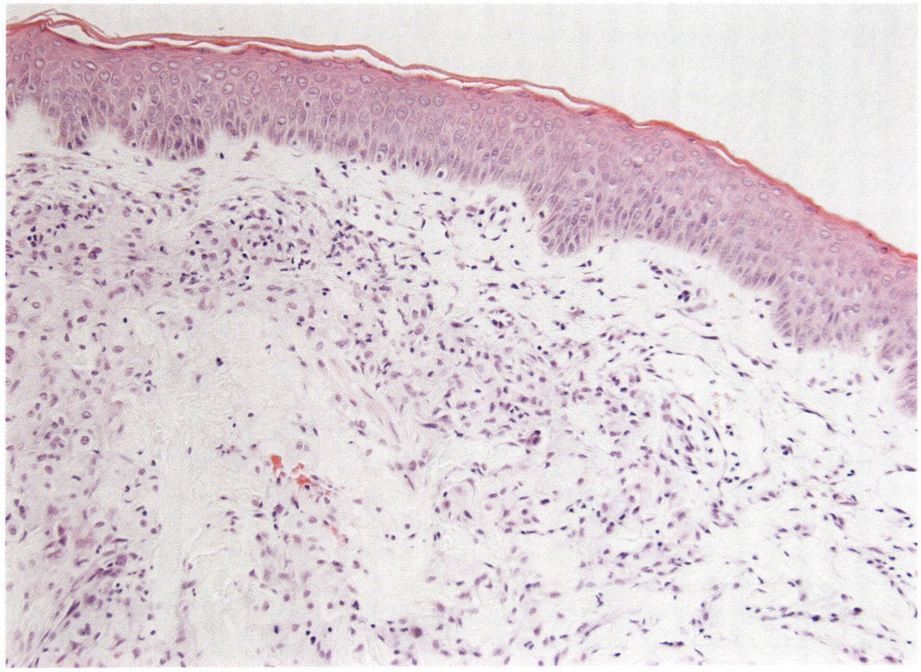

Figure 31.4. High power detail with perivascular foamy histiocytes and neutrophils.

References

1. Parker F. Xanthomas and hyperlipidemias. *J Am Acad Dermatol* 1985; 13: 1.
2. Parker F. The hyperlipidemias. In BH Thiers, RL Dobson (eds.), *Pathogenesis of Skin Diseases*. New York: Churchill Livingstone, 1986, 358–362.
3. Maher-Wiese V, Marmer E, Grant-Kels J. Xanthomas and the inherited hyperlipoproteinemias in children and adolescents. *Pediatr Dermatol* 1990; 7: 166.
4. Barr R, Fujita W, Graham J. Eruptive xanthomas associated with intravenous miconazole. *Arch Dermatol* 1978; 114: 1544.
5. Dicken C, Connolly S. Eruptive xanthomas associated with isotretinoin. *Arch Dermatol* 1980; 116: 951.
6. Jaber P, Wilson B, Johns D, et al. Eruptive xanthomas during pregnancy. *J Am Acad Dermatol* 1992; 27: 300.
7. Archer C, MacDonald D. Eruptive xanthomata in Type V hyperlipoproteinemia associated with diabetes mellitus. *Clin Exp Dermatol* 1984; 9: 312.
8. Brunzell J, Bierman E. Chylomicronemia syndrome. *Med Clin North Am* 1982; 66: 455.
9. Vermeer B, Van Gent C, Goslings B, et al. Xanthomatosis and other clinical findings with elevated levels of very low density lipoproteins. *Br J Dermatol* 1979; 100: 657.
10. Cooper P. Eruptive xanthoma: A microscopic simulant of granuloma annulare. *J Cutan Pathol* 1986; 13: 207.

32
Graft-versus-Host Disease

■ Synonyms:	Autologous graft vs. host disease, graft-vs-host reaction, cutaneous eruption of lymphocyte recovery syndrome
■ Etiology:	Cytotoxic T-cells attack antigens on keratinocytes
■ Associations:	Bone marrow transplantation
■ Clinical:	Erythematous patches, and papules progressing in some cases to bullae; associated with fevers, diarrhea, elevated liver function tests
■ Histology:	Dying keratinocytes within epidermis, mild perivascular and interface lymphocytic infiltrate
■ IHC repertoire:	Not usually necessary; CD8+ lymphocyte predominate
■ Staging:	Based upon degree of involvement in the gastrointestinal tract, liver, and skin
■ Prognosis:	Correlated with histologic grade of lesions and overall clinical stage; in general, poor
■ Adverse variables:	Histologic subtype of high-grade GVHD
■ Treatment:	Increased corticosteroids

GVHD is a common consequence of allogeneic bone marrow transplantation. Approximately 3 weeks following complete marrow eradication and the transplantation of allogeneic donor marrow cells, a cutaneous eruption is seen in up to 20% to 80% of patients, and may result in the death of the patient (1,2). The cutaneous manifestations may be the first indication of evolving GVHD.

GVHD is arbitrarily divided into acute and chronic forms. The acute form of the disease ordinarily occurs between 21 and 60 days following bone marrow transplantation. Patients develop maculopapular or scarlatiniform eruptions (Figure 32.1). In the more severe forms of the disease, bullae may develop and progress to widespread desquamation in a toxic epidermal necrolysis-like pattern. The palms and soles are often involved early in the disease, while the trunk, neck, cheeks, and ears are commonly affected as the disease progresses (Figure 32.2).

The chronic form of the disease occurs more than 100 days following bone marrow transplantation. The histologic features consist of a band-like lymphocytic infiltrate similar to lichen planus in the early chronic phase. Well developed lesions of chronic GVHD show epidermal atrophy with a thickened basement membrane and dermal fibrosis simulating morpheal scleroderma.

GVHD, or a virtually identical process, has been reported in patients receiving autologous blood transfusions (3). The process is much milder and does not ordinarily lead to adverse consequences, but suggests that even the host's own lymphocytes are capable of causing disease in these immunocompromised patients. The responsible cell is an immunocompetent T cell derived from the bone marrow, be it autologous or allogeneic (4).

The cutaneous eruption of lymphocyte recovery is a similar process that occurs in patients who have not received a transfusion of blood products. This eruption occurs during the time of bone marrow reconstitution, in patients who have had marrow ablative therapy. Again, several weeks following chemotherapy and radiation therapy, patients develop fevers and a cutaneous eruption indistinguishable from that seen in GVHD. The eruption coincides directly with an increasing lymphocyte count and abates as the marrow fully recovers (5).

The histologic features of each of these entities are similar and differ only in degree. There is a well-recognized grading scheme for evaluating histologic changes of GVHD in the skin (Table 32.1).

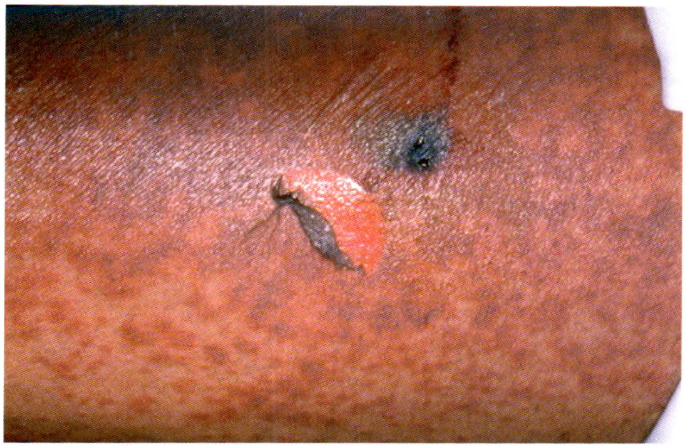

FIGURE 32.1. Acute graft-versus-host disease with erythematous macular rash and blister formation.

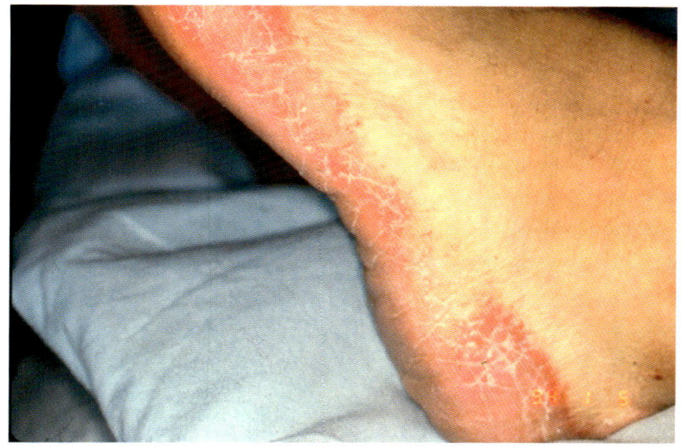

FIGURE 32.2. Acral erythematous plaques seen in acute graft-versus-host disease.

In all cases, a mild infiltrate of lymphocytes is present surrounding the vessels of the superficial vascular plexus. Scattered lymphocytes are present within the lower levels of the epidermis, and in grades II–IV, these lymphocytes are present around dying keratinocytes (Figures 32.3 and 32.4).

The histologic differential diagnosis includes an erythema multiforme-like drug eruption and a viral exanthem.

A rigorous staging classification has been developed for acute GVHD (7). Higher-stage disease is associated with increased risk for transplant-related mortality (8).

TABLE 32.1. Histologic Grading Scheme for GVHD

Histologic Grade	Histologic Features
I	Basal vacuolization, mild lymphocytic infiltrate with exocytosis—nondiagnostic
II	Basal vacuolization, dyskeratotic keratinocytes, mild lymphocytic infiltrate with exocytosis and satellitosis
III	Focal clefting at dermal epidermal junction due to basal keratinocyte necrosis; mild lymphocytic infiltrate with satellitosis
IV	Epidermis completely separated from dermis, mild lymphocytic infiltrate with exocytosis and satellitosis

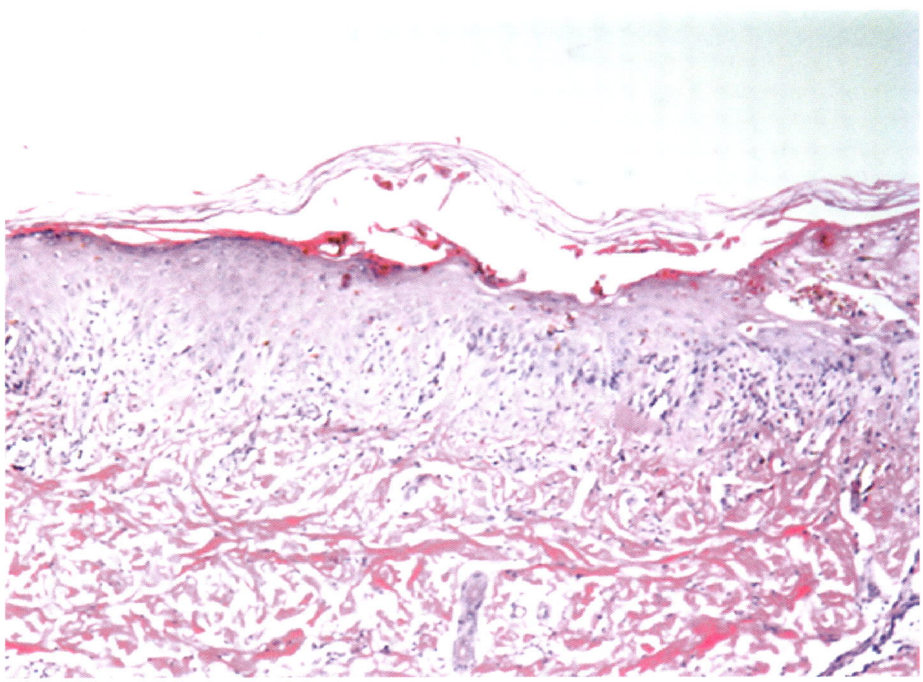

FIGURE 32.3. Medium power detail of subacute interface dermatitis with epidermal necrolysis.

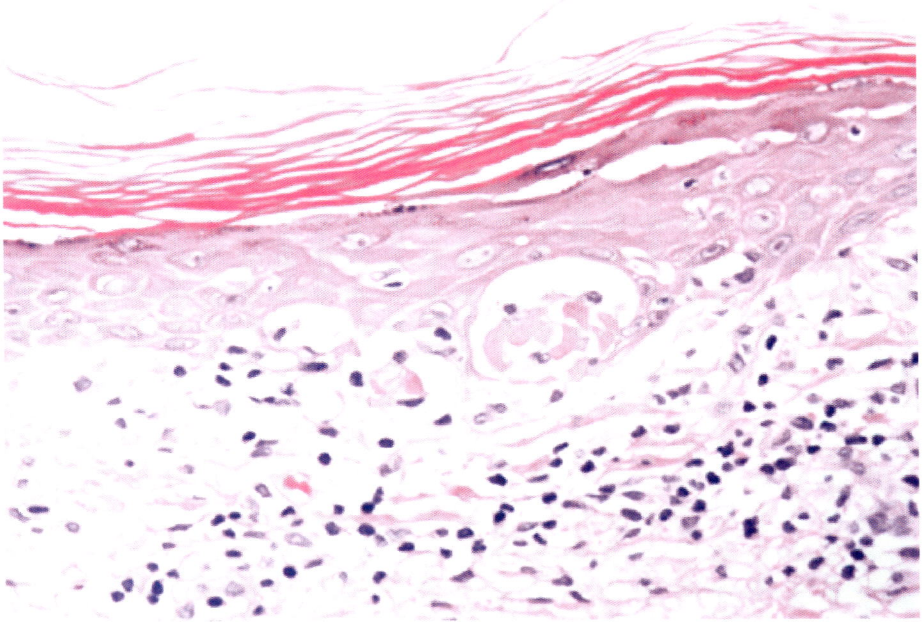

FIGURE 32.4. High power detail showing clusters of necrotic keratinocytes with adjacent lymphocytes (satellitosis) typical of acute graft-versus-host disease.

Patients who develop GVHD have been shown to have a lower risk for relapse of their primary neoplastic disease.

References

1. Thomas ED, Storb R, Clift RA, Fefer A, Johnson FL, Neiman PE, Lerner KG, Glucksberg H, Buckner CD. Bone marrow transplantation. *N Eng J Med* 1975; 292: 832–843, 895–902.
2. Deeg HJ, Storb R. Graft-versus-host disease: Pathophysiological and clinical aspects. *Ann Rev Med* 1984; 35: 11–24.
3. Anderson KC, Weinstein HJ. Transfusion-associated graft-vs.-host disease. *N Eng J Med* 1990; 323: 315–321.
4. Billingham RE. The biology of graft-versus-host reactions. *Harvey Lect* 1966–67; 62: 21–78.
5. Bauer DJ, Hood AF, Horn TD. Histologic comparison of autologous graft-vs.-host reaction and cutaneous eruption of lymphocyte recovery. *Arch Dermatol* 1993; 129: 855–858.
7. Zhou Y, Barnett MJ, Rivers JK. Clinical significance of skin biopsies in the diagnosis and management of graft-vs.-host disease in early postallogeneic bone marrow transplantation. *Arch Dermatol* 2000; 136: 717–721.
8. Storb R, Prentice RL, Buckner CD, Clift RA, Appelbaum F, Deeg J, Doney K, Hansen JA, Mason M, Sanders JE, Singer J, Sullivan KM, Witherspoon RP, Thomas ED. Graft-versus-host disease and survival in patients with aplastic anemia treated by marrow grafts from HLA-identical siblings: Beneficial effect of a protective environment. *N Eng J Med* 1983; 308: 302–307.

33
Paraneoplastic Pemphigus and Pemphigus Vulgaris

■ Synonyms:	None
■ Etiology:	Circulating antibodies (IgG) against keratinocyte cell surface peptides desmogleins (PV/PP), also envoplakin, periplakin, and desmoplakin in PP
■ Associations:	PV—Myasthenia gravis, thymoma, penicillamine, and captopril PP—Non-Hodgkin's lymphoma, chronic lymphocytic leukemia, Castleman's disease
■ Clinical:	Both variants show flaccid blisters with erosions and oral ulceration, PP associated with variable features including targetoid- and lichenoid-appearing lesions with tendency toward severe oral ulceration
■ Histology:	Intraepidermal acantholysis with bullae formation, PP may show a lichenoid/interface dermatitis or rarely, subepidermal bullae; both show intraepidermal IgG and C3 on immunofluorescence
■ IHC repertoire:	Not applicable
■ Staging:	None
■ Prognosis:	Overall: PV—5-year ~90% survival, PP—5-year ~50%
■ Adverse variables:	PV—Delay in diagnosis, advanced age, high-dose corticosteroids, associated infection PP—Non-Hodgkin's lymphoma and chronic lymphocytic leukemia
■ Treatment:	PV—Corticosteroids, cyclophosphamide, mycophenolate mofetil, plasmapheresis, IVIG PP—Problematic, treat underlying malignancy and corticosteroids

The disease pemphigus encompasses a group of related blistering conditions characterized by circulating antibodies against keratinocyte cell surface antigens important in mediating cell-to-cell adhesion (1,2). Of the various types and forms of the disease including pemphigus foliaceus, pemphigus erythematosus, IgA pemphigus, and pemphigus vegetans, it is pemphigus vulgaris (PV) and paraneoplastic pemphigus (PP) that constitute the most important causes of mortality. Overall, these disorders are quite rare, with an estimated prevalence of between 1 in 100,000 for PV to less than 1 in 1,000,000 for PP. Both disorders are seen principally in aged adults with a near equal gender distribution. PV is more commonly observed among Jews and individuals of Mediterranean descent, whereas there is no known ethnic predilection for PP.

The etiology of both disorders involves circulating IgG antibody against specific adhesion molecules present on the cell surface of keratinocytes that mediate cell-to-cell adhesion and are localized to the desmosome apparatus (3,4). These antigens are transmembrane glycoproteins and include the desmogleins pathogenically important in PV and the plakins that are important in pathogenesis of PP. Antibodies directed against these peptides disrupt cell-to-cell adhesion or desmosome assembly, resulting in acantholysis and blister formation. Despite a similarly evoked mechanism of blister formation, it is thought that

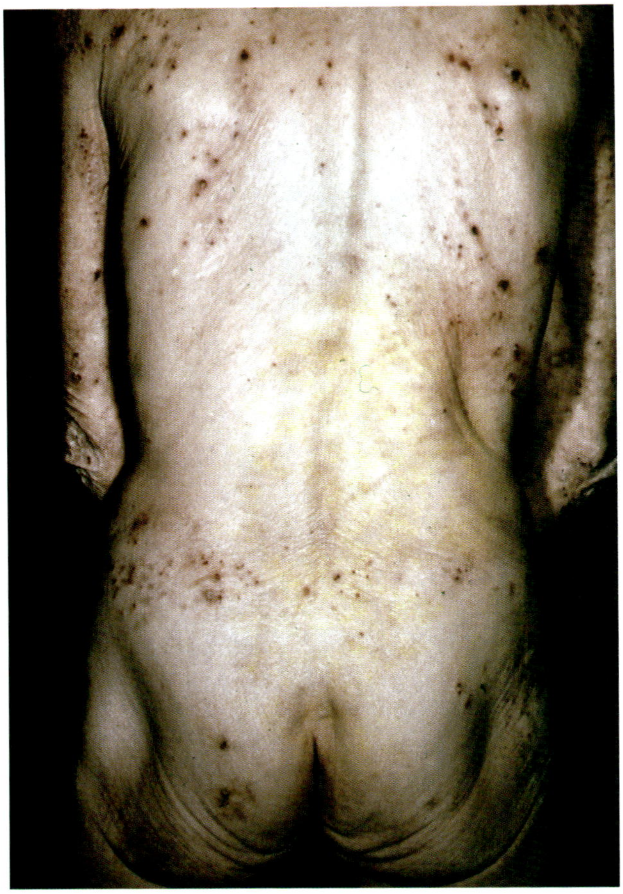

FIGURE 33.1. Widespread superficial ulcers in an elderly man with pemphigus vulgaris

the pathogenesis of antibody induction is different among these disorders. Patients with PV have a markedly increased frequency of certain class II major histocompatibility complex antigens including HLA-DR4 that predispose to antibody induction against desmogleins. In contrast, antibody induction in patients with PP is thought to involve tumor antigen cross-reactivity to normal cell surface constituents and dysregulated immune modulation mediated by host and tumor cytokine production (5). There are distinct disease associations with these disorders as well. PV is associated with myasthenia gravis, as well as the administration of certain medications including penicillamine and captopril (6). PP is invariably associated with the lymphoproliferative disorders, most commonly non-Hodgkin's lymphoma, followed by chronic lymphocytic leukemia, Castleman's disease, and Waldenstrom's macroglobulinemia. Interestingly, both disorders are associated with thymoma. There is no association between PP and the more common solid organ malignancies such as beast, lung, colorectal, or prostate adenocarcinoma.

The clinical manifestations of PV consist of flaccid blisters with erosions that develop anywhere on the skin surface (7,8). The blisters may develop on normal appearing or erythematous skin (Figure 33.1). Vegetative lesions with excessive granulation tissue may be seen in the intertriginous areas. Mucous membrane involvement, most importantly of the oral cavity, is present in nearly all cases of PV and is often a heralding symptom. It may antedate the development of skin lesions for several months and often persists following skin resolution. The most common presentation is of painful shallow ulcerations most frequently involving the buccal mucosa, palate, floor of mouth, tongue, and less commonly the pharynx, larynx, conjunctiva, vagina, penis, or anus. The clinical findings in PP are more varied, although mucous membrane involvement is characteristic of the disorder (Figure 33.2). The skin lesions often occur episodically as waves of tense or flaccid blisters surmounted on an erythematous base situated on the trunk or extremities. Individually, the lesions may appear as shallow ulcerations similar to PV, tense blisters similar to bullous pemphigoid, as confluent and erosive patches similar to erythema multiforme/toxic epidermal necrolysis, or flat-topped papules similar to lichen planus (9–12). Lichenoid-appearing lesions may be observed on the palms and soles as well as the paronychial skin in established cases, constituting an important means of clinically distinguishing this disorder from PV. The most important facet of the clinical presentation is stomatitis. It is usually the earliest sign of the disorder, often persisting throughout the course of the disease, and is usually refractory to therapy. Painful erosions and ulceration is typically encountered throughout the oropharynx, although lateral tongue involvement with extension to and involvement of the vermilion border of the lips is characteristic of this disorder.

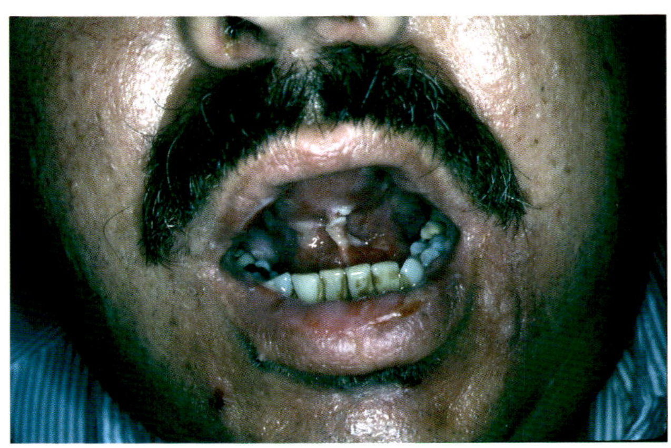

FIGURE 33.2. Severe mucositis seen in paraneoplastic pemphigus. Note involvement of the nasal mucosa.

The histopathology of PV is distinctive. Early lesions show exocytosis of neutrophils with accompanying intercellular spongiosis and focal acantholysis. Established lesions show a mixture of dermal and epidermal neutrophils and eosinophils with conspicuous epidermal acantholysis and bullae formation (Figure 33.3). The acantholyis characteristically spares the basilar layer of epithelium, imparting an appearance likened to that of "tombstones." Chronic lesions, in particular derived from intertriginous areas, are apt to show acanthosis with neutrophilic and eosinophilic abscesses. Although the histopathology of PP may be identical to that of PV, more often, considerable histologic variation capable of simulating lichenoid/interface dermatitis or bullous pemphigoid is encountered. This histologic diversity may be seen in disparate lesions biopsied synchronously or in metachronous lesions from the same individual. The lichenoid interface pattern often shows striking dyskeratosis with a tendency toward confluent basilar necrolysis (Figure 33.4). The inflammatory infiltrate of PP often shows a predominance of lymphocytes. Oral biopsies obtained from patients with both disorders show a variable degree of acantholysis with intramucosal or submucosal vesiculation. The inflammatory infiltrate characteristically shows a predominance of neutrophils. The direct immunofluorescence (DIF) findings are similar and consist of interepithelial staining with antibodies to IgG and C3 of lesional skin (13,14). DIF is more likely to be negative among patients with PP or to additionally show basement membrane staining. Distinction of these disorders can also be attained with indirect immunofluorescence involving cell extract immunoblotting or incorporating a rat bladder substrate with IgG antibodies directed toward the plakins.

The prognosis of PV is generally favorable, particularly since the advent of noncorticosteroid immunosuppressive therapy (15). Historically, corticosteroid-induced iatrogenesis, and in particular, predisposition for opportunistic infection, was the principal mechanism responsible for a 15%–25% mortality rate. Today, the 5-year mortality rate is much lower and is due to more effective steroid-reducing therapies such as cyclophosphamide, mycophenolate mofetil, and intravenous immunoglobulin. Although infection, in particular with *Staphylococcus aureus*, remains the most important risk, the mortality rate still remains close to 10%. The prognosis of younger patients with PV or those cases associated with medications, myasthenia gravis, and/or thymoma is generally more favorable. Overall, the prognosis of PP is grave with a 5-year mortality rate of 50%. More favorable outcomes are observed among patients with resectable tumors including thymoma or among patients with indolent lymphoproliferative disorders such as chronic lymphocytic leukemia. The treatment of this disorder tends to be more difficult with the oral and skin lesions often refractory to most therapies. Oral corticosteroids alone or in combination with cyclosporine will usually result in partial improvement of lesions.

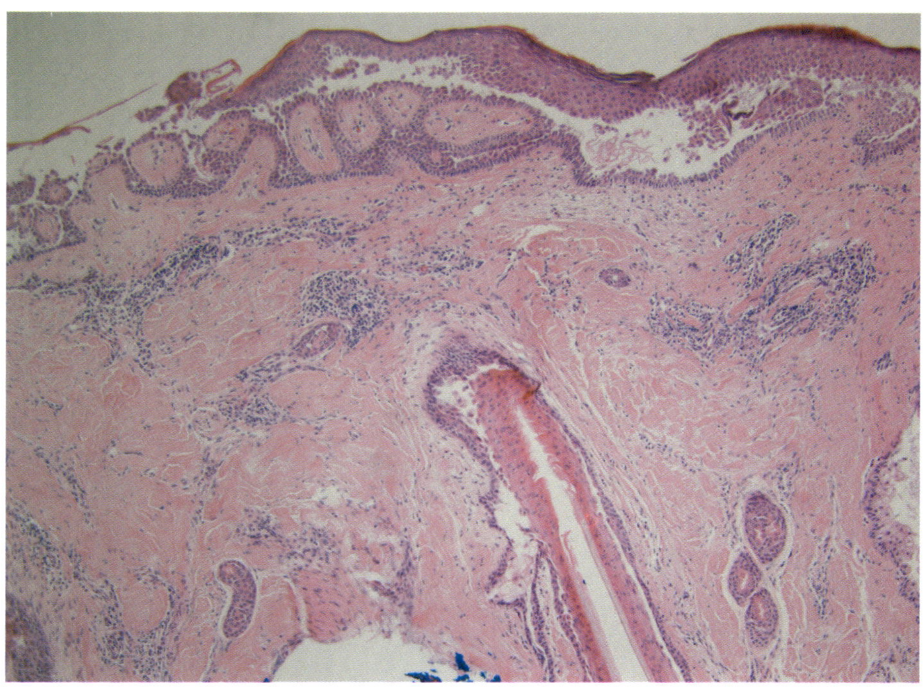

FIGURE 33.3. Low power photomicrograph depicting suprabasilar acantholysis with follicular involvement.

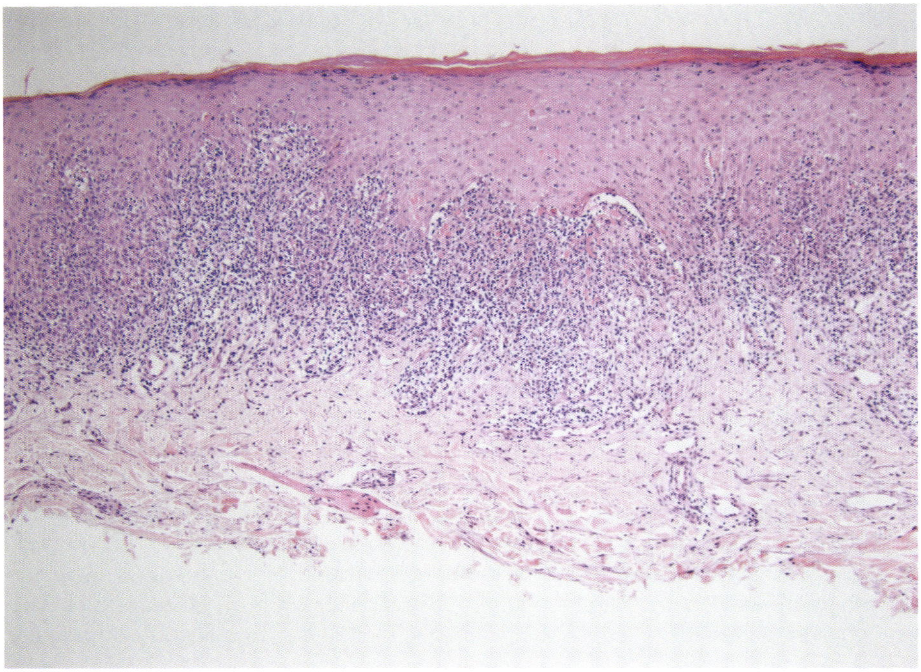

FIGURE 33.4. Dense lichenoid inflammatory infiltrate with increased necrotic keratinocytes and incipient subepidermal blister formation seen in paraneoplastic pemphigus.

References

1. Becker B, Gaspari A. Pemphigus vulgaris and vegetans. *Dermatol Clin* 1993; 11: 429.
2. Lever W. Pemphigus and pemphigoid. *J Am Acad Dermatol* 1979; 1: 2.
3. Judd K, Lever W. Correlation of antibodies in skin and serum with disease severity in pemphigus. *Arch Dermatol* 1979; 115: 428.
4. Fellner M, Fukuyama K, Moshell A, et al. Intercellular antibodies in blood and epidermis. *Br J Dermatol* 1973; 89: 115.
5. Joly P, Thomine E, Gilbert D, et al. Overlapping distribution of autoantibody specificities in paraneoplastic pemphigus and pemphigus vulgaris. *J Invest Dermatol* 1994; 103: 65.
6. Pisani M, Ruocco V. Drug-induced pemphigus. *Clin Dermatol* 1986; 4: 118.
7. Ahmed A. Clinical features of pemphigus. *Clin Dermatol* 1983; 1: 13.
8. Meurer M, Milns J, Rogers R, et al. Oral pemphigus vulgaris: A report of ten cases. *Arch Dermatol* 1977; 113: 1520.
9. Camisa C, Helm T. Paraneoplastic pemphigus is a distinct neoplasia-induced autoimmune disease. *Arch Dermatol* 1993; 129: 883.
10. Mutasim D, Pelc N, Anhalt G. Paraneoplastic pemphigus. Dermatol Clin 1993; 11: 473.
11. Fried R, Lynfield Y, Vitale P, et al. Paraneoplastic pemphigus appearing as bullous pemphigoid-like eruption after palliative radiation therapy. *J Am Acad Dermatol* 1993; 29: 815.
12. Tankel M, Tannenbaum S, Parekh S. Paraneoplastic pemphigus presenting as an unusual bullous eruption. *J Am Acad Dermatol* 1993; 29: 825.
13. Rongioletti F, Truchetet F, Rebora A. Paraneoplastic pemphigoid-pemphigus? Subepidermal bullous disease with pemphigus-like direct immunofluorescence. *Int J Dermatol* 1993; 32: 48.
14. Moy R, Jordan R. Immunopathology in pemphigus. *Clin Dermatol* 1983; 1: 72.
15. Ahmed A, May R. Death in pemphigus. *J Am Acad Dermatol* 1982; 7: 221.

34
Relapsing Polychondritis

■ Synonyms:	None
■ Etiology:	Unknown, antibodies against type II collagen are common; HLA-DR4 association
■ Associations:	Myelodysplastic syndromes, systemic vasculitis, connective tissue/autoimmune diseases
■ Clinical:	Erythematous, painful ear(s), nose, arthropathy, respiratory, ocular symptoms
■ Histology:	Frequently nonspecific, degenerative changes of cartilage with fibrosis and lymphocytic infiltrate at chondrofibrous junction
■ IF:	Immunoglobulin and C3 at chondrofibrous junction
■ Evaluation:	CBC, creatinine, urinalysis, ESR, RF, PFTs, ophthalmological evaluation, EKG, possible biopsy of involved ear
■ Treatment:	Systemic corticosteroids, nonsteroidal anti-inflammatory drugs, colchicine, methotrexate
■ Prognosis:	>55% 10-year survival

In 1923, Jaksch-Wartenhorst described a 32-year-old man with polyarthritis and fever who subsequently developed bilateral auricular and nasal chondritis. He applied the term *polychondropathia* to this entity (1). In 1960, Pearson and colleagues added four more cases, and coined the term *relapsing polychondritis*, which has become the accepted terminology for this disease (2).

Relapsing polychondritis (RP) is a systemic disease of unknown etiology, associated with the formation of antibodies to type II collagen, the type of collagen predominating in cartilage. This results in inflammation of the cartilage of the ears, nose, tracheobronchial tree, and joints (3). Involvement of inner ear and heart may be explained by evidence suggesting that type II collagen exists in those tissues (4,5). Murine models suggest that tissue-specific antibody and complement activation are both necessary for expression of the disease (6). The presence of circulating antibody to type II collagen is not specific to RP. In one investigation, these antibodies were found in 50% of RP patients, 15% of rheumatoid arthritis patients, and 4% of normal controls (7). Reactivity against different epitopes probably results in different disease manifestations. Antibodies in the sera of normal controls are specific to bovine or chick type II collagen, suggesting that they are induced by dietary exposure to antigen. These antibodies do not cross-react with human type II collagen (7). Genetic susceptibility to RP is associated with expression of HLA-DR4, but no predominant subtype is present in patients with the disease (8). Further evidence of a genetic component to RP is seen in its association with multiple autoimmune diseases.

The most common presentation of RP is auricular chondritis or arthritis. Other relatively frequent presentations include nasal chondritis, laryngotracheal symptoms, ocular inflammation, auditory or vestibular dysfunction, or cutaneous eruption. The onset of disease is usually abrupt, and most commonly is manifested as a tender, erythematous, indurated ear (Figure 34.1). Bilateral involvement is common. Acute episodes of chondritis last from days to several weeks, and resolve spontaneously. Repeated episodes result in a distorted auricular contour, with a "cauliflower ear" deformity, and a similar nasal deformity, resulting in a "saddle nose." Arthropathy is also a common presenting manifestation of RP, and is usually migratory, asymmetric, non-nodular, nonerosive, and seronegative. Joint sizes involved are variable and include parasternal articulations (9). Anemia and an elevated erythrocyte sedimentation rate may be present. Noncutaneous manifestations of RP are catalogued in Table 34.1 (10–12).

Cutaneous involvement in RP is divided into two categories: that consisting of changes overlying areas of auric-

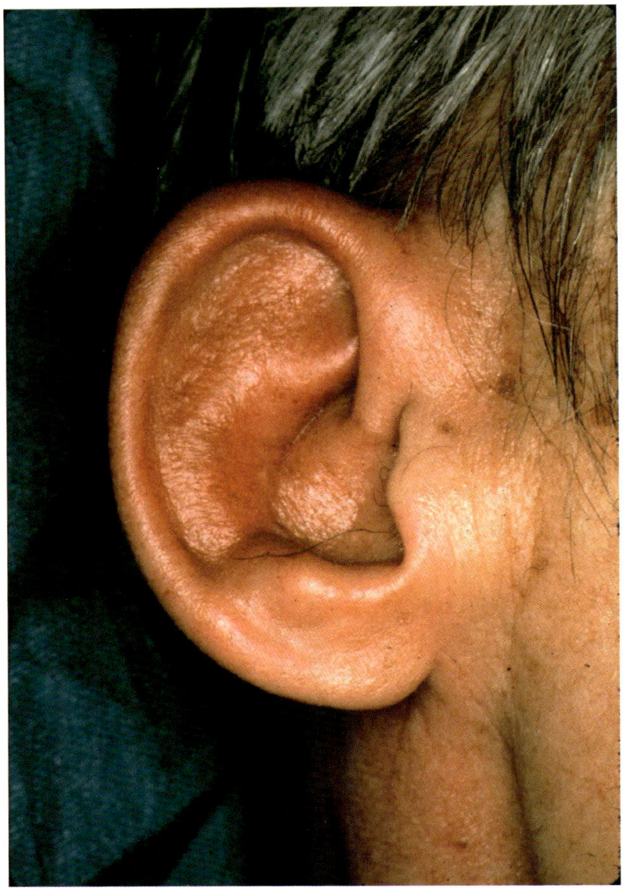

FIGURE 34.1. Erythema and induration of the ear, with sparing of the lobe.

TABLE 34.1. Clinical Features of Relapsing Polychondritis

Auricular and nasal chondritis
Laryngotracheal inflammation (throat pain, cough, hoarseness, dyspnea, stridor, wheezing, choking)
Arthritis
Ocular (episcleritis, scleritis, iritis, keratoconjunctivitis sicca, keratitis, optic neuritis, retinopathy, cataracts, proptosis, eyelid edema)
Neurologic (headaches, cranial nerve palsies, cerebellar ataxia, hemiplegia, encephalopathy, seizures)
Audiovestibular (hearing loss, tinnitus, vertigo, dizziness, nausea, vomiting)
Cardiovascular (aortic or mitral regurgitation, aortic aneurysm, myocarditis, pericarditis, silent myocardial infarction, conduction system abnormalities)
Renal (mesangial proliferation, focal and segmental necrotizing glomerulonephritis, glomerulosclerosis, IgA nephropathy, tubulointerstitial nephritis)
Constitutional (fever, malaise, weight loss)

ular or nasal chondritis, and those cutaneous manifestations not directly associated with chondritis. Typical ear and nasal involvement with cutaneous erythema and induration occurs in the majority of patients with RP at some time during the course of their disease, frequently at the outset. Other cutaneous findings attributable to RP occur in approximately 35% of patients. However, the actual percentage of patients with skin disease in RP is greater than that because of the cutaneous manifestations of co-morbidities. Cutaneous, nonchondritic presentations of RP represent approximately 10% of the total (13). The more common mucocutaneous lesions seen in a series of 200 patients with RP include oral and genital aphthosis, acral subcutaneous nodules resembling erythema nodosum, and purpura, most of which is due to small vessel neutrophilic vasculitis. A summary of cutaneous findings excluding skin changes superficial to chondritis reported in this case series is given in Table 34.2 (13).

Cutaneous lesions have not been found to correlate with disease severity, or specific organ system involvement, but occur with higher frequency in patients with coexistent disease, particularly those with myelodysplastic syndromes. Cutaneous disease activity correlates with systemic disease activity in approximately 50% of cases.

RP is a multisystem disease with a wide array of clinical manifestations, potentially delaying diagnosis. This is further complicated by its occurrence with other diseases in 25%–35% of cases (11). The most common disease associations are myelodysplastic syndromes, in approximately 10% of cases, other connective tissue and autoimmune disease, and systemic vasculitis. Disease associations with RP are summarized in Table 34.3 (10,11,13).

There is no specific diagnostic test for RP. Criteria for diagnosis as suggested by McAdam include presence of three of the following clinical features and histologic confirmation: (1) bilateral auricular chondritis, (2) non–erosive seronegative inflammatory polyarthritis, (3) nasal chondritis, (4) ocular inflammation, (5) respiratory tract chondritis, (6) audiovestibular damage (11). In an attempt to diagnose RP, biopsy specimens of areas suspected to represent chondritis are frequently taken, the ear being the most common site. Sampling of posterior auricular

TABLE 34.2. Mucocutaneous Findings in RP (in Approximate Order of Frequency)

Aphthosis, oral and genital
Acral subcutaneous nodules (septal panniculitis, neutrophilic vasculitis, neutrophilic panniculitis, vascular thrombosis)
Purpura (neutrophilic predominating over lymphocytic vasculitis)
Papular eruption (urticarial, or blue-gray)
Sterile pustules
Superficial phlebitis
Livedo reticularis
Digital necrosis

TABLE 34.3. Relapsing Polychondritis: Associated Diseases (in Approximate Order of Frequency)

Hematologic (myelodysplastic syndrome, IgA myeloma, lymphoma, acute leukemia)
Connective tissue disease (rheumatoid arthritis, juvenile rheumatoid arthritis, systemic lupus erythematosus, scleroderma, dermatomyositis, Sjogren's syndrome, Reiter's syndrome, psoriatic arthritis)
Autoimmune diseases (Grave's disease, hypothyroidism, Hashimoto's thyroiditis, ulcerative colitis, Crohn's disease, myasthenia gravis, primary biliary cirrhosis, pernicious anemia, diabetes mellitus)
Systemic vasculitis (Wegener's granulomatosis, polyarteritis nodosa, Behçet's disease, Churg-Strauss syndrome, temporal arteritis, Takayasu's arteritis)
Dermatologic disease (psoriasis, lichen planus, vitiligo, atopic dermatitis, Sweet's syndrome (14), erythema nodosum, erythema elevatum diutinum (15))
Infection (hepatitis C infection (16), HIV infection (17))

skin and underlying cartilage is preferred to prevent accentuation of any contour deformities. Histopathologic changes of affected ear are not specific, and may include perichondrial fibroplasia, collagen hyalinization, angioplasia, hemosiderin deposits, vacuolated or pyknotic chondrocytes, loss of cartilaginous matrix basophilia, and lymphohistiocytic and plasmacytic inflammation (Figure 34.2A and 34.2B) (18). Given the distinctive clinical pattern of RP in most cases and nonspecific histologic findings, it has been suggested that performing a biopsy is usually unnecessary to make the diagnosis (19). Direct immunofluorescence of affected areas may show granular deposits of immunoglobulins and C3 at the chondrofibrous junction (20).

The differential diagnosis of relapsing polychondritis is extensive because of the wide variety of disease manifestations. In the classic presentation with auricular chondritis, the differential diagnosis includes auricular cellulitis associated with otitis externa, systemic vasculitis, trauma, frostbite, phototoxic reaction, and arthropod bite reaction. Chondritis is usually distinguished by its frequent bilateral occurrence and typical sparing of the lobe because of its lack of cartilage. With repeated episodes, distortion of the auricular contour may be noted, and there may be radiographic evidence of dystrophic calcification. Joint presentations may mimic other forms of arthritis, including rheumatoid arthritis, septic arthritis, and crystal-induced arthritis. Other organ system involvement may result in clinical presentations resembling Behçet's disease, Wegener's granulomatosis, sarcoidosis, asthma, posterior circulation stroke, or Ménière's disease.

TABLE 34.4. Evaluation of the Patient with Relapsing Polychondritis

1. Complete blood count
2. Erythrocyte sedimentation rate
3. Urinalysis
4. Serum creatinine
5. Rheumatoid factor
6. Pulmonary function tests, with CT of chest if abnormal
7. Ophthalmological examination
8. Electrocardiogram
9. Echocardiography if abnormal cardiac physical examination

Patients with RP should undergo diagnostic evaluation because of the possibility of multisystem disease and coexistent diseases. While evaluation should be directed by clinical symptoms and signs, general guidelines are suggested in Table 34.4. Additional diagnostic evaluation may be necessary if preliminary evaluation suggests the presence of coexistent disease.

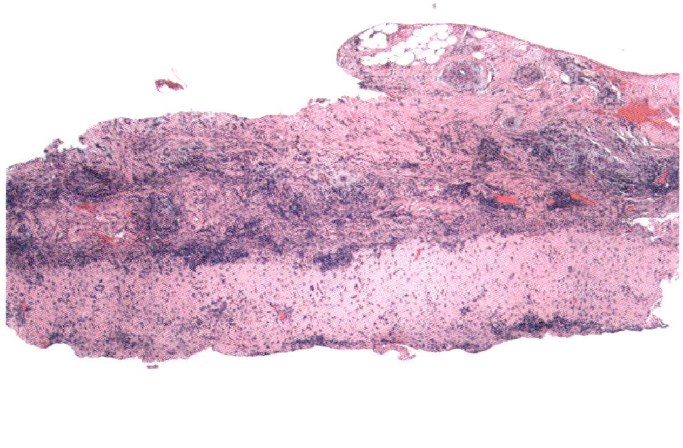
A

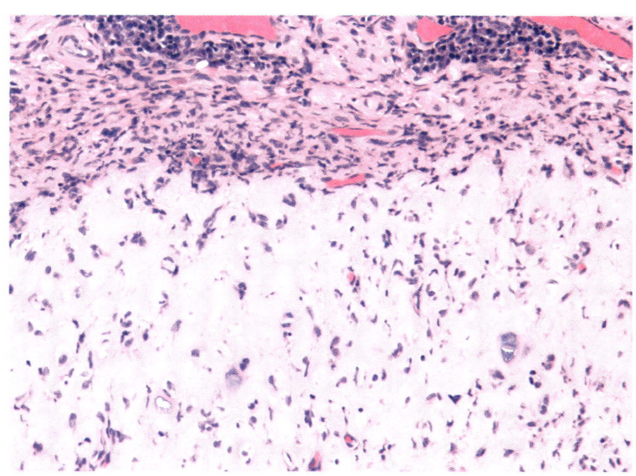
B

FIGURE 34.2. (A and B) Prominent degenerative changes of ear cartilage with perichondral scarring and lymphoplasmacytic inflammation.

Mortality in RP is most frequently due to complications of respiratory tract involvement, either respiratory collapse or infection. Other causes of death include cardiovascular involvement (vasculitis, aneurysm, or valve rupture), and malignancy (11). Ten-year survival in a group of 112 patients followed at one institution was 55%, but a more recent series of 66 patients had a survival rate of 94% with a mean follow-up of eight years (10,12). Anemia at the time of diagnosis predicts decreased survival. In patients less than 51 years old, saddle-nose deformity and systemic vasculitis are the worst prognostic signs, and in older patients, only anemia correlates with worse clinical outcomes (12).

The mainstay of treatment for RP is systemic corticosteroids. Doses of 10 to 20 mg of prednisone per day may be sufficient. Higher doses are usually required for respiratory, audiovestibular, and ocular involvement (19). Low-dose colchicine and methotrexate may be useful as steroid-sparing agents. Nonsteroidal anti-inflammatory agents may help with mild flares of inflammation. Other treatments have included azathioprine, dapsone, cyclosporine, penicillamine, cyclophosphamide, minocycline, and plasma exchange (10). Recently, infliximab has been reported to be of benefit in two patients with refractory RP (21). A novel treatment using oral type II collagen as a tolerogen has been described in a child with RP (22). Adjunctive treatments may include airway stent placement, cardiac valve replacement, or surgical repair of aneurysms. Long-term follow-up is indicated because of a propensity for disease persistence, recurrences, and evolution of coexistent diseases.

References

1. Jaksch-Wartenhorst R. Polychondropathia. *Wien Arch Int Med* 1923; 6: 93–100.
2. Pearson CM, Kline HM, Newcomer VD. Relapsing polychondritis. *New Engl J Med* 1960; 263: 51–58.
3. Foidart JM, Abe S, Martin GR, et al. Antibodies to Type II collagen in relapsing polychondritis. *New Engl J Med* 1978; 299: 1203–1207.
4. Rahkonen O, Savontaus M, Abdelwahid E, Vuorio E, Jokinen E. Expression patterns of cartilage collagens and Sox9 during mouse heart development. *Histochem Cell Biol* 2003; 120: 103–110.
5. Dreiling FJ, Henson MM, Henson OW Jr. Immunolabeling type II collagen in the basilar membrane: A pre-embedding approach. *Hear Res* 2002; 166: 181–191.
6. Hansson AS, Johannesson M, Svensson L, Nandakumar KS, Heinegard D, Holmdahl R. Relapsing polychondritis, induced in mice with matrilin 1, is an antibody- and complement-dependent disease. *Am J Pathol* 2004; 164: 959–966.
7. Terato K, Shimozuru Y, Katayama K, et al. Specificity of antibodies to type II collagen in rheumatoid arthritis. *Arthritis Rheum* 1990; 33: 1493–1500.
8. Lang B, Rothenfusser A, Lanchbury JS, et al. Susceptibility to relapsing polychondritis is associated with HLA-DR4. *Arthritis Rheum* 1993; 36: 660–664.
9. O'Hanlan M, McAdam LP, Bluestone R, Pearson CM. The arthropathy of relapsing polychondritis. *Arthritis Rheum* 1976; 19: 191–194.
10. Trentham DE, Le CH. Relapsing polychondritis. *Ann Intern Med* 1998; 129: 114–122.
11. McAdam LP, O'Hanlan MA, Bluestone R, Pearson CM. Relapsing polychondritis: Prospective study of 23 patients and a review of the literature. *Medicine* 1976; 55: 193–215.
12. Michet CJ, McKenna CH, Luthra HS, O'Fallon WM. Relapsing polychondritis: Survival and predictive role of early disease manifestations. *Ann Intern Med* 1986; 104: 74–78.
13. Frances C, El Rassi R, Laporte JL, Rybojad M, Papo T, Piette JC. Dermatologic manifestations of relapsing polychondritis. *Medicine* 2001; 80: 173–179.
14. Fujimoto N, Tajima S, Ishibashi A, Ura-Ishikou A, Manaka I. Acute febrile neutrophilic dermatosis (Sweet's syndrome) in a patient with relapsing polychondritis. *Br J Dermatol* 1998; 139: 930–931.
15. Bernard P, Bedane C, Delrous JL, Catanzano G, Bonnetblanc JM. Erythema elevatum diutinum in a patient with relapsing polychondritis. *J Am Acad Dermatol* 1992; 26: 312–315.
16. Herrera I, Concha R, Molina EG, Schiff ER, Altman RD. Relapsing polychondritis, chronic hepatitis C infection, and mixed cryoglobulinemia. *Semin Arthritis Rheum* 2004; 33: 388–403.
17. Dolev JC, Maurer TA, Reddy SG, Ramirez LE, Berger T. Relapsing polychondritis in HIV-infected patients: A report of two cases. *J Am Acad Dermatol* 2004; 51: 1023–1025.
18. Feinerman LK, Johnson WC, Weiner J, Graham JH. Relapsing polychondritis: A histopathologic and histochemical study. *Dermatologica* 1970; 140: 369–377.
19. Kent PD, Michet CJ, Luthra HS. Relapsing polychondritis. *Current Opinion Rheum* 2003; 16: 56–61.
20. Valenzuela R, Cooperrider PA, Gogate P, Deodhar SD, Bergfeld WF. Relapsing polychondritis: Immunomicroscopic findings in cartilage of ear biopsy specimens. *Human Pathol* 1980; 11: 19–22.
21. Saadoun D, Deslandre CJ, Allanore Y, Charlier C, Pham XV, Kahan A. Sustained response to infliximab in 2 patients with refractory relapsing polychondritis. *J Rheumatol* 2003; 30: 1394–1395.
22. Navarro MJ, Higgins GC, Lohr KM, Myers LK. Amelioration of relapsing polychondritis in a child treated with oral collagen. *Am J Med Sci* 2002; 324: 101–103.

Part V
Vascular Diseases

35
Calciphylaxis (Calcific Uremic Arteriolopathy)

■ Synonyms:	Calcifying panniculitis, subcutaneous calcific arteriolopathy, uremic small artery disease with medial calcification and intimal hyperplasia, metastatic calcinosis cutis
■ Etiology:	Multifactorial, including hyperphosphatemia, hypercalcemia, hyperparathyroidism, hypoalbuminemia, rapid weight loss, obesity
■ Associations:	Chronic renal insufficiency
■ Histopathology:	Subcutaneous vascular calcification and epidermal necrosis
■ Evaluation:	Serum blood urea nitrogen, creatinine, calcium, phosphate, albumin, parathyroid hormone, quantitative and functional protein C and S, skin biopsy, possible soft tissue radiographic evaluation for subcutaneous calcification, arterial large vessel evaluation in distal variant
■ Treatment:	Reduction of calcium and phosphorous levels, treatment of secondary hyperparathyroidism if severe, hyperbaric oxygen

Calciphylaxis is a syndrome of subcutaneous vascular calcification resulting in painful ulcers on the legs, thighs, or abdomen. The disease develops almost exclusively in patients with end-stage renal disease, and is frequently fatal due to infectious complications. Calciphylaxis was described in 1962 by Hans Selye. He made rats hypercalcemic with "sensitizers" vitamin D or parathyroid hormone. "Challengers" were then administered. These included skin injury by hair-plucking, or injections of various sorts. Injured areas calcified and became ulcerated. Injection of "challengers" intravenously resulted in systemic necrotic lesions associated with tissue calcification (1). The concept of calciphylaxis has been imperfectly applied to cutaneous ulcerations that develop in patients with end-stage renal disease due to vascular calcification and subsequent occlusion. While this clinical scenario has some parallels with Selye's experiments, his experimental subjects were not uremic, and the calcifications were not vascular. Therefore, "calciphylaxis" does not accurately describe the syndrome. Because this disease does not conform to the model of calciphylaxis as described by Selye, many advocate eliminating that label in favor of "calcific uremic arteriolopathy."

The pathogenesis of calciphylaxis is likely multifactorial. The precise process has remained elusive. Most patients developing calciphylaxis have end-stage renal disease, but some have milder renal insufficiency. Other cases have occurred in association with Crohn's disease (2), alcoholic cirrhosis (3), acute renal failure (4), metastatic breast cancer (5), and primary hyperparathyroidism (6). Most earlier literature on the subject regarded the disease as a form of metastatic calcification due to secondary hyperparathyroidism of end-stage renal disease. This view is not supported by data that show that only one third of patients with calciphylaxis have an elevated calcium-phosphate product. Additionally, the calcium-phosphate product of calciphylaxis patients and a control group of patients with end-stage renal disease without skin lesions is similar (7). Evidence of hyperparathyroidism is often lacking in patients with calciphylaxis, and treatment by parathyroidectomy results in clinical improvement in only a subset of patients. A group of patients with calciphylaxis has been described in which low turnover of renal bone disease is present, with low intact parathyroid hormone levels and a low calcium-phosphate product, favoring other inciting factors (8).

Earlier descriptions of calciphylaxis attribute its cause to metastatic calcification resulting from an elevated calcium-phosphate product and secondary hyperparathyroidism. However, the pathogenesis is likely multifactorial. Vascular calcification, the hallmark of calciphylaxis, is a complex process regulated by many factors. Medial arterial calcification is a feature characteristic of both diabetes mellitus and end-stage renal disease. This calcification involves a phenotype switch of the vascular myofibroblast to one of an osteoprogenitor, a process influenced by osteotropic hormones and inhibitors. In pathologic states, the end result is vascular calcification. Local paracrine control of the process involves bone morphogenetic protein-2, parathyroid hormone-related peptide, osteopontin, osteoprotegerin, Pit-1 (a sodium-dependent phosphate cotransporter), and matrix Gla protein, all of which respond to various metabolic and inflammatory stimuli (summarized in Figure 35.1) (9,10). Osteopontin production likely contributes to mineralization, and can be induced by hyperglycemia, uremia, and hyperphosphatemia, all common features in patients with calciphylaxis (9). Matrix Gla protein (MGP) may be an inhibitor of vascular calcification. Warfarin, which is a risk factor for calciphylaxis, inhibits gamma-carboxylation of MGP, rendering it nonfunctional, theoretically tipping the balance toward vascular calcification (11). Parathyroid hormone-related peptide is an endogenous inhibitor of vascular calcification that is suppressed by vitamin D3, another mechanism by which vascular calcification may occur (12). The activity of Pit-1, a sodium-dependent phosphate cotransporter, is enhanced by exposure to calcium and phosphorous, as may occur in patients with chronic renal insufficiency. Pit-1 transports phosphorous into vascular smooth muscle cells, causing mineralization of matrix vesicles that provide nuclear elements for mineralization of the extracellular matrix. Intracellular phosphorous also induces phenotypic switching toward an osteoprogenitor cell (10).

In addition to vascular calcification, tissue calcification due to precipitation of calcium phosphate may occur. Such calcification is normally suppressed by mineralization inhibitors, such as fetuin-A, a circulating glycoprotein, and tissue pyrophosphates. Fetuin-A production may be suppressed by vitamin D, another factor favoring calcification in some patients with end-stage renal disease (9). Matrix metalloproteinases, which can be associated with the catabolic state of rapid weight loss, partially digest elastic tissue, which then avidly binds calcium. This process may contribute to the pathogenesis of calciphylaxis in patients with recent weight loss (13). Some of the factors involved in tissue calcification are summarized in Figure 35.2. While the above observations do not elucidate a specific pathogenesis of calciphylaxis, they indicate that vascular and tissue calcification is induced in a certain metabolic milieu. Many of the forces that favor this process are found in patients with renal disease.

In addition to metabolic factors that may be involved in the pathogenesis of calciphylaxis, there may also be physical factors. Obesity is known to be a risk factor for the development of disease, and it is noted that skin lesions tend to occur in areas of greatest adipose tissue deposition, such as the abdomen, hips, and thighs. With fixed subcutaneous fibrous septae, there may be considerable tensile stress that compromises blood flow in these areas, predisposing to vascular stasis, associated ischemia, and dystrophic lesions (14). Another predisposing factor may be reduced cutaneous oxygen tension. Patients with calciphylaxis have been shown to have reduced transcu-

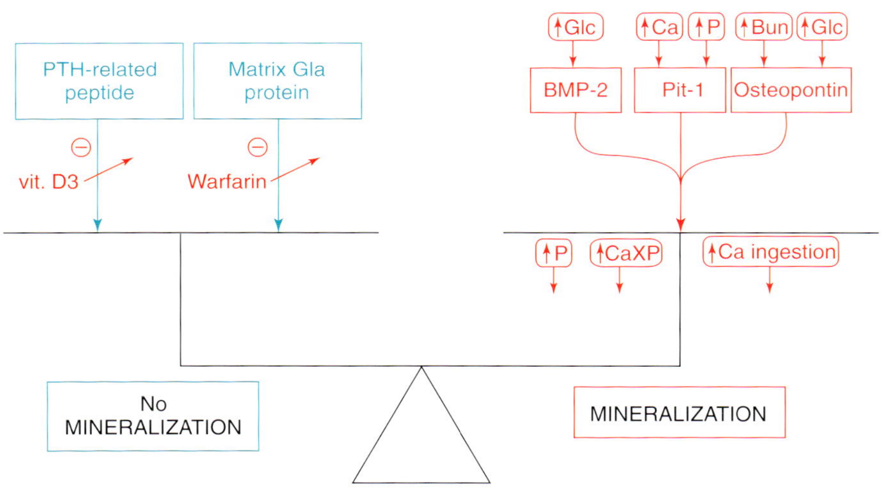

Glc = glucose Bun = blood urea nitrogen Ca = calcium
P = phosphate PTH = parathyroid hormone
BMP-2 = bone morphogenetic protein-2

FIGURE 35.1. Vascular calcium homeostasis.

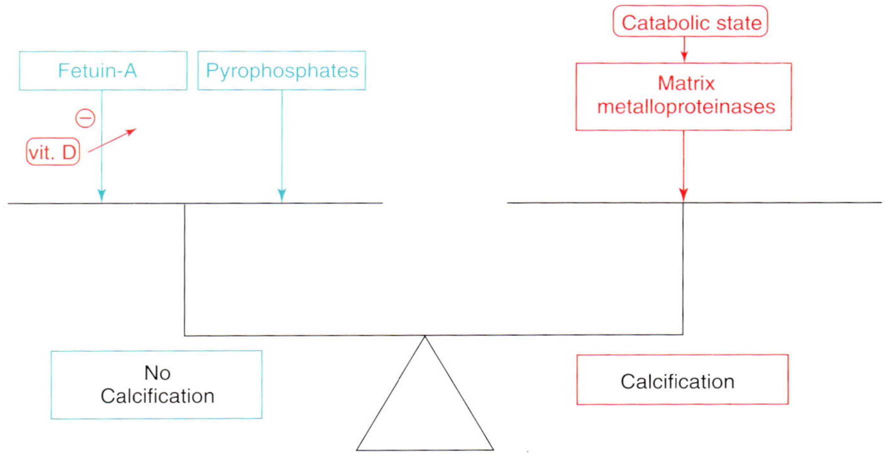

FIGURE 35.2. Tissue calcification homeostasis.

taneous oxygen tension in multiple body regions, in areas with, and without, ulcers (15). This phenomenon may be explained by background vascular calcification of subcutaneous vessels that precedes the onset of clinical lesions. This has been referred to as the "primary lesion" of calciphylaxis (14). It is in this background setting that patients are susceptible to developing ischemic necrosis and tissue calcification. Hypercoagulable states such as protein C or S deficiency or functional impairment may further contribute to precipitation of the disease (16).

Risk factors for calciphylaxis tend to be those that induce a metabolic or physical state favoring vascular and tissue calcification in an already susceptible patient with renal insufficiency. In addition to those factors, the influence of vascular stasis as may be seen in obesity, hypotension, and hypercoagulable states may contribute to precipitation of lesions of calciphylaxis. The risk factors for the development of calciphylaxis are summarized in the following:

Risk Factors for Calciphylaxis

1. Renal insufficiency
2. Obesity
3. Female sex
4. Caucasian
5. Hypotensive episode
6. Recent period of rapid weight loss
7. Diabetes mellitus
8. Hypoalbuminemia
9. Albumin infusions
10. Increased parathyroid hormone level
11. Vitamin D use
12. Calcium carbonate use
13. Increased calcium-phosphate product
14. Warfarin use
15. Protein C or S deficiency or functional impairment

Patients with calciphylaxis usually present with painful indurated plaques or nodules of the abdomen, thigh, and hips, which frequently ulcerate (Figures 35.3 and 35.4). Livedo reticularis, purpura, and bullae may also be seen. Disease localized to the breast or penis has been described (11,17). There is also a distal form of the disease in which patients present with acral ischemia resembling that of peripheral arteriosclerotic disease. A distinguishing feature is that peripheral pulses are generally intact. These patients are reported to have higher survival rates than those with proximal disease (18).

In addition to cutaneous involvement in calciphylaxis, myopathy may develop secondary to skeletal muscle involvement. This usually occurs in areas of skin involvement, and may result in rhabdomyolysis. Other less common areas of involvement are heart, joints, lungs, pancreas, eyes, and gastrointestinal tract (11).

Histopathologic features of calciphylaxis are vascular calcification and varying degrees of necrosis and inflammation, depending on timing and location of the biopsy specimen. Calcification occurs in small to medium-sized venules, and arterioles, in the subcutaneous tissue, and in some instances, the dermis (Figure 35.5A and 35.5B) (18,19). Calcification of subcutaneous septate and adipocytes may also occur (14). The inflammatory infiltrate consists of lymphocytes, neutrophils, and occasional eosinophils. Early lesions devoid of necrosis may have a dermal inflammatory infiltrate. The subcutaneous component is predominantly septal. Calcifications are usually readily seen, but occasionally require histochemical staining with von Kossa or Alizarin red. The degree of calcium deposition identified microscopically does not appear to

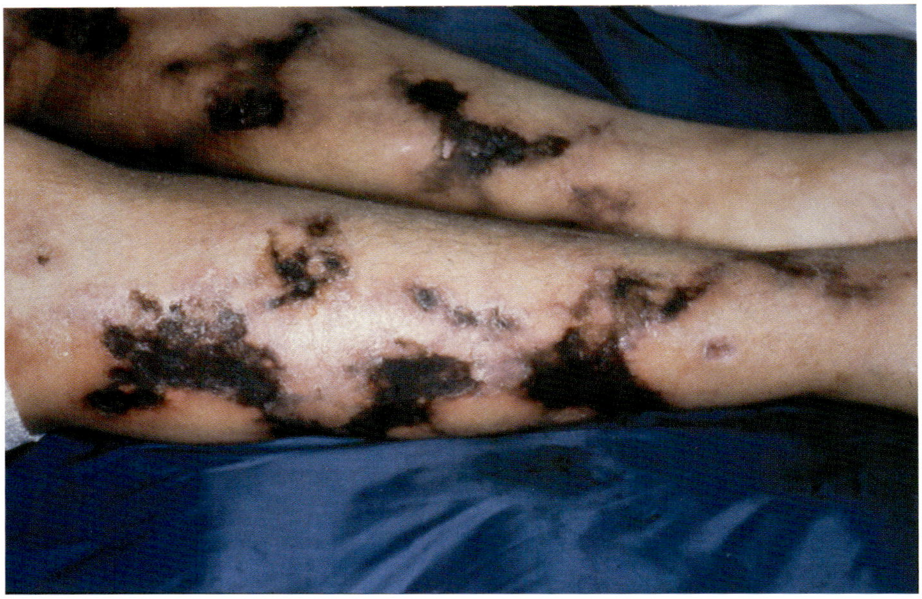

FIGURE 35.3. Reticulated and stellate pattern of ulceration with eschar formation on the legs.

correlate with clinical severity. Vascular thrombi are seen in the minority of cases (19). Necrosis is variable. Subcutaneous calciphylaxis-like calcifications have been reported in biopsy specimens from patients with nephrogenic fibrosing dermopathy, a morphea-like cutaneous sclerosing disorder occurring in some patients with renal failure. This finding was not accompanied by clinical evidence of calciphylaxis (20). These calcifications may correspond to the "primary lesion" of calciphylaxis that represents the setting in which clinical lesions develop. The histologic differential diagnosis of subcutaneous calcifications includes pancreatic panniculitis and Mönckeberg's medial calcific sclerosis. Pancreatic panniculitis has diffuse subcutaneous necrosis with "ghost" cells and an infiltrate of neutrophils, without vascular calcification. Mönckeberg's medial calcific sclerosis occurs as an incidental finding in cutaneous biopsy specimens from the leg, and correlates with underlying arteriosclerotic disease.

The differential diagnosis of calciphylaxis depends upon the distribution of lesions, but may include warfarin

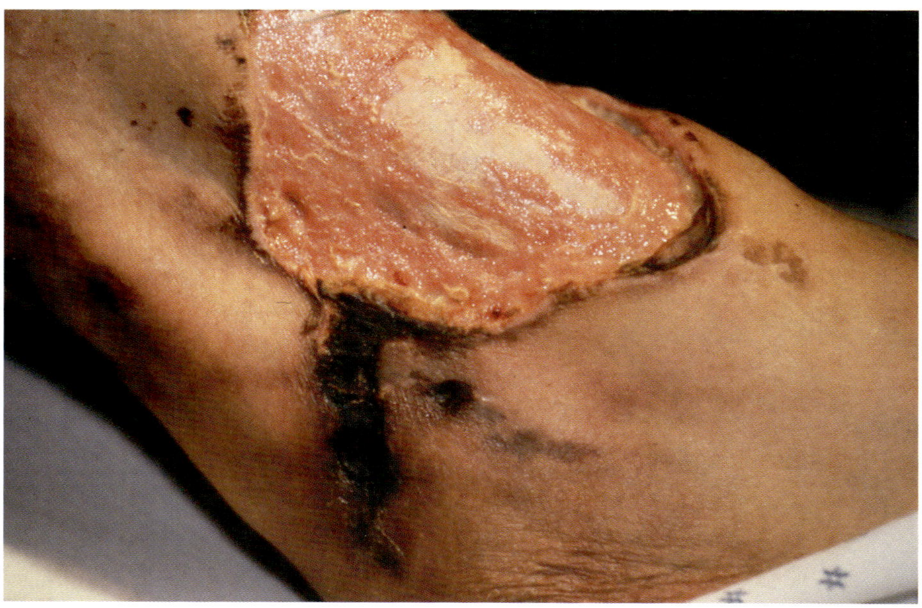

FIGURE 35.4. Later-stage deep ulceration of the thigh with peripheral eschar.

A 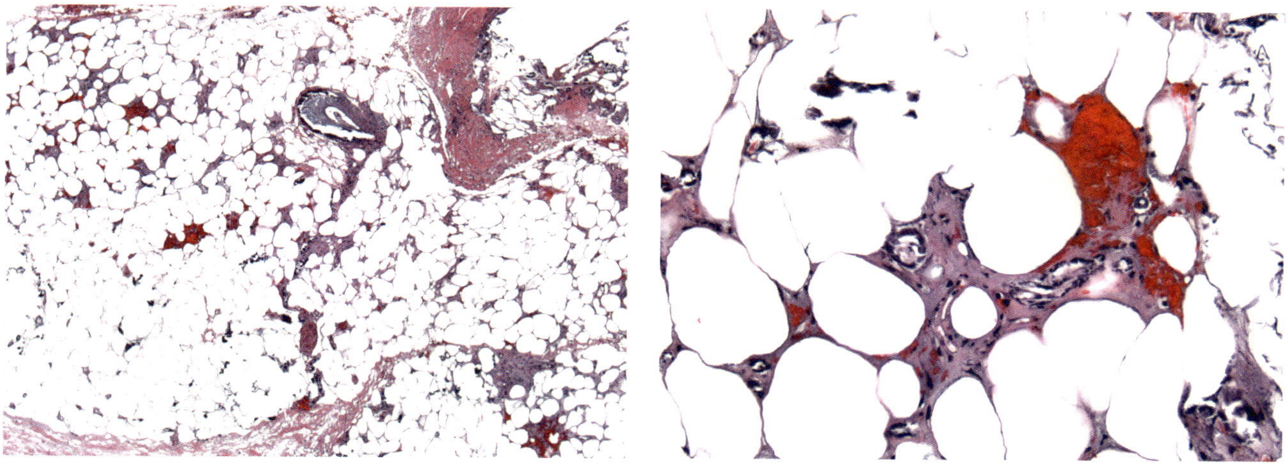 B

FIGURE 35.5. (A) Subcutaneous vascular and interstitial calcification. (B) Stippled vascular and lipocyte calcification.

necrosis, primary hyperoxaluria, peripheral arteriosclerotic disease, vasculitis, emboli, cryoglobulinemia, and cryofibrinogenemia. The diagnosis of calciphylaxis in the right clinical setting is usually apparent. However, some evaluation is indicated for confirmation, and perhaps more importantly, to gather data that will help direct management. A diagnostic evaluation is suggested in the following:

Diagnostic Evaluation of Suspected Calciphylaxis

1. Serum calcium, phosphate, blood urea nitrogen, creatinine, glucose.
2. Serum albumin.
3. Serum intact parathyroid hormone.
4. Protein S and C levels, quantitative and functional.
5. Skin biopsy of indurated plaque or ulcer margin.
6. Evaluation for large vessel arterial disease (in distal subset).
7. Consider radiographic evaluation of soft tissue for subcutaneous calcifications.

Treating calciphylaxis is far more challenging than establishing the diagnosis. Treatment is directed at reversing metabolic derangements favoring calcification. In early series, the focus of treatment was parathyroidectomy. Literature favoring parathyroidectomy reported higher survival rates in surgically treated patients, but these were uncontrolled studies with limited follow-up (18). Use of parathyroidectomy is likely to be beneficial only in cases with striking elevations in parathyroid hormone. It may be that secondary hyperparathyroidism is less relevant than it was in earlier reports because of ever-improving metabolic control in patients with end-stage renal disease. The incidence of calciphylaxis appears be increasing, and this may be, in part, due to a switch from aluminum-containing phosphate binders to those containing calcium. In the patient with calciphylaxis, calcium-containing phosphate binders should be changed to non-calcium ones such as sevelamer. Increased frequency of dialysis from three to five times a week with a low calcium bath has been advocated to reduce calcium burden (21). This requires careful monitoring for hypocalcemia. While the use of vitamin D would be expected to worsen disease based on Selye's model, it has a theoretical advantage of suppressing parathyroid hormone levels while limiting gastrointestinal absorption of calcium and phosphorous in the patient with secondary hyperparathyroidism (21). Hyperbaric oxygen has been reported to be of benefit in healing of cutaneous ulcers (22). Even oxygen administration by nasal cannula may increase cutaneous oxygen tension in patients with calciphylaxis (11). Bisphosphonates have been found to suppress experimental calciphylaxis, and intravenous treatment with the bisphosphonate, pamidronate, was reported to result in dramatic disease resolution in a case report (23,24). Intravenous sodium thiosulfate, which may solubilize tissue calcium deposits, was used with striking beneficial effect in a case report (25). Another case report noted good response to low-dose tissue plasminogen activator in a patient with calciphylaxis, history of deep venous thrombosis, low protein C and antithrombin III, and elevated fibrinogen levels, suggesting that this is a therapy to consider in calciphylaxis patients with evidence of a hypercoagulable state (26). A summary of possible tools in calciphylaxis treatment is suggested:

Management of Calciphylaxis

1. Eliminate calcium-containing phosphate binders and other oral calcium intake.

2. Avoid excessive calcium-phosphate product.
3. Low or no-calcium dialysate.
4. Increased frequency of dialysis.
5. Parathyroidectomy in cases with severe secondary hyperparathyroidism.
6. Consider IV vitamin D in low doses in nonsurgical candidates with hyperparathyroidism.
7. Hyperbaric oxygen, consider oxygen by nasal cannula.
8. Weight loss in obese patients.
9. Nutritional supplementation to reverse catabolic state in those with precipitous weight loss.
10. Serum glucose control in diabetics.
11. In patients on warfarin, attempt switch to a different anticoagulant.
12. Gentle wound debridement.
13. Consider sodium thiosulfate, bisphosphonates, low-dose tissue plasminogen activator based on anecdotal reports.

The prognosis in calciphylaxis has been poor, with most patients succumbing to sepsis because of extensive cutaneous ulceration. Severe debilitation from co-morbidities also contributes to a poor outcome. While the disease has a grave prognosis, elucidation of the pathways of metabolic control of vascular and tissue calcification give hope for effective management and treatment of these patients in the future.

References

1. Selye H. *Calciphylaxis*. Chicago, IL: University of Chicago Press, 1962.
2. Barri YM, Graves GS, Knochel JP. Calciphylaxis in a patient with Crohn's disease in the absence of end-stage renal disease. *Am J Kidney Dis* 1997; 29: 773–776.
3. Fader DJ, Kang S. Calciphylaxis without renal failure. *Arch Dermatol* 1996; 132: 837–838.
4. Chavel SM, Taraszka KS, Schaffer JV, Lazova R, Schechner JS. Calciphylaxis associated with acute, reversible renal failure in the setting of alcoholic cirrhosis. *J Am Acad Dermatol* 2004; 50: S125–S128.
5. Mastruserio DN, Nguyen EQ, Nielsen T, Hessel A, Pellegrini AE. Calciphylaxis associated with metastatic breast carcinoma. *J Am Acad Dermatol* 1999; 41: 295–298.
6. Mirza I, Chaubay D, Gunderia H, Shih W, El-Fanek H. An unusual presentation of calciphylaxis due to primary hyperparathyroidism. *Arch Pathol Lab Med* 2001; 125: 1351–1353.
7. Llach F. Calcific uremic arteriolopathy (calciphylaxis): An evolving entity? *Am J Kidney Dis* 1998; 32: 514–518.
8. Mawad HW, Sawaya BP, Sarin R, Malluche HH. Calcific uremic arteriolopathy in association with low turnover bone disease. *Clin Nephrol* 1999; 52: 160–166.
9. Vattikuti R, Towler DA. Osteogenic regulation of vascular calcification: An early perspective. *Am J Physiol Endocrinol Metab* 2004; 286: E686–E696.
10. Giachelli CM. Vascular calcification mechanisms. *J Am Soc Nephrol* 2004; 15: 2959–2964.
11. Wilmer WA, Magro CM. Calciphylaxis: emerging concepts in prevention, diagnosis, and treatment. *Semin Dialysis* 2002; 15: 172–186.
12. Jono S, Nishizawa Y, Shioi A, Morii H. 1,25-Dihydroxyvitamin D3 increases *in vitro* vascular calcification by modulating secretion of endogenous parathyroid hormone-related peptide. *Circulation* 1998; 98: 1302–1306.
13. Munavalli F, Reisenauer A, Moses M, Kilroy S, Arbiser JL. Weight loss-induced calciphylaxis: potential role of matrix metalloproteinases. *J Dermatol* 2003; 30: 915–919.
14. Janigan DT, Hirsch DJ, Klassen GA, MacDonald AS. Calcified subcutaneous arterioles with infarcts of the subcutis and skin ("calciphylaxis") in chronic renal failure. *Am J Kidney Dis* 2000; 35: 588–597.
15. Wilmer WA, Voroshilova O, Singh I, Middendorf DF, Cosio FG. Transcutaneous oxygen tension in patients with calciphylaxis. *Am J Kidney Dis* 2001; 37: 797–806.
16. Mehta RL, Scott G, Sloand JA, Francis CW. Skin necrosis associated with acquired protein C deficiency in patients with renal failure and calciphylaxis. *Am J Med* 1990; 88: 252–257.
17. Karpman E, Das S, Kurzrock EA. Penile calciphylaxis: analysis of risk factors and mortality. *J Urol* 2003; 169: 2206–2209.
18. Hafner J, Keusch G, Wahl C, et al. Uremic small-artery disease with medial calcification and intimal hyperplasia (so-called calciphylaxis): A complication of chronic renal failure and benefit from parathyroidectomy. *J Am Acad Dermatol* 1995; 33: 954–962.
19. Essary LR, Wick MR. Cutaneous calciphylaxis: An underrecognized clinicopathologic entity. *Am J Clin Pathol* 2000; 113: 280–287.
20. Edsall LC, English JC, Patterson JW. Calciphylaxis and metastatic calcification associated with nephrogenic fibrosing dermopathy. *J Cutan Pathol* 2004; 31: 247–253.
21. Don BR, Chin AI. A strategy for the treatment of calcemic uremic arteriolopathy (calciphylaxis) employing a combination of therapies. *Clin Nephrol* 2003; 59: 463–470.
22. Basile C, Montanaro A, Masi M, Pati G, De Maio P, Gismondi A. Hyperbaric oxygen therapy for calcific uremic arteriolopathy: A case series. *J Nephrol* 2002; 15: 676–680.
23. Price PA, Omid N, Than TN, Williamson MK. The amino bisphosphonate ibandronate prevents calciphylaxis in the rat at doses that inhibit bone resorption. *Calcif Tissue Int* 2002; 71: 356–363.
24. Monney P, Nguyen QV, Perroud H, Descombes E. Rapid improvement of calciphylaxis after intravenous pamidronate therapy in a patient with chronic renal failure. *Nephrol Dial Transplant* 2004; 19: 2130–2132.
25. Cicone JS, Petronis JB, Embert CD, Spector DA. Successful treatment of calciphylaxis with intravenous sodium thiosulfate. *Am J Kidney Dis* 2004; 43: 1104–1108.
26. Sewell LD, Weenig RH, Davis MDP, McEvoy MT, Pittelkow MR. Low-dose tissue plasminogen activator for calciphylaxis. *Arch Dermatol* 2004; 140: 1045–1048.

36
Kawasaki Disease

- Synonyms: Mucocutaneous lymph node syndrome
- Etiology: Unknown
- Associations: None
- Histology: Coronary arteritis with macrophages, plasma cells, lymphocytes, and occasionally eosinophils; skin nonspecific with dermal edema and perivascular lymphocytes
- Evaluation: Throat culture, serologic testing for viral infections, urinalysis, complete blood count with differential, electrocardiogram, transthoracic echocardiography in younger patients, magnetic resonance angiography in older patients
- Treatment: Intravenous gammaglobulin and aspirin
- Prognosis: Good with treatment, 1%–2% cardiac sudden death due to coronary arteritis

Kawasaki disease, or mucocutaneous lymph node syndrome, was first described in Japan in the late 1960s as an illness characterized by persistent fever, conjunctivitis, mucous membrane changes, acral erythema with desquamation, and cervical adenopathy, associated with coronary arteritis (1,2). While earlier descriptions of the disease were limited to Asia and Hawaii, the disease is now known to occur worldwide. The disease is primarily one of young children, with 85% of cases occurring in children under five years. It is uncommon in children less than 6 months. There have been some epidemiologic investigations linking Kawasaki disease to freshly cleaned carpets, humidifier use, and living near a body of water, but these associations have not been observed consistently (3).

The etiology of Kawasaki disease is unknown. There are seasonal peaks in the winter and spring months, with occasional epidemics. There are only rare cases of the disease occurring in infants less than three months, suggesting protection via passive maternal antibodies. These findings have suggested an infectious agent, yet extensive investigations have failed to detect one. There is a recently described association between Kawasaki disease and a novel coronavirus in a small series, but further study will be required to evaluate the strength of this association (4). IgA plasma cells have been found in early and subacute lesions of Kawasaki vasculitis, suggesting the possibility of an immune response to a gastrointestinal or respiratory tract pathogen (5). Furthermore, the IgA response is oligoclonal rather than polyclonal, favoring an antigen-driven response over nonspecific B-cell activation (6). The incidence of Kawasaki disease is greater in the Asian population and in siblings and parents of those with the disease, suggesting a genetic predisposition (3).

Patients with Kawasaki disease present with persistent fever despite antibiotics, conjunctival congestion, oral dryness, redness, fissuring of the lips, strawberry tongue, and mucosal erythema (Figures 36.1 and 36.2). These findings are accompanied by acral erythema and edema, followed by desquamation in the convalescent stage (Figure 36.3). The acral erythema spreads to a truncal exanthem within three to five days (Figure 36.4). Cervical adenopathy is also a relatively constant feature. Other symptoms may include diarrhea, arthralgia or arthritis, and aseptic meningitis (2). A feature found in the majority of patients, but not emphasized in early descriptions, is perineal erythema and subsequent desquamation (Figure 36.5) (7). Small sterile pustules have also been described in some patients with Kawasaki disease, occurring symmetrically on erythematous skin on the buttocks, axillae, genitalia, and extensor surfaces (8).

Diagnostic criteria for Kawasaki disease are as follows (3):

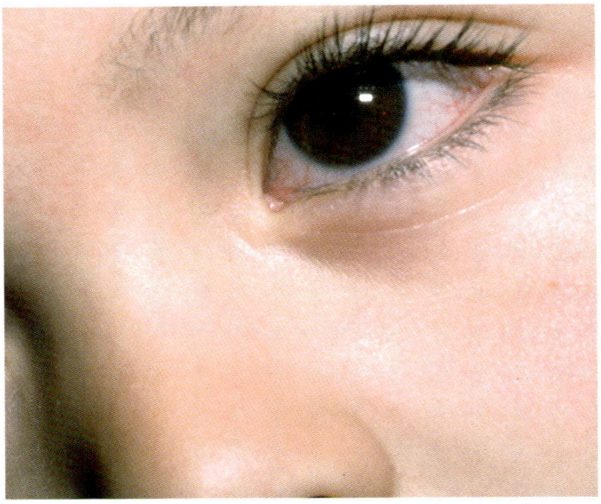

FIGURE 36.1. Conjunctival injection. Courtesy of Nancy Esterly, MD.

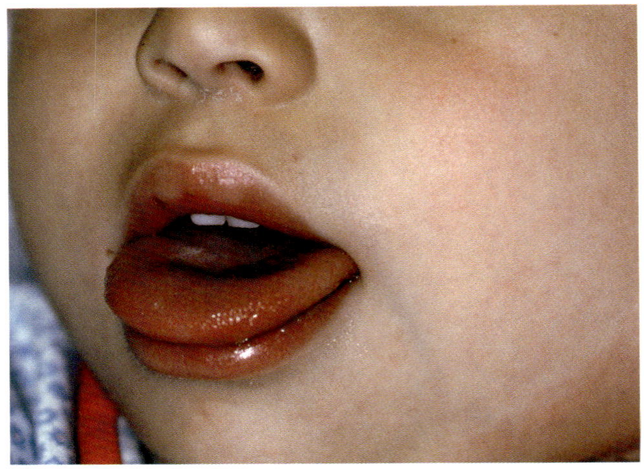

FIGURE 36.2. Lip and tongue erythema and edema. Courtesy of Nancy Esterly, MD.

Diagnostic Criteria for Kawasaki Syndrome

Presence of fever for at least 5 days, 4 of the 5 criteria below, and lack of another known disease process to cause the illness:

1. Bilateral conjunctival injection
2. Changes of the mucous membranes of the upper respiratory tract: injected pharynx; injected, fissured lips; strawberry tongue
3. Polymorphous rash
4. Changes of the extremities: peripheral edema, peripheral erythema, periungual desquamation
5. Cervical adenopathy

Strict use of these criteria will miss cases of Kawasaki disease, so-called "atypical" or "incomplete" Kawasaki disease. These are patients in whom coronary arteritis is present, in association with persistent fever, and fewer than four other diagnostic criteria. Vigilance for these cases is mandated because of the potential for disastrous consequences in untreated coronary arteritis. In cases of suspected Kawasaki disease, imaging of the coronary vessels is indicated. In young children, transthoracic echocardiography can be used to diagnose coronary artery changes with high specificity, but in older children and in adults, visualization of the vessels is more difficult. Coronary X-ray angiography has been the

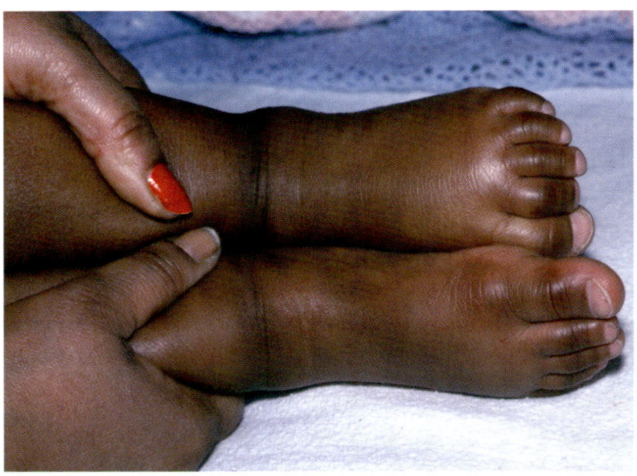

FIGURE 36.3. Acral edema and erythema. Courtesy of Nancy Esterly, MD.

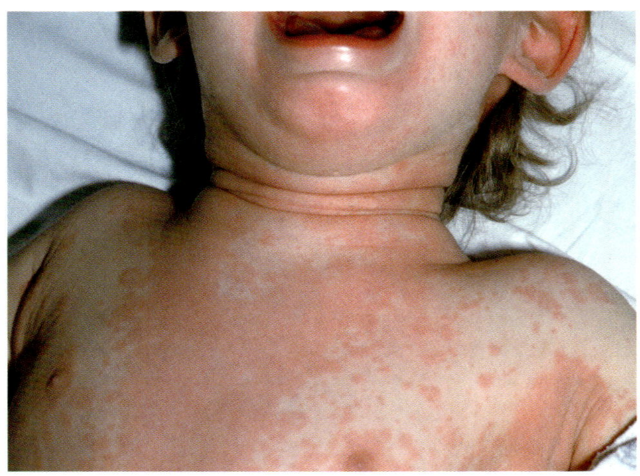

FIGURE 36.4. Morbilliform exanthem. Courtesy of Nancy Esterly, MD.

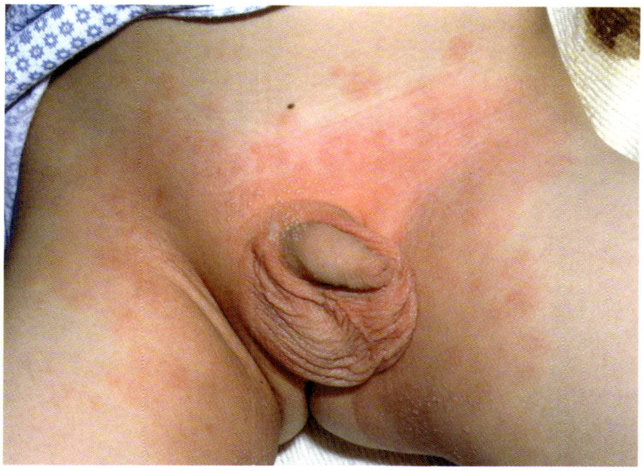

FIGURE 36.5. Inguinal and genital accentuation of exanthem with minute pustules. Courtesy of Nancy Esterly, MD.

mainstay of evaluation. However, recently, magnetic resonance angiography has been shown to be comparable to X-ray angiography, and is likely to become the future standard for evaluation of coronary abnormalities in older children and in adults (9). Laboratory findings may include elevated erythrocyte sedimentation rate and C-reactive protein, leukocytosis with left shift, pyuria, proteinuria, or anemia. In cases of suspected Kawasaki disease, a suggested diagnostic evaluation is given.

Diagnostic Evaluation in Suspected Kawasaki Disease

1. Complete blood count and differential
2. Throat and nasal cultures
3. Nasopharyngeal swab for adenovirus, rapid direct fluorescent antigen test
4. Urinalysis
5. Erythrocyte sedimentation rate, C-reactive protein
6. Electrocardiogram
7. Echocardiogram or magnetic resonance angiography
8. BUN, creatinine, SGOT, SGPT

The principal differential diagnosis of Kawasaki syndrome includes scarlet fever, Staphylococcal scalded skin syndrome, toxic shock syndrome, and adenovirus infection. A summary of important features of each is given in Table 36.1.

TABLE 36.1. Differential Diagnosis of Kawasaki Disease

	Kawasaki Disease	SS	Scarlet Fever	Toxic Shock Syndrome	Adenovirus (10)
Age group	>3 months, <5 years	<3 months most common, but any age	2–10 years most common	Menstruating women, uncommon in children	Usually <10 years
Conjunctival involvement	+, injection	+, purulent	–	+/–, injection	Usually present
Strawberry tongue	+	–	+, white early on	+/–	rare
Lip involvement	+	–	–	–	–
Acral	+	+, but part of diffuse involvement	–	+, but part of diffuse involvement	–
Perineal	+	+, but part of diffuse involvement	+/–	+/–	–
Bullae	–	+	–	–	–
Other	Cervical adenopathy, may have aseptic meningitis, pyuria	May be able to culture *Staphylococcus aureus*	+throat culture, group A *Streptococcus*, truncal exanthem accentuated in skin folds, "sandpaper" texture on skin	+culture for *Staphylococcus aureus*, sometimes group A *Streptococcus*, from primary site of infection, scarlatiniform eruption, rhabdomyolysis, liver dysfunction, thrombocytopenia	May have exudative pharyngitis and conjunctivitis

The typical pathologic finding in Kawasaki disease is that of a vasculitis, occurring most commonly in the coronary arteries, but also occurring in renal, iliac, femoral, and mesenteric arteries. There are initially subendothelial cell collections of macrophages, lymphocytes, and neutrophils (11). Plasma cells and eosinophils are also constituents of the infiltrate (5,12). The inflammation eventually becomes transmural, and can extend along the adventitia as in polyarteritis nodosa. In Kawasaki disease, in contrast to polyarteritis nodosa, there are fewer neutrophils, and fibrinoid necrosis is not prominent (11). Biopsy specimens of skin in Kawasaki disease do not have specific findings, but in those with sterile pustules, the location is subcorneal (8).

The mainstay of treatment of Kawasaki disease is intravenous gammaglobulin, with aspirin. A comparison of treatment with aspirin alone versus aspirin with gammaglobulin reveals a striking reduction in the development of coronary aneurysms in the gammaglobulin group, and greater resolution of existing coronary lesions over time in the same group (13). Treatment with gammaglobulin is generally given using 2 mg/kg as a single infusion (3). High-dose aspirin is recommended early on in the disease to prevent thrombotic events, 80–100 mg/kg per day, divided in four doses, for up to 14 days, and then 3–5 mg/kg as a single daily dose for seven weeks or longer (14). Some authors advocate lower doses of aspirin (15). Aspirin does not reduce aneurysm formation (16). A recent retrospective study has called into question the benefit of aspirin therapy, but for the present, it remains part of the standard treatment (17). Eighty-nine percent of patients respond to a single dose of gammaglobulin, but the remainder will remain febrile. A second dose of gammaglobulin has been advocated in those remaining febrile for the 48 to 72 hours following the first dose. Of these, two-thirds will become afebrile with the second dose (18). Patients with persistent fever after one dose of gammaglobulin, who receive additional gammaglobulin, have a decrease in cardiac complications (19). Treatment options for those refractory to two doses of intravenous gammaglobulin include additional doses of gammaglobulin, pulse methylprednisolone, infliximab, cyclosporine, cyclophosphamide, and plasmapheresis (3,20). A small trial of pulse methylprednisolone in addition to gammaglobulin and aspirin revealed more rapid resolution of symptoms in the group treated with steroids compared to the standard treatment group (gammaglobulin and aspirin), but no differences in cardiac outcome between the two groups (21).

The principal complication of Kawasaki disease is coronary artery disease. Sudden death occurs in 1%–2% of patients in the acute phase of the disease, and coronary aneurysms develop in 25% of patients with the disease; 55% eventually regress, but some are complicated by stenosis or occlusion (22). Patients with giant aneurysms (those greater than 8 mm in diameter) are at considerably higher risk for complications (3). Lifelong follow-up is warranted in those with cardiac abnormalities. Recent data suggest that persistent coronary lesions tend to occur in patients with persistently elevated indices of inflammation, such as C-reactive protein, serum amyloid-A, interleukin-6, and soluble intercellular adhesion molecule-1 (23). This potential functional relationship may have implications for long-term treatment. Recurrent skin peeling has been described in patients with a history of Kawasaki disease, without any other evidence of disease reactivation. Some of these episodes have been associated with respiratory tract infections (24).

Kawasaki disease may resemble several bacterial toxin-mediated diseases, and, less likely, viral infections. Early diagnosis is important because of the ability to dramatically decrease the risk of complications with gammaglobulin treatment.

References

1. Kawasaki T. Mucocutaneous lymph node syndrome: Clinical observation of 50 cases. *Jpn J Allerg* 1967; 16: 178–222 (in Japanese).
2. Kawasaki T, Kosaki F, Okawa S, Shigematsu I, Yanagawa H. A new infantile acute febrile mucocutaneous lymph node syndrome (MLNS) prevailing in Japan. *Pediatrics* 1974; 54: 271–276.
3. Burns JC, Glode MP. Kawasaki syndrome. *Lancet* 2004; 364: 533–544.
4. Esper F, Shapiro ED, Weibel C, Ferguson D, Landry ML, Kahn JS. Association between a novel human coronavirus and Kawasaki disease. *J Infect Dis* 2005; 191: 499–502.
5. Rowley AH, Eckerly CA, Hans-Martin J, Shulman ST, Baker SC. IgA plasma cells in vascular tissue of patients with Kawasaki syndrome. *J Immunol* 1997; 159: 5946–5955.
6. Rowley AH, Shulman ST, Spike BT, Mask CA, Baker SC. Oligoclonal IgA response in the vascular wall in acute Kawasaki disease. *J Immunol* 2001; 166: 1334–1343.
7. Friter BS, Lucky AW. The perineal eruption of Kawasaki syndrome. *Arch Dermatol* 1988; 124: 1805–1810.
8. Kimura T, Miyazawa H, Watanabe K, Moriya T. Small pustules in Kawasaki disease: A clinicopathological study of four patients. *Am J Dermatopathol* 1988; 10: 218–223.
9. Greil GF, Stuber M, Botnar RM, et al. Coronary magnetic resonance angiography in adolescents and young adults with Kawasaki disease. *Circulation* 2002; 105: 908–911.
10. Barone SR, Pontrelli LR, Krilov LR. The differentiation of classic Kawasaki disease, atypical Kawasaki disease, and acute adenoviral infection: Use of clinical features and a rapid direct fluorescent antigen test. *Arch Pediatr Adolesc Med* 2000; 154: 453–456.
11. Jennette JC. Implications for pathogenesis patterns of injury in small- and medium-sized-vessel vasculitis. *Cleveland Clin J Med* 2003; 69: SII-33–38.

12. Terai M, Yasukawa K, Honda T. Peripheral blood eosinophilia and eosinophil accumulation in coronary microvessels in acute Kawasaki disease. *Pediatr Infect Dis J* 2002; 8: 777–781.
13. Newburger JW, Takahashi M, Burns JC, et al. The treatment of Kawasaki syndrome with intravenous gamma globulin. *N Engl J Med* 1986; 315: 341–347.
14. Monagle P, Chan A, Massicotte P, Chalmers E, Michelson AD. Antithrombotic therapy in children: The Seventh ACCP conference on antithrombotic and thrombolytic therapy. *Chest* 2004; 126: 645S–687S.
15. Brogan PA, Bose A, Burgner D, et al. Kawasaki disease: An evidence based approach to diagnosis, treatment, and proposals for future research. *Arch Dis Child* 2002; 86: 286–290.
16. Terai M, Shulman ST. Prevalence of coronary artery abnormalities in Kawasaki disease is highly dependent on gamma globulin dose but independent of salicylate dose. *J Pediatr* 1997; 131: 888–893.
17. Hsieh KS, Weng KP, Lin CC, Huang TC, Lee CL, Huang SM. Treatment of Kawasaki disease: Aspirin's role in the febrile stage revisited. *Pediatrics* 2004; 114: 689–693.
18. Freeman AF, Shulman ST. Refractory Kawasaki disease. *Pediatr Infect Dis J* 2004; 23: 463–464.
19. Miura M, Ohki H, Tsuchihashi T, et al. Coronary risk factors in Kawasaki disease treated with additional gammaglobulin. *Arch Dis Child* 2004; 89: 776–780.
20. Weiss JE, Eberhard BA, Chowdhury D, Gottlieb BS. Infliximab as novel therapy for refractory Kawasaki disease. *J Rheumatol* 2004; 31: 808–810.
21. Sundel RP, Baker AL, Fulton DR, Newburger JW. Corticosteroids in the initial treatment of Kawasaki disease: Report of a randomized trial. *J Pediatr* 2003; 142: 611–616.
22. Kato H, Sugimura T, Akagi T, et al. Long term consequences of Kawasaki disease. *Circulation* 1996; 94: 1379–1385.
23. Mitani Y, Sawada H, Hayakawa H, et al. Elevated levels of high-sensitivity C-reactive protein and serum amyloid-A late after Kawasaki disease: Association between inflammation and late coronary sequelae in Kawasaki disease. *Circulation* 2005; 111: 38–43.
24. Michie C, Kinsler V, Tulloh R, Davidson S. Recurrent skin peeling following Kawasaki disease. *Arch Dis Child* 2000; 83: 353–355.

37 Polyarteritis Nodosa

■ Synonyms:	Periarteritis nodosa, macroscopic polyarteritis nodosa, polyarteritis
■ Etiology:	Unknown
■ Associations:	Hepatitis B and C infection; rarely HIV, hairy cell leukemia
■ Histology:	Medium-sized vessel arteritis, lesser involvement of smaller vessels
■ Evaluation:	Serologic assessment for hepatitis B, C virus, creatinine, erythrocyte sedimentation rate or C-reactive protein, urinalysis; may include muscle, nerve biopsy, visceral arteriography
■ Treatment:	Systemic steroids, plasma exchange, antiviral therapy in HBV and HCV-associated cases, pulse cyclophosphamide
■ Prognosis:	Poor without treatment, 75% survival with immunosuppressive treatment

Polyarteritis nodosa is a systemic vasculitis that involves predominantly medium-sized vessels. In 1852, Rokitansky described a man who presented with fever, abdominal pain, and bloody diarrhea, and shortly thereafter expired. Autopsy findings included small aneurysms of the arterial system, sparing the arteries of the brain and the large arteries. The aneurysms were identified as inflammatory and the disease was named *periarteritis nodosa* by Kussmaul and Maier in 1866. The term *polyarteritis nodosa* was introduced by Ferrari in 1903 to emphasize the transmural inflammation that characterizes this vasculitis (1). Because polyarteritis nodosa has overlapping features with other forms of systemic vasculitis, the nosology has been confusing. Interpretation of data from case series in the literature is difficult because many series are comprised of patients now regarded as having had different diseases. This summary of polyarteritis nodosa will describe the disease in its classic form and briefly discuss the other entities that may have a similar pattern of vasculitis.

The etiology of polyarteritis nodosa is unknown, but many cases occur in individuals infected with hepatitis B virus (HBV), and, occasionally, hepatitis C virus (2). Cases associated with hepatitis B are immune complex-mediated. HBV surface antigen may be found in active lesions, implicating a role in pathogenesis. HBV-associated cases usually manifest in the first six months of infection and may be the presenting sign of the infection (3). Benign cutaneous PAN is a subset of the disease in which disease appears to remain limited to the skin. This variant has been described in a small series of patients with hepatitis C infection. None of the patients were infected with HBV (4). In another larger series of 79, no patients had evidence of hepatitis B infection, and one patient had hepatitis C infection (5). PAN unassociated with viral hepatitis is probably not immune complex-mediated (3). Other viruses reported to be associated with polyarteritis nodosa include HIV (6) and herpes zoster (7). PAN has also been reported to be associated with hairy cell leukemia (8).

Polyarteritis nodosa may present without specific features early in its evolution. Typically, symptoms slowly arise over a period of months—fever, weight loss, malaise, arthralgias without arthritis, and myalgias. Cutaneous findings generally do not occur at the outset, but eventually develop in many patients with PAN. Cutaneous manifestations include livedo reticularis, which is reticulated violaceous erythema usually occurring on the lower extremities, due to cutaneous arterial insufficiency. This finding may be accompanied by stellate necrosis, nodules, ulcers, and acral ischemia, which may include necrosis (Figure 37.1). These changes are most frequently present on the lower extremities. Mononeuritis multiplex, caused by neural infarcts, occurs in the majority of patients with PAN and is directly caused by vasculitis. The long peripheral nerves are involved most prominently, especially the sural and superficial peroneal nerves. The neuritis usually

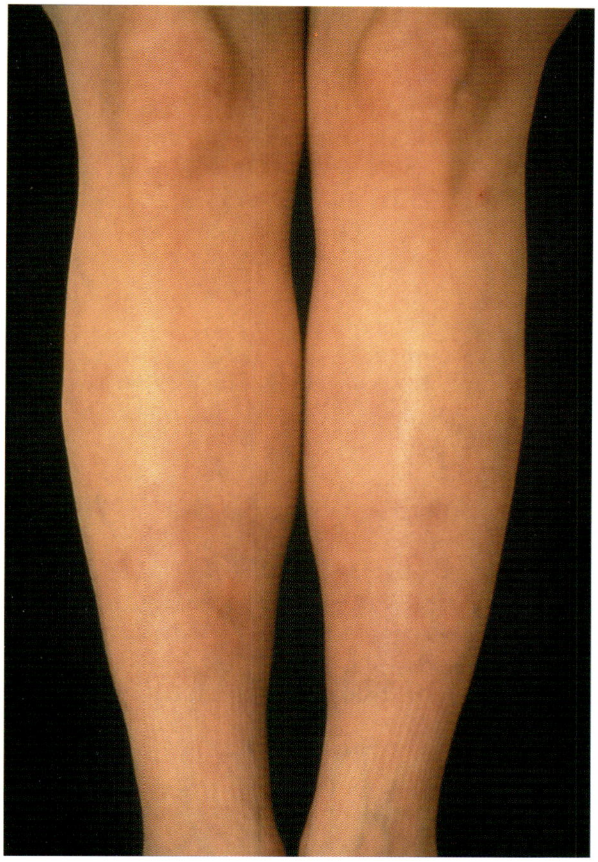

FIGURE 37.1. Multiple bilateral pretibial erythematous and slightly violaceous nodules.

starts asymmetrically, but as the vasculitis progresses, it may become more symmetric and mimic other peripheral neuropathies. Gastrointestinal manifestations due to arterial insufficiency include abdominal pain and bloody diarrhea. These symptoms indicate the presence of mesenteric arteritis and are associated with high mortality. Renal vasculitis is common in PAN, and results in wedge-shaped infarcts. Cardiac involvement occurs in the majority of cases, but frequently cannot be diagnosed clinically. Tachycardia occurs in a considerable number of patients. Coronary thrombosis is one of the more important complications of PAN. It may occur without any antecedent symptoms. Other organ systems that may be involved are the pancreas, brain, testes, ovaries, breast, and eyes. Lungs are typically spared.

Localized variants of polyarteritis are also known, including the cutaneous variant, benign cutaneous PAN. This localized form is frequently limited to a region or even a single extremity. These patients tend to present with painful nodules on the lower extremities, associated with edema and, occasionally, neuropathy. Ulceration occurs in approximately 50%, and may be associated with a more prolonged course (5). Other organ systems may have localized PAN, examples of which include appendix, bowel, breast, testis, gallbladder, and uterus (9). Clinical follow-up is warranted in cases that appear to be localized because some will eventually develop systemic disease.

The pathologic changes in polyarteritis nodosa involve medium-sized and small arteries, sometimes arterioles (Figure 37.2A and 37.2B). Aortic and other large vessel

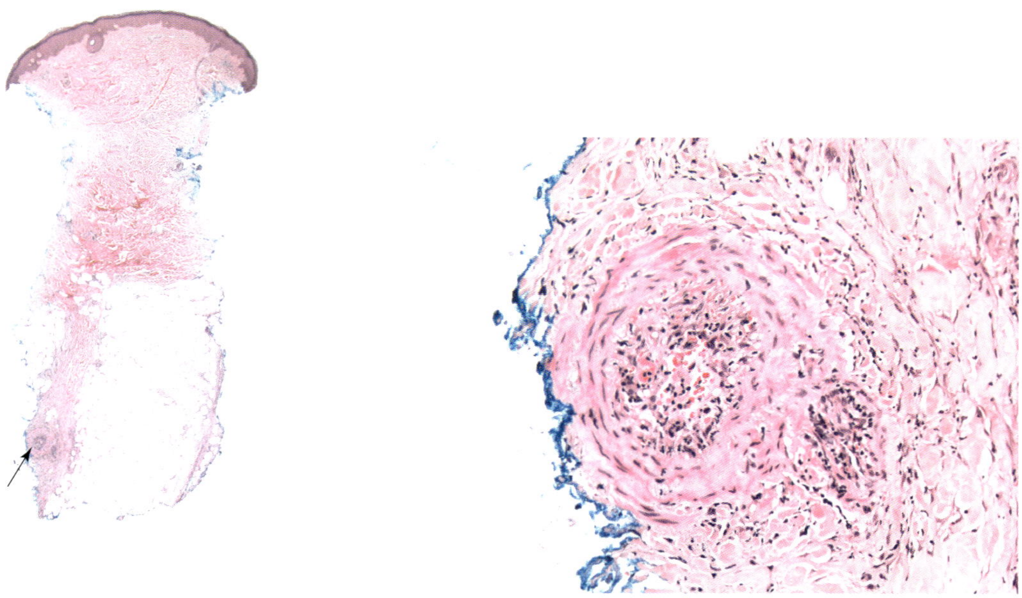

A

B

FIGURE 37.2. (A) Inflamed artery deep within subcutaneous interlobular septum. (B) Subcutaneous artery infiltrated by lymphocytes and neutrophils.

involvement is rare. Biopsy specimens of skin are frequently not specific, and thus biopsy specimens taken from sural nerve, kidney, testis, liver, skeletal muscle, or rectum are preferable. The arteritis of PAN is typically segmental. In acute lesions, there is a necrotizing vasculitis with fibrinoid necrosis. Transmural lymphocytes, neutrophils, eosinophils, and rarely granulomas are seen. Microaneurysms with nodule formation are typical, giving the disease its name. Acute lesions frequently coexist with proliferative fibrotic healing lesions (10).

The diagnosis of polyarteritis nodosa is frequently delayed because initial manifestations of the disease are generally nonspecific and may not display clinical findings that point to a vasculitis. The American College of Rheumatology 1990 criteria for the classification of polyarteritis nodosa include the following features:

1. Weight loss greater than or equal to 4 kg
2. Livedo reticularis
3. Testicular pain or tenderness
4. Mononeuropathy or polyneuropathy
5. Diastolic blood pressure >90 mm Hg
6. Elevated blood urea nitrogen or serum creatinine levels
7. Presence of hepatitis B reactants in the serum
8. Arteriographic abnormality
9. Presence of granulocyte or mixed leukocyte infiltrate in an arterial wall on biopsy
10. Myalgias

The presence of three or more yields a diagnostic sensitivity of 82% and a specificity of 87% (11). The Chapel Hill Consensus Conference on the Nomenclature of Systemic Vasculitis restricts the classification of polyarteritis nodosa to those cases with vasculitis limited to medium-sized and small arteries without involvement of smaller vessels, after exclusion of cryoglobulinemic vasculitis, Henoch-Schönlein purpura, and other forms of immune complex vasculitis (12). Depending on the classification scheme used, patients may be labeled as having microscopic polyangiitis or polyarteritis nodosa.

The clinical presentation of systemic vasculitis is frequently nonspecific. Accurate classification requires a working knowledge of different forms of vasculitis, including clinical, laboratory, and pathological features. Polyarteritis nodosa frequently presents in the skin as a medium-vessel arteritis. The differential diagnosis includes other vasculitides that typically involve smaller vessels, but occasionally present in a manner virtually indistinguishable from polyarteritis nodosa. These entities include microscopic polyangiitis, Churg Strauss syndrome, Wegener's granulomatosis, rheumatoid vasculitis, systemic lupus erythematosus vasculitis, and mixed cryoglobulinemia. Of these, microscopic polyangiitis (MPA) and PAN have been grouped together most closely in the literature. Distinguishing clinical features of MPA not generally seen in PAN include palpable purpura, pulmonary involvement, and lack of gastrointestinal tract and neuropathy early in the disease (13). Evidence further supporting a distinction between these two entities is the presence of circulating IgG and IgM antibodies to endothelial cell antigens, which cannot be detected in PAN or other forms of small- and medium-sized vessel systemic vasculitis (14), and the presence of circulating anti-neutrophil cytoplasmic antibodies (ANCA) in MPA, but rarely in PAN (15). Differences between PAN and MPA are highlighted in Table 37.1.

Laboratory evaluation is a useful tool in narrowing the differential diagnosis in the vasculitides. Circulating anti-neutrophil cytoplasmic antibodies (ANCA) are an important part of the evaluation. These may occur in cytoplasmic, perinuclear, or atypical patterns. A screening ANCA is performed by indirect immunofluorescence, and if positive, confirmed with enzyme immunoassays for anti-proteinase 3 (PR3, cytoplasmic-ANCA) and anti-myeloperoxidase (MPO, perinuclear-ANCA). Negative studies for ANCA do not completely exclude any form of systemic vasculitis, but typical ANCA profiles can be helpful in the classification of vasculitis. These patterns are included in Table 37.1.

A histologically distinctive feature of several forms of systemic vasculitis is the so-called "Churg Strauss granuloma," also referred to as Winkelmann's granuloma, cutaneous necrotizing extravascular granuloma, or palisaded neutrophilic and granulomatous dermatitis. This lesion most commonly presents as persistent papules or plaques on extremities, sometimes ulcerating. Microscopically, a diffuse dermal infiltrate of some combination of neutrophils, eosinophils, and granulomas is found, sometimes palisaded, and most commonly without frank vasculitis. The Churg Strauss granuloma may occur in many disorders, including Churg Strauss syndrome, Wegener's granulomatosis, systemic lupus erythematosus, and rheumatoid arthritis. It is not, however, a feature of PAN, MPA, or cryoglobulinemia. Table 37.1 summarizes some of the important clinical, laboratory, and pathological features of forms of vasculitis that may present in a manner similar to that of PAN.

In addition to systemic vasculitis, the clinical differential diagnosis for polyarteritis nodosa includes other arterial occlusive diseases such as cholesterol emboli, lupus anticoagulant, monoclonal cryoglobulinemia, septic emboli, coumadin necrosis, and calciphylaxis. These can sometimes be distinguished based on clinical setting, but histopathologic evaluation in each will provide ready distinction from PAN.

Laboratory findings in polyarteritis nodosa may include serologic evidence of hepatitis B or hepatitis C infection, elevated blood urea nitrogen and creatinine, increased erythrocyte sedimentation rate and C-reactive protein, leukocytosis, proteinuria, pyuria, and hematuria. Anti-

TABLE 37.1. Differential Diagnosis of Polyarteritis Nodosa and Vasculitides Affecting Medium-sized Arteries (2,3,16–18)

	Clinical	Laboratory	Pathology	
Polyarteritis nodosa	Neuropathy 60%, Renal 25%–50%, Skin 30%–40%, Pulmonary rare	Serologic evidence of HBV or HCV; p-ANCA rare; Decreased complement levels in hepatitis-associated cases; Aneurysms by arteriography	**Skin**—medium-vessel involvement predominates, particularly in benign cutaneous form	**Renal**—arteritis with glomerular sparing
Microscopic polyangiitis	Renal 90%, Skin 40%, Pulmonary 50%, Neurologic 30%, ENT 35%	MPO p-ANCA 60%, PR3 c-ANCA 30%, Normal complement	**Skin**—panvasculitis most common	**Renal**—necrotizing glomerular lesions, crescents
Churg-Strauss syndrome	History of atopy, asthma; drug or allergy shot trigger; Skin 60%—nodules, PAN-like lesions, necrotizing vasculitis, Churg-Strauss granuloma; Pulmonary 70%, Neurologic 70%, ENT 50%	Peripheral eosinophilia >10%, Normal complement, MPO p-ANCA—70%	**Skin**—vasculitis of different-sized vessels, tissue-eosinophils, Churg-Strauss granuloma	**Renal**—segmental necrotizing glomerulonephritis
Wegener's granulomatosis	Skin 40%, Renal 80%, Pulmonary 90%, ENT 90%	PR3 c-ANCA > 90%, occasional p-ANCA, Normal complement; CXR—nodules, cavities, fixed infiltrates	**Skin**—pandermal vasculitis, nonspecific chronic and granulomatous inflammation with diffuse pattern, Churg-Strauss granuloma	**Renal**—segmental necrotizing glomerulonephritis
Rheumatoid arthritis	Deforming erosive arthritis	ANCA negative RF+, decreased complement	**Skin**—pandermal vasculitis, Churg-Strauss granuloma	**Renal**—spared
Systemic lupus erythematosus	Arthritis, nephritis, malar erythema	ANCA negative ANA+, decreased complement	**Skin**—may have pandermal vasculitis, Churg-Strauss granuloma	**Renal**—mesangial, diffuse or focal proliferative, or membranous glomerulonephritis
Mixed cryoglobulinemia	Skin 90%, Renal 55%, Musculoskeletal 70%; may have connective tissue disease, malignancy, infection including HBV, HCV	ANCA negative circulating cryoglobulins, polyclonal	**Skin**—pandermal vasculitis	**Renal**—membranoproliferative glomerulonephritis

MPO = myeloperoxidase
PR3 = proteinase 3
c-ANCA = cytoplasmic antineutrophil cytoplasmic antibody
p-ANCA = perinuclear antineutrophil cytoplasmic antibody
CXR = chest X-ray
HBV = hepatitis B virus
HCV = hepatitis C virus

neutrophil cytoplasmic antibodies are found only rarely in PAN, but can be used to help differentiate PAN from other forms of systemic vasculitis.

Tissue evaluation to identify vasculitis is important in establishing a diagnosis of PAN. Site selection for biopsy should be based upon clinical evidence of involvement of that site, possibly including data from visceral arteriography and nerve conduction studies. Multiple biopsy specimens from different sites in addition to angiography are more likely to detect evidence of PAN, but are associated with considerable morbidity. Using a decision analysis model, a more conservative approach of biopsy has been advocated. Electromyography and nerve conduction studies should be used to localize potential areas of muscle or nerve involvement. If no abnormal areas are identified or if biopsy specimens are not diagnostic, then visceral angiography should be performed. If arteriography is normal, then blind muscle biopsy is recommended (19, 20).

Treatment of polyarteritis nodosa includes systemic corticosteroids and immunosuppressives. A remission rate of approximately 50% is established with the use of prednisone, but significant liver dysfunction may be a consequence of treatment in patients with coexistent viral hepatitis (21). In HBV-associated cases, one treatment regimen includes a combination of prednisone and plasma exchange, with rapid tapering of prednisone to minimize liver damage, followed by initiation of antiviral therapy (22). Monthly pulse cyclophosphamide is useful in patients refractory to systemic steroids or those with severe systemic disease. A clinical trial of 6 versus 12 pulses of cyclophosphamide in a group of patients with poor prognostic factors with PAN and MPA found the group with 12 pulses to have similar survival to the group with 6, but with lower relapse rates (23).

With the exception of benign cutaneous polyarteritis nodosa, prognosis in polyarteritis nodosa is poor without treatment. However, survival may be 75%–80% with immunosuppressive therapy (2). Poor prognostic indicators are presence of nephropathy, age greater than 50 years, gastrointestinal tract involvement, cardiomyopathy, and central nervous system involvement (22).

References

1. Matteson EL. Historical perspective of vasculitis: polyarteritis nodosa and microscopic polyangiitis. *Curr Rheum Rep* 2002; 4: 67–74.
2. Bonsib SM. Polyarteritis nodosa. *Semin Diag Pathol* 2001; 18: 14–23.
3. Stone JH. Polyarteritis nodosa. *JAMA* 2002; 288: 1632–1639.
4. Soufir N, Descamps V, Crickx B, et al. Hepatitis C virus infection in cutaneous polyarteritis nodosa: A retrospective study of 16 cases. *Arch Dermatol* 1999; 135: 1001–1002.
5. Daoud MS, Hutton KP, Gibson LE. Cutaneous periarteritis nodosa: A clinicopathological study of 79 cases. *Br J Dermatol* 1997; 136: 706–713.
6. Calabrese LH, Estes M, Yen-Lieberman B, et al. Systemic vasculitis in association with human immunodeficiency virus infection. *Arthritis Rheum* 1989; 32: 569–576.
7. Rodriguez P, Suarez P, del Rio E, et al. Cutaneous granulomatous vasculitis after herpes zoster infection showing polyarteritis nodosa-like features. *Clin Exp Dermatol* 1997; 22: 274–276.
8. Elkon KB, Hughes GR, Catovsky D, et al. Hairy-cell leukaemia with polyarteritis nodosa. *Lancet* 1979; i: 678.
9. Burke, AP, Virmani R. Localized vasculitis. *Semin Diag Pathol* 2001; 18: 59–66.
10. Lie JT. Illustrated histopathologic classification criteria for selected vasculitis syndromes. *Arthritis Rheum* 1990; 33: 1074–1087.
11. Lightfoot RW, Michel BA, Bloch DA, et al. The American College of Rheumatology 1990 criteria for the classification of polyarteritis nodosa. *Arthritis Rheum* 1990; 33: 1088–1093.
12. Jennette JC, Falk RJ, Andrassy K, et al. Nomenclature of systemic vasculitides. Proposal of an international consensus conference. *Arthritis Rheum* 1994; 37: 187–192.
13. Agard C, Mouthon L, Mahr A, Guillevin L. Microscopic polyangiitis and polyarteritis nodosa: how and when do they start? *Arthritis Rheum* 2003; 49: 709–715.
14. Chanseaud Y, Pena-Lefebvre PG, Guilpain P, et al. IgM and IgG autoantibodies from microscopic polyangiitis patients but not those with other small- and medium-sized vessel vasculitides recognize multiple endothelial cell antigens. *Clin Immu*nol 2003; 109: 165–178.
15. Hughes LB, Bridges SL. Polyarteritis nodosa and microscopic polyangiitis: Etiologic and diagnostic considerations. *Curr Rheum Reports* 2002; 4: 75–82.
16. Crotty CP, DeRemee, Winkelmann RK. Cutaneous clinicopathologic correlation of allergic granulomatosis. *J Am Acad Dermatol* 1981; 5: 571–581.
17. Jennette JC, Falk RJ. Small-vessel vasculitis. *N Engl J Med* 1997; 337: 1512–1523.
18. Seo P, Stone JH. The antineutrophil cytoplasmic antibody-associated vasculitides. *Am J Med* 2004; 117: 39–50.
19. Albert DA, Rimon D, Silverstein MD. The diagnosis of polyarteritis nodosa, I: A literature-based decision analysis approach. *Arthritis Rheum* 1988; 31: 1117–1127.
20. Albert DA, Silverstein MD, Paunicka K, Reddy G, Chang RW, Derus C. The diagnosis of polyarteritis nodosa, II: Empirical verification of a decision analysis model. *Arthritis Rheum* 1988; 31: 1128–1134.
21. Lam KC, Lai CL, Trepo C, Wu PC. Deleterious effects of prednisolone in hepatitis B surface antigen-positive chronic active hepatitis. *N Engl J Med* 1981; 304: 380–386.
22. Guillevin L, Lhote F, Gayraud M, et al. Prognostic factors in polyarteritis nodosa and Churg-Strauss syndrome: A prospective study in 342 patients. *Medicine* 1996; 75: 17–28.
23. Guillevin L, Cohen P, Mahr, et al. Treatment of polyarteritis nodosa and microscopic polyangiitis with poor prognosis factors: A prospective trial comparing glucocorticoids and six or twelve cyclophosphamide pulses in sixty-five patients. *Arthritis Rheum* 2003; 49: 93–100.

Index

Printed in China